MAKING AND MARKETING MEDICINE IN RENAISSANCE FLORENCE

THE WELLCOME SERIES
IN THE HISTORY OF MEDICINE

MAKING AND MARKETING MEDICINE IN RENAISSANCE FLORENCE

James Shaw and Evelyn Welch

Amsterdam – New York, NY 2011

First published in 2011
by Editions Rodopi B.V., Amsterdam – New York, NY 2011.

Editions Rodopi B.V. © 2011

Design and Typesetting by Mike Laycock,
The Wellcome Trust Centre for the History of Medicine at UCL.
Printed and bound in The Netherlands by Editions Rodopi B.V.,
Amsterdam – New York, NY 2011.

Index by Rosemary Anderson and James Shaw.

British Library Cataloguing in Publication Data
A catalogue record for this book is available from the British Library

ISBN 978-90-420-3156-2
E-Book ISBN 978-90-420-3157-9

'Making and Marketing Medicine in Renaissance Florence' –
Amsterdam – New York, NY:
Rodopi. – ill.
(Clio Medica 89 / ISSN 0045-7183;
The Wellcome Series in the History of Medicine)

The Wellcome name is used under licence from the Wellcome Trust.

Front cover:
'Christ the Pharmacist with Adam and Eve',
from *Chants royaux sur la Conception couronnee du Puy de Rouen.*
Bibliotheque Nationale, Paris, Ms Fr 1537,
Archives Charmet/The Bridgeman Art Library.

© Editions Rodopi B. V., Amsterdam – New York, NY 2011
Printed in The Netherlands

All titles in the Clio Medica series (from 1999 onwards) are available to
download from the IngentaConnect website: http://www.ingentaconnect.co.uk

Contents

List of Images

List of Tables

3

List of Charts

Abbreviations

Estranei	Archivio dell'Ospedale degli Innocenti (Florence), Estranei (series 144)
E541	Estranei 541
E878	Estranei 878
E882	Estranei 882
Tratte	Online Tratte of Office Holders 1282–1532 (online database)[1]
ASF	Archivio di Stato di Firenze
OED	Oxford English Dictionary (online edition)[2]
BNF	Biblioteca Nazionale di Firenze
MdP	Medici Archive Project (online database)[3]
RF	*Ricettario fiorentino*, 1499[4]
m.f.	*more fiorentino*[5]
fl	fiorino (pl. fiorini), ie. 'florin'
L	lira (pl. lire)
s	soldo (pl. soldi)
d	denaro (pl. denari)
lb(s)	libbra (pl. libbre)
oz	oncia (pl. oncie)
sc	scrupolo (pl. scrupoli)
dr	dramma (pl. dramme)
gr	grano (pl. grani)

Notes

1. The reference numbers refer to the RECKEY field used in this online database. See http://www.stg.brown.edu/projects/tratte/
2. http://dictionary.oed.com/
3. http://documents.medici.org/
4. *Ricettario fiorentino* (Florence: Compagnia del Drago, 1499). This source is available at http://gallica2.bnf.fr/ark:/12148/bpt6k59447x
5. The Florentine year began on 25 March. In the main text, dates have been converted to the standard calendar. In the endnotes, the Florentine calendar has been preserved.

Glossary

(All Florentine terms are in italics. Florentine spellings were variable in this period and have been adjusted in some cases to conform to modern Italian standards)

Agaric: type of funghi growing on trees, particularly the larch.

Albarello: ceramic pharmacy jar, available in various sizes, used at the Giglio for retail of electuaries.

Ampoule (*ampolla*): glass or ceramic pharmacy vessel used to store liquids.

Archomento, argomento: see Clyster.

Aromatico Rosato: type of 'sweet electuary' containing red roses, syrups, various gums and spices.

Azure: type of blue precious stone, in the Renaissance used as an artist's pigment.

Bath (*bagno*): mixtures of dried flowers and herbs added to hot water.

Berrichucholo: cake made from flour, honey and various spices, a speciality of Siena.

Bicchiere: drinking glass, used at the Giglio for retail of purges.

Bole Armeniac (*bolo armeno*): a type of astringent earth used in pharmacy as a poison antidote and styptic.

Braccio: measure of length, approximately an 'arm', the Florentine *braccio* was equivalent to 0.58m.

Camphor (*canfera*): aromatic substance obtained from the wood of the camphor laurel, native to Asia.

Cassia: *Cassia solutiva* or *Cassia fistula* refers to the 'pudding pipe', the pods of the golden shower tree. Cassia pulp (*polpa di cassia*) was the pulp extracted from these pods commonly used in medicine. *Cassia linea* refers to an inferior variety of cinnamon, *Cinnamomum Cassia*.

Cerate (*cerotto*): stiff variety of ointment made with wax or spread on strips of leather.

Cero: type of heavy devotional candle.

Clyster (*archomento*): enema, a liquid medicine inserted into the rectum with a syringe.

Collation (*colazione*): light repast served between meals, usually consisting of sweets, fruits and nuts.

Comfit (*confetto*): sweet consisting of a spice, seed or nut coated in several hard layers of sugar.

Composite Electuary: see Electuary.

Confection (*confetto*): complex medicinal sweet combining various drugs, simples and sugar. See also Comfit above.

Confettiera: tray for serving sweets.

Coralline (*corallina*): type of calcareous seaweed, considered an effective vermifuge.

Cordial: medicine considered good for the heart.

Cotognato: 'quiddany' or quince jelly.

Date (*dattero*): type of fruit, the term was also used to describe a solid form of purge, referred to elsewhere in Italy as a *bolus*.

Decoction (*dicozione*): a liquid vehicle made by boiling simples in water.

Diacassia: also known as 'confected cassia', a drug based principally on Cassia.

Diacatholicon: drug containing a variety of purgative simples, but chiefly senna, pudding pipe, tamarinds and rhubarb.

Diamanna: drug based principally on manna.

Diaradon Abbatis: type of 'sweet electuary' made from various spices combined with syrup of red roses.

Diapenidion: a medicinal confection of ground pennets, spices and nuts.

Diaphœnicon: drug containing a variety of purgative simples, but principally dates.

Diasenna: drug based on senna leaves.

Doppiere: type of candle made from several candles twisted together.

Dragée, dredge (*treggiea*): type of small comfit; some varieties were also made for medical purposes.

Dragon's Blood (*sangue di drago*): type of red gum or resin, used in painting, dyeing and medicine.

Dram (*dramma, drachma*): apothecary measure of weight; the Florentine *dramma* was equivalent to 3.54g.

Drugs: a term we have reserved for compound preparations whose recipes are found in medical textbooks like the *Ricettario fiorentino*.

Electuary (*lattovare*): type of drug in the form of a thick syrup. We have used the term 'Composite Electuary' to refer to combinations of several different drugs.

Epithem (*pittima*): powdered drugs mixed with a liquid for external application to the body with cloth or sponge.

Falcola: taper, a type of candle.

Fomentation: liquid preparations for external application to the body with cloth or sponge. Similar to epithems but without the powdered drugs.

Gonfaloniere di giustizia: the chief official of the city of Florence, elected for a two-month term of office.

Grain (*grano*): apothecary measure of weight; the Florentine *grano* was equivalent to 0.05g.

Inbrattato, imbrattato: a type of 'smeared' or 'dirtied' comfit with rough rather than smooth coatings of sugar.

Julep: type of sugary drink, much thinner than a syrup.

Lattovare: see Electuary.

Libbra: measure of weight, literally a 'pound'; the Florentine *libbra* was equivalent to 339.5g.

Loc: type of thicker syrup, midway between standard syrups and electuaries.

Manipolo: 'handful', a measure used for dried herbs and flowers.

Manna: sap forming on the leaves of a type of ash, found mostly in Calabria.

Manuschristo: type of medicinal sweet made from sugar, rose water and other ingredients.

Marzipan: type of cake made of sugar, almond paste and sometimes rose-water.

Medicina: medicine; used specifically at the Giglio to refer to a Purge (short for *medicina solutiva*)

Mithridate: compound drug famous as a drug and poison antidote.

Moccolo: candle stub.

Morselletto: 'little morsel', type of confection (see above), a medicinal electuary combining drugs with sugar in the form of a ball.

Musk: strong smelling substance obtained from gland of the male musk-deer.

Myrobalan: fruit of various species of *Terminalia.*

Ointment (*unguento, unzione*): medicine for external application, usually containing oils.

Oncia: measure of weight, literally an 'ounce'; the Florentine *oncia* was equivalent to 28.3g.

Oxymel: combination of vinegar and honey used in medicine.

Pannicle: fleshy membrane attaching the skin to the tissue beneath.

Pennet: medicinal sweet, consisting of twisted sticks of pulled sugar, mixed with starch and oil of sweet almonds.

Peverada: type of spicy meat sauce.

Pill (*pillola*): form of drug coated with sugar or wax, designed to be ingested easily.

Pinochiato: type of small cake made from pine-nuts and sugar.

Pittima: see Epithem.

Pizzicata: type of small comfit made from coriander seeds

Plaster (*empiastro*): a stiff variety of ointment made with gums or resins.

Populeon: medicinal ointment made from buds of the black poplar.

Pudding Pipe: see Cassia.

Purge: type of medicine designed to purge the body of excess humours. In Florence, 'medicina' was a term specifically used for a purge.

Quarro: quarter ounce.

Rhubarb: root of a variety of medicinal rhubarb imported from China.

Rob (*robbo*): type of medicinal syrup.

Rosato Colato: honey of roses, purified by straining.

Savonia: sweet made from sugar boiled with rose-water, combined with starch to give a soft consistency.

Scruple (*scrupolo*): apothecary measure of weight; the Florentine *scrupolo* was equivalent to 1.18g.

Senna: leaves of a type of shrub of the *Cassia* genus, used in medicine as a purgative.

Simple: an individual medicinal commodity that could be consumed alone, or more commonly in combination with other drugs and simples.

Speziale: apothecary/spicer.

Spezie: spices, available in standard mixtures as 'fine' or 'camelline' spices; the term was also used to refer to drugs in powdered form.

Spike (*spigo*): French lavender.

Spikenard (*spigo nardo*): costly aromatic substance obtained from an oriental plant, *Nardostachys Jatamansi.*

Staio: measure of volume, typically used for grain, the Florentine staio was equivalent to 24.4 litres.

Stomachic: medicine for the stomach, sometimes confused in the sources with stomatic, medicine for the mouth.

Sugo Rosato: electuary of roses.

Tamarind (*tamerindo*): fruit of the tree *Tamarindus indica.*

Tamarisk (*tamerigia*): plant of the genus *Tamarix.*

Terra Sigillata: an astringent bole, a type of reddish earth used in medicine, imported from Lemnos, and bearing a seal guaranteeing its quality.

Theriac (*triaca, teriaca*): compound drug famous as a drug and poison antidote.

Trebbiano: aromatic white wine local to Tuscany.

Treggiea: see Dragée.

Trochisks, Troches (*torcisci*): dried tablets of drugs and simples, a form used to preserve perishable ingredients.

Turpeth (*turbitti*): a cathartic simple prepared from the root of East Indian jalap, *Ipomœa Turpethum.*

Unction: a type of ointment.

Waters: distilled waters used to prepare essences of herbs and flowers.

Wormwood: the plant *Artemisia Absinthium.*

Currencies, Weights and Measures

In the text, all metric measures are modern usage; all 'imperial' measures and their abbreviations (oz, lbs etc.) are Florentine measures.

Apothecary measures:

1 libbra = 339.5 g = 12 oncie
1 oncia = 4 quarri (quarter ounce) = 8 dramme
1 dramma = 3 scrupoli
1 scrupolo = 24 grani
A manipolo, or 'handful', was a measure typically used for dried herbs and flowers.[1]

Currency:

1 lira (pl. lire) = 20 soldi
1 soldo (pl. soldi) = 12 denari
The conversion rate between the gold florin and the silver money of account varied over time. In 1493–4, one florin was approximately equal to L6s10; by 1500–2, one florin was approximately equal to L7.[2]

Length and Volume:

1 braccio = 0.58 m
1 staio (pl. staia) = 24.4 litres (typically used for grain)[3]

Notes

1. *Ricettario fiorentino* (Florence: Compagnia del Drago, 1499), 'Manipolo e' tanto quanto si puo pigliare co' una mano'.
2. R.A. Goldthwaite, *The Building of Renaissance Florence: An Economic and Social History* (Baltimore: Johns Hopkins University Press, 1980), 301, 429–30, on lira–florin conversion rates over time.
3. A. Martini, *Manuale di metrologia ossia misure, pesi e monete in uso attulamente ed anticamente presso tutti i popoli* (Turin: Loescher, 1883), 207–8.

1

Introduction and Acknowledgements

This project was funded by the Wellcome Trust Grant 064962/Z/01: 'Selling Health in Renaissance Italy: Consumers and Consumption in the Tuscan Apothecary, 1350–1600'.

In 1996, the British artist Damien Hirst sold the Tate Gallery in London an installation he had created four years earlier. Entitled 'Pharmacy', this was a mid-sized space designed to evoke a local chemist's shop.[1] Empty packets emulating medicines stood in glass cabinets; glass jars containing coloured water stood on the desk at which sales were meant to take place. The next year, in 1997, Hirst opened an eponymous restaurant, *Pharmacy*, in London's Notting Hill. Food critics were hostile, but more interestingly, he was quickly attacked by the Royal Pharmaceutical Society of Great Britain.[2] They objected to his use of the name, and to his display of bottles and medical paraphernalia for fear that it could confuse customers (see Image 1.1 overleaf).

When describing the rationale behind his long-standing theme of the pharmacist and his shop, Hirst commented:

> They were believing in medicine in exactly the same way I wanted them to believe in art... I still get a kick out of the fact that there is no medicine involved in *Pharmacy*. It's a very simple way to look at how this confidence works with medicine companies. The packaging is the power.[3]

Hirst was articulating a commonly held contemporary view: that drug companies use visual means, advertising and a sense of confidence in the curative powers of their products to persuade consumers that they will get well if they buy these goods. The Royal Pharmaceutical Society's response was also typical. It wanted to protect its monopoly over not only the name but also the 'look' of the pharmacy, in order to protect consumers from fraud. Although there was considerable local press attention in the UK to this dispute and to the eventual, highly profitable sale of the restaurant's interior fittings in 2004, few noted the traditional nature of this debate.[4] There is a long history of attempts to cure illness through manufactured means, by taking pills, syrups, distillates, lotions, creams or enemas. There has been an almost equally long tradition of trying to oversee and control

Image 1.1

Damian Hirst, Pharmacy,
Installation, Tate Modern, 1992.
© Damien Hirst.

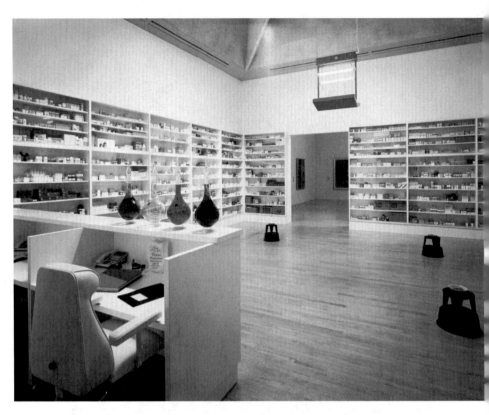

their makers and sellers. Yet the terms used today for over-the-counter or prescription drug sales: 'pharmacy' or 'chemist' represent a relatively recent development.[5] Pharmacy comes from the Greek word, *pharmakos* or drug; chemist is taken from the Latin term *chemista* an abbreviation of alchemist. But this nomenclature was not generally used for the sale of medical products before the end of the sixteenth century. Instead, shopkeepers and customers usually referred to spice shops as *spezierie* or simply to an *apotheke*, a term derived from the Greek word for storehouse and from which we take the label, 'apothecary'. The latter was a particularly apposite Renaissance description for the fifteenth- and early sixteenth-century apothecary's shop, which was indeed a storehouse and manufacturing site for a remarkable range of products. While these included medicines, they also ranged from sugar and spice to wax, savoury sauces, sweet biscuits, candied nuts, artists' pigments, house paints and the ingredients for perfume. A century later, there was much greater specialisation, with stronger divisions between the sale of pharmaceutical items and other goods. Even though the boundaries were still far from fixed, most of the work on pharmacies and apothecaries has concentrated on this later period, particularly on the seventeenth- and eighteenth-century innovations in the sales and marketing of medicines through shops, and street-sellers such as charlatans.[6] But the transitions and traditions of the later centuries are impossible to appreciate without an understanding of the role played by the apothecary or *spezieria* of the fifteenth and sixteenth centuries.

The archive of the Ospedale degli Innocenti in Florence contains the records of a number of apothecary shops for this earlier period, with seemingly dry, but often very complete, accounts of retail sales arranged by customer. They record the names, and above all the debts and payments, of clients who entered the shop. These range from those who came in only once to those who stopped by on a daily basis. They usually indicate what was sold and for how much; more rarely they tell us why the purchase was made. Amongst the most complete of these records are the forty-nine registers of the Speziale al Giglio, which run from 1464 to 1568, serving Florence's community from the same site for over a century. Although it passed through three generations during this period, each descendent kept the records of the previous owner before eventually passing them all on to the Ospedale, which inherited the possessions of the last *speziale*, (Images 1.2 and 1.3, overleaf). These records have been used by, amongst others, Julia DeLancey as part of her examination of where artists obtained pigments in fifteenth-century Florence.[7] But they, and indeed the many other shop accounts that survive, have not been fully exploited by cultural historians or historians of science. This must be in part because they were never designed to tell us about the history of an apothecary's shop, the transition period from one type of retailing to another, or about medical practices. Instead, they were kept as a legal record in case of disputes over credit, payment and taxes. Nonetheless, those keeping the books at the Speziale al Giglio were as interested in carefully recording to whom they sold their products, where they obtained their ingredients, and even why these items were sold, as they were in the money they might make. Indeed, perhaps with the tax inspector in mind, they made it particularly difficult to determine the latter.

Although prosperous, the Speziale al Giglio was not a particularly special shop; that in itself makes these records of interest. They reveal a fairly typical business at the height of the Renaissance in Florence, immediately prior to

19

Image 1.2

Archivio dell' Ospedale degli Innocenti, Speziale al Giglio *accounts,*
E882 ff. 355v–356r.
Photo: Donato Pineider.

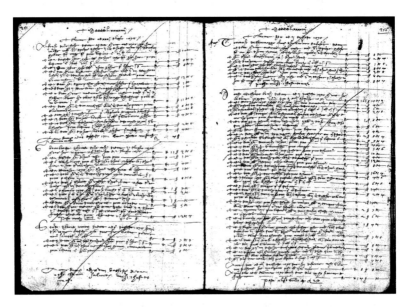

the period of instability and change that was to begin in November 1494
with the arrival of the French army and the collapse of Medici control. The
political turmoil of the 1490s marked the end of an era symbolically, but the
sixteenth century would also see important changes medically and
institutionally, with new diseases (syphilis), growing public regulation of the
trade, and extensive revision of the accepted pharmacological tradition.
Furthermore, there were dramatic changes in trading patterns following the
opening up of the Cape Route and the Americas, with the appearance of new
medicinal commodities such as guaiac (see Chapter 8). Despite all this,
apothecaries continued to sell many of the same goods. The most important
effects of an expanding commercial network were to widen the range of
exotic goods on sale and to make these cheaper – prices generally fell across
the fifteenth and sixteenth centuries – but without transforming the retail
market: many of the pills, potions and medications on offer in the Giglio in
the 1490s would have been quite acceptable to a client in the 1590s. The
apothecary's practice grew, not in revolutionary leaps, but in adaptations and
accretions. Understanding the daily life of the mid-sized Florentine

Image 1.3

Archivio dell' Ospedale degli Innocenti, account of 'Benedetto di Bartolomio degli Alesandri', E882 fo. 55v.
Photo: James Shaw.

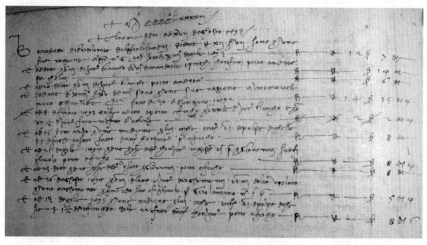

operation, therefore, provides important insights into the overlaps between the theories which survived from the medieval period and the practices that went on well into the eighteenth century.

The issues raised in this book concerning sociability, information networks and commercial practice have only recently been posed when examining medical practice in Renaissance Italy.[8] Indeed, most of the work on apothecaries has been antiquarian in nature, emphasising description over historical analysis. Many studies simply consist of transcriptions of the surviving documentary material.[9] There has been considerable work on guild statutes, for example; yet although these documents can tell us much about the institutional context, they provide little reliable data for retailing. Price limits on medicines and other goods were not necessarily respected in practice; nor can regulations tell us anything about the volume of sales. Similarly, while statutes dedicate much attention to the regulation of poisons, they generally neglect more innocuous products such as sweets that were the staple of many Renaissance apothecaries.

Thus, simply *reading* the accounts is insufficient – there is so much information that it is impossible to extract general patterns from the data without employing a more rigorous analysis.[10] We therefore adopted a quantitative approach, using a database to organise the raw material recorded in the accounts. The results detail the purchase of over 16,000 individual items in nearly 12,000 transactions by 2,247 clients. Only in this way is it possible to extract key trends such as the total retail sales in a year, the relative importance of different products within that, and patterns of consumer behaviour. Although one consequence of adopting this 'quantitative microhistory' approach has been to focus the study on a relatively short span of time, it has enabled us to extract information that reveals clear patterns of consumer and medical behaviour and so make significant contributions to our understanding of the apothecary trade. In this book we have also tried to relate this economic analysis to the ways that consumers chose, paid for, consumed and described the various products on sale.

This combination of efforts allows an investigation of how the theoretical precepts of social, medical and economic behaviour were put into practice. The time frame chosen avoids unusual events in its attempt to map the norm and for most of 1493, and well into 1494, there was relative calm. There were no particular problems with the harvest and prices remained relatively stable. Over one year, from August 1493 to July 1494, we can follow the vagaries of running a mid-sized business in late fifteenth-century Florence, an experience that was very different from that undertaken by the bankers, silk and wool merchants on whom historians have generally focused. The core of this book, the Speziale al Giglio is remarkable only in the survival of its many account books. With forty-nine volumes documenting daily transactions, ranging from the most mundane to the most complex, these detailed records offer an evocative glimpse into a world often hidden from historians: the common, everyday experiences of seemingly 'ordinary' Florentines. In the Speziale al Giglio, we see individuals trying to manage their health, their diet and even their spiritual welfare. At the same time, we can also see a businessman and his family negotiating the difficulties of making a living in a tense political climate at the end of the century.

The data we have collected confirm the need for a nuanced approach in applying the widely used concept of the 'medical marketplace' to early modern society. This has rightly emphasised the way that consumers could employ a wide range of therapies as alternatives or in parallel, be they pharmacological, dietary, magical or religious (see Chapter 7). Nevertheless, it is important not to imply a proto-modern environment of free competition, where consumers chose from a range of different products and suppliers who competed to satisfy their needs, a capitalist model that leads smoothly into Damien Hirst's twentieth-century critique. The late fifteenth-century marketplace was solidly embedded in social relations; the free circulation of goods, credit and information that characterises the capitalist market economy was to appear at a much later stage.[11] As Sandra Cavallo's work on barber–surgeons in seventeenth-century Turin and Giovanna

Pomata's investigation of Bologna in the same period have both shown, markets for medical cures offered a more complex social and economic arena than we might first expect.[12] It was a marketplace, but it did not correspond to the modern ideal of an impersonal, freemarket economy. On the consumer side, obtaining access to medicines and other goods was not so much a matter of cost, but rather of *being connected.* On the retailer side, like most of Florence's shopkeepers, apothecaries, who could be expected to act as competitors, turn out to collaborate effectively. They prove willing to supply each other with goods when supplies run short and agree to avoid overlaps in specialisations. They train each others' children, marry each others' relatives and mourn each others' deaths. More intriguingly, they work closely not only with other medical practitioners but also with associated professionals, providing financial as well as social support. This is not the competitive market that was increasingly envisaged in seventeenth- and eighteenth-century England, but one where the aim was to work collectively to survive and prosper in an unstable and unprotected political and financial environment. As we will show, it was not the institutional guild affiliations that provided security, but the social networks created by long-term associations, family, neighbourhood and the intricate system of credit.

Studying small-scale trade and social networks is a task that has only recently attracted attention.[13] Although Florence prided itself on a prosperity based on trade, its sixteenth-century historians such as Francesco Guicciardini were dismissive of low-level commerce. The great Florentine families, the Medici, Strozzi, Acciaiuoli, Tornabuoni, had made their fortunes from international businesses, lending money to princes and Popes, importing wool and silk threads and exporting fine cloths and brocades. They might invest in the importation of spices or sugar but they would not serve in shops, however valuable the products that were on offer. Florence's political histories, therefore, generally overlook or simply ignore the city's shopkeepers. This is despite the fact that many of the narrators, such as Matteo Palmieri, author of the *Vita Civile*, the Lucchese writer, Giovanni Sercambi, or the loquacious diarist, Luca Landucci, were all apothecaries, while others adapted the language of the pharmacist to their writings.[14] The philosopher Marsilio Ficino's brothers were both apothecaries and there are references in his *Three Books on Life* which reflect these family links. He uses the metaphor of the 'shop' to describe his own book, describing his offerings as a range of cures on offer to the reader, who is invited to pick and choose from among them:

> This shop of ours displays various antidotes, drugs, fomentations, ointments, and remedies, according to the differing mental capacities and natures of

men. If in some way they happen to displease you, pass over these, by all means, but do not for that reason repudiate the rest.[15]

But if contemporaries rarely reflected on the history of small-scale commerce, recent economic historians such as Richard Marshall have turned to this topic to demonstrate the dense networks of credit and sociability of such 'middling figures'.[16] As they provided services and products, loaned money to their clients and their colleagues and took on debts in turn, their patterns of exchange made it possible to survive in an economically challenging climate. Apothecaries or pharmacists were particularly important links in these networks, acting as informal bankers as well as providers of essential and luxury products.[17] Travellers stopped off in the city's main apothecaries to hear the latest news or to gamble; these were spaces to find information as well as products.[18] Research on Renaissance pharmacies in Venice has demonstrated that they were key sites for the exchange of political and other ideas, while work on later outlets in Europe has demonstrated their importance in developing new forms of botanical expertise.[19]

Thus, Part One of this book considers the shop itself and its spatial geography, tracing the customers who made purchases and examining what they bought. Most relied on credit and this key form of trust is discussed in detail in Part Two. From the people we then move to the products. Part Three offers separate chapters on each of the most important commodities sold at the Speziale al Giglio: wax, sugar, spices and sweets, and medicines. We conclude with a glance at what happened to the Giglio as Florence moved into the sixteenth century and from a republic to a court community.

We first investigated these ideas and the account books as part of Evelyn Welch's research on Renaissance shopping practices,[20] but the sheer amount of material available meant that they, and the Speziale al Giglio itself, deserved an independent study in its own right. This project was funded by a three-year Wellcome Trust Project for which James Shaw, a specialist in the institutions of market justice,[21] originally undertook postdoctoral work. He became a co-investigator in 2003, and we are very grateful to Philippa Woodcock, who stepped in to help finalise the database he originally created and analysed in detail throughout this project. This work has been heavily dependent upon developments in the technology and access to material: in addition to the database, we have employed digital photography in the archive of the Ospedale degli Innocenti (for which we are particularly grateful to Dr Lucia Sandri), and made use of key primary sources that have been digitised and made available to the public, such as the 1499 edition of the *Ricettario fiorentino* provided by the Bibliothèque Nationale de France.[22] The research for this book was delivered in seminars at The Wellcome Trust

Centre for the History of Medicine at UCL; the Universities of Warwick, Cambridge, and Oxford; the Institute of Historical Research; and at the conferences organised by the Renaissance Society of America in Toronto and Cambridge and by the Society for Renaissance Studies in Edinburgh. The authors wish to thank those who invited them to speak and their audiences for the opportunities to test their ideas. Particular thanks go to Andrea Mozzato, Julia DeLancey, Reinhold Mueller, Filippo de Vivo, John Henderson, Katherine Park, David Gentilcore and Sandra Cavallo for their help in realising this project. Finally, we would like to thank the Wellcome Trust for its support, without which this work would not have been possible.

Notes

1. C. Lury, 'Contemplating a Self-Portrait as a Pharmacist', *Theory, Culture and Society*, 22 (2005), 93–110; I. Szmigin, 'The Aestheticization of Consumption: An Exploration of "Brand New" and "Shopping"', *Marketing Theory*, 6 (2006), 107–18.

2. N. Reynolds, 'Pickled Sheep off the Menu as Hirst Opens', *The Daily Telegraph*, 15 January 1998; L. Barton, 'The Drugs Didn't Work', *The Guardian*, 24 September 2003, http://www.guardian.co.uk/news/2003/sep/24/food.foodanddrink

3. http://www.tate.org.uk/pharmacy/

4. J. Styles, 'Product Innovation in Early Modern London', *Past & Present*, 148 (2000), 124–69.

5. E. Kremers, G. Sonnedecker, and G. Urdang, *Kremers and Urdang's History of Pharmacy*, 4th edn (Madison: American Institute of the History of Pharmacy, 1986).

6. Styles, *op. cit.* (note 4).

7. J. DeLancey, 'Dragonsblood and Ultramarine: The Apothecary and Artists' Pigments in Renaissance Florence', in M. Fantoni, L.C. Matthew, and S.F. Matthews-Grieco (eds), *The Art Market in Italy : 15th–17th Centuries. Il mercato dell'arte in Italia (secc. XV–XVII)* (Modena: Franco Cosimo Panini, 2003), 141–50.

8. F. De Vivo, 'Pharmacies as Centres of Communication in Early Modern Venice', *Renaissance Studies*, 21, 4 (2007), 505–21; E.S. Cohen, 'Miscarriages of Apothecary Justice: Un-separate Spaces of Work and Family in Early Modern Rome', *Renaissance Studies*, 21, 4 (2007), 480–504.

9. A. Nannizzi, 'L'arte degli speziali in Siena', *Bollettino senese di storia patria*, n.s. 10 (1939), 93–131 and 260; *Speziali aromatari e farmacisti in Sicilia. Convegno e mostra sulla storia della farmacia e del farmacista in Sicilia dal secolo XIII al secolo XIX*, (Palermo: Associazione Culturale Apotheke, 1990).

10. S. Gaddoni and B. Bughetti, *Giornale di una spezieria in Imola nel sec. XIV* (Imola: University Press Bologna, 1995) well illustrates the problem of simply transcribing this sort of data.

11. C. Jones, 'The Great Chain of Buying: Medical Advertisement, the Bourgeois Public Sphere and the Origins of the French Revolution', *American Historical Review* 101, 1 (1996), 13–40.

12. S. Cavallo, *Artisans of the Body in Early Modern Italy: Identities, Families, Masculinities* (Manchester: Manchester University Press, 2007); G. Pomata, *Contracting a Cure: Patients, Healers, and the Law in Early Modern Bologna,* (Baltimore: Johns Hopkins University Press, 1998).

13. A. Astorri, 'Appunti sull'esercizio dello speziale a Firenze nel quattrocento', *Archivio storico italiano,* 147 (1989), 31–62: 33; R. Ciasca, *L'arte dei medici e speziali nella storia e nel commercio fiorentino dal secolo XII al XV* (Florence: Leo S. Olschki, 1927), 746.

14. E. Coturri, 'Spunti di medicina e di farmacia nelle novelle di uno speziale toscano del trecento, Giovanni Sercambi (1348–1424)', in *Atti del IV convegno di studi AISF, Varese: 3–4 Ottobre 1959* (Pisa: Arti grafiche Pacini Mariotti, 1959); S. Calonacci, 'Luca Landucci', in *Dizionario biografico degli italiani* (Rome: Istituto della Enciclopedia Italiana, 2004), 543–6; E. Conti (ed.), *Matteo Palmieri. Ricordi fiscali, 1427–1474* (Rome: Istituto storico italiano per il medio evo, 1983).

15. M. Ficino, *Three Books on Life,* C.V. Kaske and J.R. Clark (trans.), (Binghampton: Medieval and Renaissance Texts and Studies, 1989), 239.

16. R.K. Marshall, *The Local Merchants of Prato: Small Entrepreneurs in the Late Medieval Economy* (Baltimore: Johns Hopkins University Press, 1999).

17. I. Ait, *Tra scienza e mercato: gli speziali a Roma nel tardo medioevo* (Rome: Istituto Nazionale di Studi Romani, 1996); G. Carra, 'Speziali e spezierie nella Mantova dei Gonzaga', *Civiltà mantovana,* 12 (1978), 245–75; P. Wallis, 'Consumption, Retailing and Medicine in Early Modern London', *Economic History Review,* 61 (2008), 26–53.

18. J.-P. Bénézet, *Pharmacie et médicament en Méditerranée occidentale: (XIIIe–XVIe siècles)* (Paris: H. Champion, 1999), 263; De Vivo, *op. cit.* (note 8).

19. For Venice, see R. Palmer, 'Pharmacy in the Republic of Venice in the Sixteenth Century', in A. Wear, R.K. French, and I.M. Lonie (eds), *The Medical Renaissance of the Sixteenth Century* (Cambridge: Cambridge University Press, 1985), while P. Findlen, 'Inventing Nature: Commerce, Art and Science in the Early Modern Cabinet of Curiosities', in P.H. Smith and P. Findlen (eds), *Merchants and Marvels: Commerce, Science, and Art in Early Modern Europe* (New York: Routledge, 2002), 297–323, has tackled the topic on a broader scale. For recent work on the Dutch republic, see the key role played by apothecaries in A. Goldgar, *Tulipmania: Money, Honor and*

Knowledge in the Dutch Golden Age (Chicago: University of Chicago Press, 2007) and H.J. Cook, *Matters of Exchange: Commerce, Medicine, and Science in the Dutch Golden Age* (New Haven: Yale University Press, 2007); for Germany, see A. Burmester, V. Haller and C. Krekel, 'Pigmenta et Colores: The Artist's Palette in Pharmacy Price Lists from Liegnitz (Silesia)', in J. Kirby, S. Nash and J. Cannon, *Trade in Artisis' Materials: Markets and Commerce in Europe in 1700* (London: Archetype, 2010).

20. E. Welch, *Shopping in the Renaissance: Consumer Cultures in Italy 1400–1600* (New Haven: Yale University Press, 2005).

21. J.E. Shaw, *The Justice of Venice: Authorities and Liberties in the Urban Economy, 1550–1700* (Oxford: Oxford University Press, 2006).

22. *Ricettario Fiorentino* (Florence: Compagnia del Drago, 1499).

PART ONE

SELLING HEALTH

2

The Shop and the City

In 1493, the Speziale al Giglio or 'The Apothecary at the Lily', stood on the Canto al Giglio near the Mercato Vecchio in Florence, the heart of the city's commercial life.[1] With fishmongers and butchers' stalls in the centre of the square, and with women selling vegetables, cheese and wine, and grocery shops on its perimeter, this is where Florentine families came to get their daily provisions. The second-hand dealers' premises that surrounded the square provided used clothing, furniture and even paintings and statuary at bargain prices. Here too, laws were pronounced and criminals punished and shamed under the column topped by Donatello's figure of *Dovizia* (Image 2.1, overleaf).

By the late fifteenth century, the Giglio had probably been on this bustling central site for over thirty years. Owned by Tommaso di Giovanni Guidi, it was a well-established outlet patronised by Florentines from all walks of life. Its clients included the Ambassador of the Duke of Ferrara[2] and serving girls from local families. Unskilled labourers and fishermen might find themselves standing alongside well-known Florentine painters such as Sandro Botticelli, Domenico Ghirlandaio and Cosimo Rosselli, as well as members of the patrician élite such as Bartolomeo Scala, the city's chancellor.[3] Some customers only came into the shop once or twice a year; others arrived on a daily basis. Some came for prescription drugs, some for sweets, sugar and cordials, some wanted wax candles or simply to listen to gossip. Not all interchanges were pleasant. While waiting in another apothecary shop, the *Aromatario della Luna* in the Mercato Vecchio in early fifteenth-century Florence, the prostitute Maddalena of Ragusa hit the daughter of one of the servants of the Florentine Signoria over the head with her clog, resulting in a three-florin fine and a florin to be paid in compensation to the victim.[4]

The apothecary shop encouraged sociability, even if it resulted in arguments, partly because clients often had to wait a long time to be served, and partly because medicines were usually made up according to individual prescription, rather than being ready-made products that were kept in store. Drugs were supposed to be tailored to the individual constitution, ensuring that any drive to standardise practice had to be reconciled with the expert role of the doctor. In Renaissance Europe, practitioners and clients shared a

31

Image 2.1

Mercato Vecchio, Florence,
with view of the statue of Dovizia
nineteenth-century photographic view, © *Alinari.*

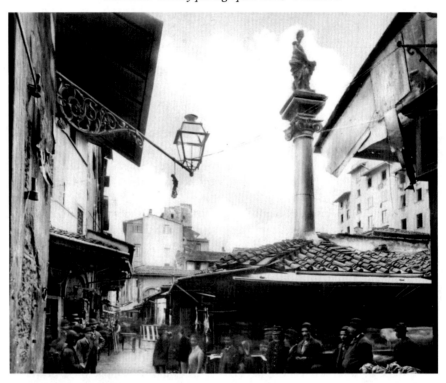

common explanatory model of the body and health derived from Greek medical tradition. This saw the body as being constituted of four humours (blood, yellow bile, black bile and phlegm). Each of these was defined in terms of two physical characteristics, which in turn were derived from the four elements (blood was 'hot' and 'humid', black bile was 'cold' and 'dry'). If these humours were properly balanced, mixed and distributed, then the person was healthy; conversely, an imbalance of humours created disease. Health, as illustrated in a figure of the four humours, was therefore essentially a function of internal factors, those that were considered 'natural' to the body[5] (see Image 2.2)

The body did not constitute a closed system; rather, the balance of humours was influenced by six 'non-naturals' (that is, factors external to the body). These 'inputs' to the system included such things as the quality of the

Image 2.2

The Four Humours
from the Guild Book of the Barber Surgeons of York, circa fifteenth century.
© British Library Board. The Bridgeman Art Library.

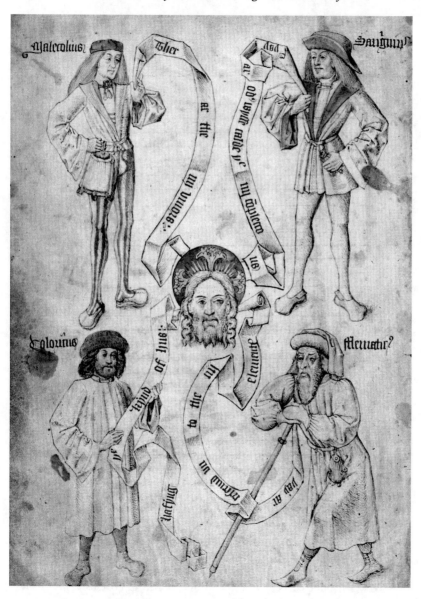

Image 2.3

'Vomiting', Italian School, fourteenth century.
Osterreichische Nationalbibliothek, Vienna, Nova 2644, Fol. 99v Austria,
© Alinari/Réunion des Musées Nationaux

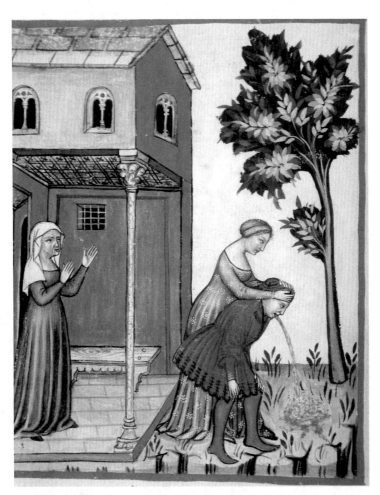

air, exposure to heat or cold, sleep, violent exercise, emotional shock, and most importantly, food and drink. The model could therefore account for seasonal patterns; for example, in winter, the cold and wet phlegm tended to increase, producing diseases such as colds, bronchitis, pneumonia and consumption. Advice, often given in a manuscript or printed 'Taccuinum sanitatis', encouraged people to adopt an holistic approach to their own

Image 2.4

'Sleep-talking', Italian School, fourteenth century.
Osterreichische Nationalbibliothek, Vienna, Nova 2644, Fol.101v Austria,
©Alinari/Réunion des Musées Nationaux

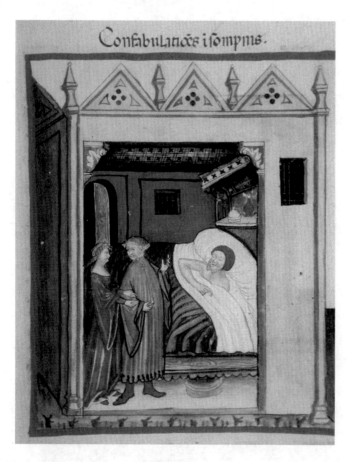

health, including when it was appropriate to vomit or how to handle sleep-talking (Images 2.3 and 2.4). Staying well meant adopting an appropriate 'regimen', including various aspects of lifestyle such as the ventilation of the bedroom, moderate exercise, getting a good sleep, eating the right food. Although there were associated systems which placed great emphasis on planetary influences, as shown in the image of the 'planetary man', this was a purely physical model of bodily health, with little room for spiritual or magical causes (see Image 2.5, overleaf). God was the ultimate source of

Image 2.5

'Planet Man' from Book of Hours, *printed by Philippe Pigouchet
for Simon Vostre, 1498, French School, fifteenth century.*
© *Lambeth Palace Library, London/The Bridgeman Art Library.*

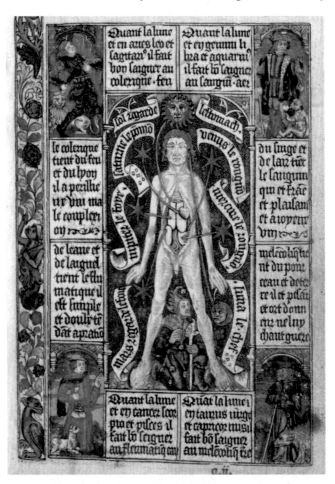

health and disease, but he worked through physical means. Miracles could
occur, but they were a matter for churchmen, not for doctors. Importantly,
both had their place, but one could not necessarily replace the other. Thus,
men and women could turn to the saints, use rings with magical invocations
and other techniques such as placing a copy of the Life of Saint Margaret on
a pregnant woman's belly to ensure safe childbirth.[6] But at the same time,

they knew that they also required much more individualised treatments. Each person had a given complexion and a tendency towards one particular humour. This was defined at birth by such factors as the stock of the parents, the circumstances of the birth and external influences such as the stars. There were obviously some general tendencies related to gender, status, and climate – women tended to be wet and cold; men were hot and dry; peasants tended to be 'sanguine'; scholars to be 'melancholy'; people from Northern Europe tended to be 'cold', those from the Mediterranean tended to be 'hot'. Men and women were also expected to change over time – people tended to 'dry out' as they got older. Individuals were therefore conceived of being of a particular humoral type – for example, a particularly 'choleric' young man – and doctors would need to take this into account. Therapy that was appropriate for a sturdy young peasant boy might prove terminal for an old aristocratic widow.

Although this model was capable of great theoretical elaboration, in its simplest form it allowed a considerable degree of popular participation. People were able to look after their own health to a considerable extent by adopting a suitable regimen. Good health began with good diet, eating foods appropriate to the person and to the season.[7] The education and status of patients and practitioners determined the extent of their engagement with medical theory, but underlying this were common assumptions about how the body worked. Many patients knew that they required an annual bloodletting in the spring as the weather began to warm up; otherwise the increase of blood in this season might result in fever. For more significant imbalances, the expert guidance of a doctor would usually be sought. The doctor's recommendations usually encompassed changes in regimen, but it also involved more decisive corrective actions. One common therapy was to remove excess humours through lancing or cupping, a task usually performed by barber-surgeons. The other main pillar of therapy was the consumption of drugs. These were intended to strengthen the humours that were lacking, and purge those in excess.[8] Most drugs were in fact cathartics, laxatives, emetics, diuretics and expectorants, designed to expel substances from the body.[9]

This meant that there were serious conflicts between the desire to standardise medicines – a long-standing need prompted by the concerns over efficacy and the potential for poisoning – and the impulse to ensure that each drug was adapted to a particular individual's requirements at the particular time, place and moment of consumption. This must have led to considerable discussion between patient, doctor and the apothecary inside or outside the shop. There is also some evidence that the shop was a space for consumption of medical products as well as for their production. For example, the stocking-maker Antonio Martelli, whose own business lay directly opposite the Giglio, bought a medicinal syrup – made from rob of scabious and water of soapwort – 'to drink in the shop' on three occasions.[10] Another client drank syrups in the shop 'on several occasions',[11] and a third also took syrup 'here in the shop'.[12] The fact that the apothecary bothered to record this detail suggests that it was an unusual practice that was limited to syrups, one perhaps prompted by the desire to avoid any need to buy a drinking glass, or to have to carry one back to the shop.[13]

Florence 1493–4

The periods of waiting and consumption meant that apothecaries' shops were often equipped with benches where people could sit, or even with chess sets, while clocks often informed clients of the passing time.[14] This may explain why apothecary shops were frequently connected with intellectual and literary activities. Thus, the apothecary Luca Landucci was described as a 'diarist and man of letters, [who] opened the Farmacia al Canto dei Tornaquinci in the late fifteenth century, where he met with other literary figures.'[15] By the sixteenth century, these shops were associated with formal literary academies such as the famous Florentine academy of the *Umidi*, a trend that was also true in seventeenth-century Venice.[16] More worryingly for the political authorities, the long periods of idleness, and the marked social mix of clientele, where gentlemen waited alongside artisans and serving girls, made these shops potentially subversive sites for political discussion and the exchange of illicit information.[17]

There was much to discuss in Florence between the summers of 1493 and 1494. First of all, there was the weather. In January 1494, Luca Landucci noted:

> The day of San Bastiano [Saint Sebastian] there was the severest snowstorm in Florence that the oldest people could remember. And amongst other extraordinary things, it was accompanied by such a violent wind that for the whole day it was impossible to open the shops, or the doors and windows.[18]

By Spring, the warming air brought fear of disease and the news that there was plague in Rome. In March, Florence's government, the Signoria created a committee or *balia* of five citizens to protect against the plague, 'per cura della peste'.[19] In April, the city's gatekeepers were warned to turn away 'scoundrels and beggars' as part of the policy of keeping the town disease-free. Bans were put in place against markets, festivals and processions, features which were lifted once the summer was over in September 1494.[20]

Along with worries about plague came concerns over an uncertain military situation. In 1493, the city government was still dominated, as it had been since the 1430s, by the Medici family and its allies.[21] Their faction was led by Lorenzo de' Medici's son, Piero di Lorenzo. Married to a daughter of an important Roman noble family, Clarice Orsini, he was viewed with some suspicion by his fellow Florentines for harbouring princely ambitions and failing to provide the same security and prosperity that his father and grandfather had offered. Urban politics was changing in other ways as well. In 1490, Girolamo Savonarola, a Dominican preacher from the Ferrarese nobility, had returned to Florence and embarked on a programme of preaching for religious renewal.[22] His preaching called for an austere lifestyle, a return to a highly moral society where women would remain indoors and men would focus on their spiritual rather than their economic and political needs. His ambitions, however, were made possible by the impending invasion of Italy by the King of France, Charles VIII, whom Savonarola welcomed as a scourge that would cleanse the corrupt republic.[23]

The friar's ideal was a return to Florence's original medieval values, for it had remained a republic in its organisational structure, despite the Medici ascendency. The city was led by a rotating magistracy chosen by lot every six months, the Priors, whose official leader was the 'Gonfaloniere di Giustizia'. At least three of these élite political figures were regular customers at the Giglio between 1493 and 1494.[24] A legislature, composed of two hundred men elected by lot, met regularly in the town hall to vote on laws and proposals posed by the Priors, while extraordinary committees called *balie* took charge of problem areas such as warfare and public health. When Piero di Lorenzo's grandfather, Cosimo de' Medici, and his allies had taken power in 1434, they had introduced a range of new institutions designed to maintain even closer control over the government.[25] Nonetheless, even after these modifications, Florence differed dramatically from other Italian cities. Landed aristocrats had been barred from government since the thirteenth century, and political participation depended on guild membership rather than military prowess. Although the Medici were regarded as prince-like in their demeanour, the family was generally careful to maintain the appearance of ordinary citizenship. Famously, Lorenzo had argued that he was simply a private individual who had to retain power in order to prevent the dissolution of his wealth and that of his supporters.[26] The attempt to assassinate Lorenzo and his family in 1478 had already revealed the rifts that lay between the competing members of the Florentine patriciate. With Lorenzo's death in 1492, rumours continued to circulate over Piero's ability to maintain his family's ascendancy.[27] A complex diplomatic web that linked the Medici and Florence to the fate of the Kings of Naples meant that the latter's enemy, the King of France Charles, VIII, who claimed the throne of Naples for himself, was eager to remove the family from power.[28]

39

Guilds and guildsmen in Florence

The eventual downfall of Piero di Lorenzo and his associates would come in 1494 with the arrival of Charles VIII's troops on the peninsula. During the year leading up to this, however, the diplomatic and military manoeuvres were followed with anxiety by all Florentines who were only too aware of what the international tensions might mean for the city. Earlier quarrels between the Medici, the Papacy and the Neapolitan rulers had led to warfare, an interdict that prevented church services from taking place in the city and most problematic, damage to international trade, something that was unthinkable for a commercial city such as Florence. Unlike cities such as Naples or Milan, Florence had built its political structures around the guild membership of its politically active, male citizens. In theory, even at the end of the fifteenth century, Florentines who wanted to be active in government needed to belong to one of the city's seven major guilds, or *Arti*.[29] These were the Bankers, the guild in which the Medici were enrolled, the Wool Merchants, the Silk Merchants, the Armourers, the Linen Drapers, the Goldsmiths and the guild of Doctors and Apothecaries. In practice, however, membership was no longer always obligatory and the numbers enrolled in these institutions had consistently dropped over the fifteenth century. Instead, the guilds were much more involved in the surveillance and monitoring of the trades themselves. The Guild of Doctors and Apothecaries, which oversaw the activities of the Speziale al Giglio, was one of the largest and most prominent of these institutions.[30] Like other Florentine guilds, it was highly heterogeneous, covering a wide range of different trades and practitioners. In addition to the doctors and apothecaries themselves, the Guild incorporated mercers, chandlers, stationers, leather-workers, metal-workers and painters. By the mid-fourteenth century, it had expanded to incorporate barbers – who undertook a considerable amount of medical interventions – and grave-diggers. This was very different from, for example, Venice, where there was a high level of guild specialisation and a clear differentiation between apothecaries who sold medicines, *speziali da medicine* and those who sold a much wider range of products such as wax and confectionery, the *speziali da grosso*.[31] In Florence, by contrast, it was not even easy to differentiate between apothecaries and grocers who dealt in spices.

But, as we shall see, the high level of capital investment required meant that a dedicated apothecary shop was not an easy business to maintain; tax records suggest a declining presence of apothecaries among the tax-paying population over the fifteenth century.[32] This is supported by declining figures for Guild membership and for the number of apothecary shops in the city.[33] Nonetheless, such trends may represent only an aggregate decline in the number of operators, while those who remained in business continued to prosper. One scholar has argued that this represents a process of consolidation of the trade in the hands of a restricted circle of wealthier operators, a closely knit community bound by family and business ties and which increasingly dominated the Guild.[34] This trend may not therefore have been symptomatic of an economic 'decline' but rather of a structural shift in favour of larger operators who possessed the capital required to stock their shops with an increasingly varied range of products while at the same time offering generous credit facilities to consumers. Thus, by the end of the century, there were around sixty-six apothecary shops in Florence and, in 1481, only forty heads of household described themselves as *speziali*. But since the apothecary at the Giglio was not even registered with the Guild of Apothecaries, this may reflect a loosening of Guild control over the marketplace in this period rather than a decline in the business itself. Indeed the owner in 1493, Tommaso di Giovanni, was repeatedly elected, not to the guild of apothecaries, but to that of the shoemakers, across a period extending from 1466 to 1496.[35] His sons Lorenzo, Marco and Cristofano were also listed as members of the Guild of Shoemakers, as was his son-in-law Lapino d'Agnolo Lapini – who also acted as a mercer and who eventually inherited the shop.[36] The family's long-standing connection to the shoemakers' guild must explain why the guild of shoemakers was itself one of the shop's biggest clients, along with a number of its key officials and also a great number of shoemaker clients.[37] Indeed, the notary at the shoemakers' guild, ser Monte di Ventura, was instrumental in arranging the rental contract for the shop of the Giglio itself, as described in the Catasto record.[38]

There is no immediately identifiable reason for Tommaso's membership of the shoemakers' guild, apart from the fact that it offered important social and commercial connections; clearly such boundaries and definitions were slippery. Despite this formal association with the shoemakers, he clearly considered himself to be an apothecary, describing himself in his will as 'aromatarius'.[39] But if the apothecary's guild appears to have been unconcerned by a man formally defined as a 'shoemaker' operating a major business in their area of oversight, other boundaries did give rise to considerable anxiety. Most worrying were the questions of intellectual and social status. In principle, the doctor or *medicus* was an educated professional who had undergone a high level of training at one of Italy or Europe's expanding universities. He – being almost always male – might have studied at Bologna, Padua or one of the smaller institutions in Pavia, Ferrara, Siena or Florence, learning theories derived from Galen, Hippocrates and Avicenna alongside practical skills such as diagnosing illness and anatomy.[40] But Florence was unusual in permitting doctors to practise without a degree as long as they could pass a Guild examination concerning their competency.[41] The Guild deliberations of 1475 refer to empirics, 'those who begin to practice medicine on their own authority, based on simple and fallible experience'.[42] This meant that a shoemaker who used his sewing skills to couch cataracts could be considered a qualified medical practitioner, a conjunction that may explain the appearance of Maestro Benedetto di Francesco di Michele who listed his profession as 'shoemaker and eye-doctor' in the 1427 Catasto.[43] It even meant that there could be migration from one status to another, as when one Piero di Bello matriculated in the Guild as an apothecary but then reappeared in later records as a doctor.[44]

Despite these examples of overlap, it was acknowledged that the apothecary required a less formal education than his medically trained counterparts. Literacy and numeracy were taught in Florence's abacus schools such as the one attended by Luca Landucci in the 1470s; these ensured that the apothecary understood weights and measures, how to calculate dosages, how to read recipe-books and prescriptions, and, above all, how to keep his books.[45] Apprenticeship was the main method of gaining experience – a division between 'knowing' and 'making' that would again become much more acute in the sixteenth century. Yet while the Guild recognised this clear divide between the skills of a university-educated doctor and those of a more empirically trained apothecary, business relationships between the two were permitted well into the fifteenth century. Although doctors were not supposed to dispense medicines and apothecaries were not supposed to give medical advice, it was common practice to establish close working relationships. Doctors might own or invest in apothecary shops. They might join with apothecaries to import expensive ingredients or an apothecary could hire a doctor to work in his shop and vica-versa.[46] In 1459, for example, Master Polidoro Bracali noted that he had entered an agreement to serve in the:

> [B]ottega of Lorenzo di ser Cortese, the apothecary, with an agreement that
> I had to order medicines from his shop and practice according to the rules of
> the physicians of Pistoia, and that he had to give me eight large Florentine
> florins per year. I made the agreement for two years.[47]

In the 1470s, each apothecary was connected with a single doctor who examined patients and wrote prescriptions within the shop itself.[48]

It is not clear if this sort of close partnership was the practice at the Giglio, but the few references to doctors in the accounts suggest a close link to one 'maestro Mingho', probably the doctor from Faenza called Mengo Bianchelli (*c.*1440–1520), a distinguished physician who mixed in the highest social circles of Florence in this period.[49] Bianchelli was the author of various medical treatises – a work on fevers including a 'head to toe' compendium of other ailments, one on the properties of the local thermal springs at Porretta, and one on the plague.[50] In the accounts he can be found prescribing drugs for nuns and monks,[51] and a 'powder for the womb' and other drugs for the wife of the Ambassador of Ferrara – which Doctor Mengo delivered in person.[52] The shop also retailed some of his patent recipes, including a 'ferrous electuary' and purgative pills made with rhubarb, which were sold to the Badia of Florence on a number of occasions.[53] However, this does not appear to have been an exclusive relationship, since the shop handled prescriptions from other doctors on occasion, as in a powder prescribed by 'Maestro Cristofano'.[54]

Katherine Park has shown how substantial a percentage of a doctor's income might come from the medicines he prescribed. In the late fourteenth century, for example, a doctor such as Maestro Ugolino da Montecatini claimed to, 'earn fl.400 or more a year with an apothecary's shop'.[55] The close financial links were usually reinforced with family ties, with considerable intermarriage between doctors and apothecaries.[56] Although there were concerns about such connections, formal business partnerships were also permitted within certain limits. Indeed, the only restriction was that doctors and apothecaries should not agree to prescribe and sell medicines in order to divide the profit. The Guild statutes were clear that doctors were not to accept 'kickbacks' from apothecaries on the price of their medications.[57] But even here the strong familial connections that often formed between the two groups meant such minor restrictions could be evaded in practice. This again was very different from other Italian cities where attempts were made to prevent any form of collaboration at all. The understandable anxiety was either that doctors and apothecaries would collude to provide medicines for maximum profit rather than patient benefit or that the differences between the two groups would evaporate altogether.[58]

In many cities such fears led to considerable civic oversight, particularly during times of plague when public health measures were led by special committees.[59] In Florence, in contrast, the Guild was given considerable liberty and tended to provide its own regulations and rules for members. Thus, in 1499, the Guild itself, rather than the newly established republican government, introduced the *Ricettario fiorentino*, the first official pharmacopoeia in Europe.[60] This was designed to establish a list of official recipes, offering a manual for pharmacists who were increasingly expected to provide standardised products. From at least the early fourteenth century, a doctor's prescription was required for the more powerful 'solutive' purges – 'medicina solutiva' – the most important category of drugs retailed at the shop.[61] By the middle of the next century, the professional association of doctors was attempting to assert full control over all health-related activities from prescriptions to midwifery. With the development of institutional authorities known as the *proto-medicato* in Tuscany and Rome, apothecaries were not allowed to sell any medicines at all except on the presentation of a doctor's prescription;[62] compound medicines were supposed to be prepared in the presence of *proto-medicato* officials. By this stage the assumption was still strong that doctors were trained at university while apothecaries were trained through apprenticeship. In practice, the divisions were not yet as sharp as the regulations would wish; but in principle, the former could achieve high social standing while the latter were restricted by the fact that they worked with their hands.[63]

But this sixteenth-century divide should not be read back onto the earlier period.[57] Far more fluid, flexible and with greater autonomy, the apothecary fulfilled a wide range of functions in the fifteenth century. Entry into the profession was through apprenticeship and Guild membership, and often facilitated by family relationships. There was a real demand for their services which were often provided twenty-four hours a day, three-hundred and sixty-five days out of the year. This was primarily because being ill was a challenging business in fifteenth-century Florence. Fevers, chest infections, unusual swellings, stomach upsets, diarrhoea, headaches, eye problems or simply a general feeling of malaise might make it impossible to earn a living and support a family. For women suffering from the after-effects of miscarriage or pregnancy, it might be difficult to look after infants and children, much less continue to work. If one were poor, there was the possibility of recourse to charitable hospitals such as Santa Maria Nuova or Sant'Egidio in Florence.[65] During the fifteenth century, Florence boasted around thirty-five hospitals where beds and care, both physical and spiritual, were provided for the indigent. But such beds tended to be occupied either by the long-term sick and elderly, who were unable to work at all, or those with acute problems that would quickly resolve themselves, with patients either dying or being discharged.[66] The majority of the patients tended to be male, often single men who were immigrants to the city and had no social network on which to fall back on. Those with strong familial links, above all women, expected to be cared for at home.

Purchasing medical help was costly and a visit from the doctor could cost as much as a gold florin. The medicines that were prescribed were often similarly expensive as were the foods that the doctor counselled the ill to digest, including chickens, capons, eggs, and fine wines. The sheer cost of conventional medicine meant that looking after one's health was a complex multi-layered process. At one level, remedies were prepared at home according to recipes that circulated amongst women and their families, many of which would be formalised in sixteenth-century printed editions. At the same time, patients and their families might buy ready-made pills and potions from travelling mountebanks who offered preventatives against poisons and all forms of diseases.[67] Many of these figures gave themselves exotic names and origins, such as the San Paolini, who presented themselves as the descendents of Saint Paul from Malta, with the ability to sell earth or bread that would prevent death from snake-bites.[68] Others simply sold incantations or prayers against illness or harm, often using dramatic spectacles. The Florentine apothecary Luca Landucci describes one such figure known as 'Lo Spagnolo', who essentially undertook a bit of fire-walking and fire-eating in order to sell his prayers. Landucci described how 'Lo Spagnolo' started his patter in the marketplace and then moved on to an oven in order to demonstrate the efficacy of his products:

> On arrival at the baker's, he said: give me some uncooked bread! and threw it on the oven to show that it was hot, and then he stripped down to his shirt and dropped his trousers to his knees, and in this way he entered until high up, and stayed there awhile, and picked up the bread and turned around inside. And note, the oven was hot, he brought out the bread and he didn't harm himself at all. When he had got out of the oven, he was given a torch and he lit it, and lighted as it was, he put it in his mouth and kept it there until it was extinguished. And many other times on the bench, over the course of several days he took a handful of lighted tapers, and held up his hand for a length of time, and then he put them burning into his mouth so that they went out. And he was seen to do many other things with fire: raising his hands into a pot of oil that was seen many times by all the people. And thus he sold as many of the prayers as he could make; and I say that among all the things I have ever seen, I have not seen a greater miracle than this, if it is a miracle.[69]

Landucci was sceptical but in a period when there were competing ways of obtaining cures, it was important to demonstrate success in a highly visible manner. Reputation was an important key to success, and in addition to charlatans, the sick could turn to empirics, wise women and men whose knowledge of herbs and remedies was well regarded in the local neighbourhood. They usually charged less than a physician but they still expected to be paid. For the poor, an official city doctor was the next step, either in hospital or at home. The wealthy might turn to the same figure but, as described above, they were expected to pay handsomely for the privilege. In addition to these figures, formal and informal, Florentines could consult a barber-surgeon who scraped and pulled teeth, cauterised wounds, set bones, cut hair and trimmed beards and moustaches and removed ear wax.[70] They could also go to an apothecary with their complaint and receive a standard treatment, visit the doctor in the apothecary's shop, or present a prescription. None of these were contradictory and as Katherine Park has shown, most patients with conditions that were not easily resolved chose to use a range of different medical sources.[71]

But while the Speziale al Giglio was a key site for medical care for fifteenth-century Florentines, it offered more than medications. In the next chapter we examine the geography and networks involved in keeping shop, intersections that were often complex and intended to offer reassurance through design and packaging as well as through the trust generated by long-standing social connections.

Notes

1. A. Astorri, 'Appunti sull'esercizio dello speziale a Firenze nel quattrocento', *Archivio storico italiano*, 147 (1989), 31–62: 52–3, the Canto del Giglio was located at the crossroads of the present-day via dei Calzaiuoli and via degli Speziali.
2. E882, ff. 61r, 339r, 'messer Manfredi inbasciadore di ferrara'.
3. E882, fo. 181r, 'Alessandro di mariano detto sandro di botticiello dipintore'; fo. 127v, 'Domenicho di tomaso di qurado dipintore'; ff. 111r, 161r, 'Chosimo di lorenzo rosselgli dipintore'; ff. 49r, 338r, 'messer Bartolomeo di [BLANK] schala'.
4. M.M. Serena, *Prostitute e lenoni nella Firenze del quattrocento* (Milan: Il Saggiatore, 1991), 367.
5. A.G. Carmichael, 'The Health Status of Florentines in the Fifteenth Century', in M. Tetel, R.G. Witt, and R. Goffen (eds), *Life and Death in Fifteenth-Century Florence* (Durham: Duke University Press, 1989), 28–45.
6. J. Musacchio, 'Conception and Birth', in M. Ajmar-Wollheim and F. Dennis (eds), *At Home in Renaissance Italy* (London: V&A Publications, 2006), 128; J. Cherry, 'Healing through Faith: The Continuation of Medieval Attitudes to Jewellery into the Renaissance', *Renaissance Studies*, 15, 2 (2001), 154–71.
7. T. Scully, 'The Sickdish in Early French Recipe Collections', in S.D. Campbell, B.S. Hall, and D. Klausner (eds), *Health, Disease and Healing in Medieval Culture* (Basingstoke: Macmillan, 1992), 132–40.
8. J.M. Riddle, *Quid Pro Quo: Studies in the History of Drugs* (Aldershot: Variorum, 1992), 158; N.G. Siraisi, *Medieval & Early Renaissance Medicine: An Introduction to Knowledge and Practice* (Chicago: University of Chicago Press, 1990), 141.
9. D.L. Cowen and W.H. Helfand, *Pharmacy: An Illustrated History* (New York: Harry N. Abrams, 1988), 28.
10. E882, fo. 116v, 'Antonio dandrea martelgli chalzaiuolo dirinpetto': 3 October 1493 'per bere in bottegha', 5 October 1493 'prese qui in bottegha'; 7 October 1493 'prese qui in bottegha'.
11. E882, fo. 150v, 'Pennone di [BLANK] da san ghallo', 27 April 1495, 'prese in bottegha in piu volte'.

12. E882, fo. 329v, 'Jachopo dant.o del cittadino', 2 June 1494, 'prese lui detto qui i' botttegha'; fo. 67r, 'ser Domenicho di Lucha Marucielgli', 4 September 1493, 'presa in bottegha'.

13. Customers had to pay for the vessels they used, which are listed as part of the bill. In some cases the lack of such payment suggests that customers brought used vessels back to the shop and exchanged them.

14. J.-P. Bénézet, *Pharmacie et médicament en Méditerranée occidentale: (XIIIe–XVIe siècles)* (Paris: H. Champion, 1999), 263–4.

15. L. Sguanci. 'Dante, l'arte dei medici e speziali e le spezierie della Firenze medioevale', *Relazione presentata al 5. Congresso della Società italiana di farmacia ospitaliera, tenuto a Firenze nel 1960* (Florence: 1960), 7.

16. *Itinerario farmaceutico di Firenze*, (Milan: I.E.I., 1969); R. Romano, 'Farmacie e farmacisti a Venezia', in R. Romano and A. Schwarz (eds), *Per una storia della farmacia e del farmacista in Italia. Vol 2. Venezia e Veneto* (Bologna: Edizioni Skema, 1981), 5.

17. F. De Vivo, 'Pharmacies as Centres of Communication in Early Modern Venice', *Renaissance Studies*, 21, 4 (2007), 505–21; W. Eamon, 'Medical Self-Fashioning, or How to Get Rich and Famous in the Renaissance Medical Marketplace', *Pharmacy in History*, 45 (2003), 123–9. For a comparative discussion, see F. Franceschi, 'La bottega come spazio di sociabilità', in F. Franceschi and G. Fossi (eds), *La grande storia dell'artigianato* (Florence: Giunti, 1999), 65–84 and J.D. Jensted, '"The City Cannot Hold You": Social Conversation in the Goldsmith's Shop', *Early Modern Literary Studies*, 8 (2002), 1–26.

18. L. Landucci, *A Florentine Diary from 1450 to 1516*, A. De Rosen Jervis (trans.), (London: J.M. Dent & Sons, 1927), 55–6, entry for 20 January 1494.

19. A.G. Carmichael, *Plague and the Poor in Early Renaissance Florence* (Cambridge: Cambridge University Press, 1986), 104–5.

20. *Ibid.*

21. R.J. Crum and J.T. Paoletti (eds), *Renaissance Florence: A Social History* (Cambridge: Cambridge University Press, 2006); N. Rubinstein, 'Oligarchy and Democracy in Fifteenth-Century Florence', in S. Bertelli and N. Rubinstein (eds), *Florence and Venice: Comparisons and Relations: Volume 1 – Quattrocento* (Florence: La Nuova Italia, 1980), 99–112.

22. L. Martines, *Scourge and Fire: Savonarola and Renaissance Italy* (London: Jonathan Cape, 2006), 19–28.

23. G. Savonarola, 'On the Renovation of the Church', in J.C. Olin (ed.), *The Catholic Reformation: Savonarola to Ignatius Loyola* (New York: Fordham University Press, 1992).

24. Online tratte records: http://www.stg.brown.edu/projects/tratte/search/office.php3, searches for 1493 and 1494. At least three of the

gonfalonieri across the two-year period 1493–4 are listed in the shop accounts. Tratte 122842, Piero di Gino Capponi, elected 29 October 1493; tratte 116721, Filippo di Giovanni Dell'Antella, elected 29 December 1493; tratte 121734, Niccolò di Antonio Martelli, elected 28 April 1494. On these see E882, fo. 154r, 'Piero di gino chapponi'; fo. 196v, 'Filippo di giovanni dalantella'; fo. 200v, 'Niccholo dant.o martelgli'.

25. N. Rubinstein, *The Government of Florence under the Medici (1434 to 1494)*, [1966] 2nd edn (Oxford: Clarendon, 1997), 1–153.

26. A. Brown, 'Florence, Renaissance and Early Modern State: Reappraisals', in *The Medici in Florence: The Exercise and Language of Power* (Florence: L.S. Olschki, 1992), 316; Lorenzo de' Medici, 'A Memoir and a Letter', in R.N. Watkins (ed.), *Humanism and Liberty: Writings on Freedom from Fifteenth-Century Florence* (Columbia: University of South Carolina Press, 1978), 160.

27. P.C. Clarke, *The Soderini and the Medici: Power and Patronage in Fifteenth-Century Florence* (Oxford: Clarendon, 1991).

28. D. Abulafia (ed.), *The French Descent into Renaissance Italy, 1494–5: Antecedents and Effects* (Aldershot: Variorum, 1995).

29. J.M. Najemy, 'Guild Republicanism in Trecento Florence: The Successes and Ultimate Failure of Corporate Politics', *American Historical Review*, 84, 1 (1979), 53–71.

30. R. Ciasca, *L'arte dei medici e speziali nella storia e nel commercio fiorentino dal secolo XII al XV* (Florence: L.S. Olschki, 1927).

31. *Ibid.*, 347, n.3.

32. Astorri, *op. cit.* (note 1), 35–8.

33. Ciasca, *op. cit.* (note 30), 698, 323–4.

34. Astorri, *op. cit.* (note 1), 42.

35. Tratte records for 'Tommaso di Giovanni di Piero Guidi', refs. 107973–85, 107932–4.

36. Tratte records for 'Lorenzo di Tommaso di Giovanni Guidi', refs. 73022, 73029–30; 'Marco di Tommaso di Giovanni Guidi', refs. 76710–1, 76718–20; 'Cristofano di Tommaso Guidi', refs. 320815, 31162–5; 'Lapino d'Agnolo Lapini', refs. 67040–3. There are also references to 'Lorenzo di Tommaso di Piero Guidi' and 'Marco di Tommaso di Piero Guidi', elected to the Guild of Shoemakers, and these probably refer to the same people.

37. E882, fo. 30r, 'Larte de chalzolai'; fo. 167v, 'Ghuglielmo dandrea familglio al arte de chalzolai'; fo. 170v, 'Mariano di franc.o bardini proveditore al arte de chalzolai'.

38. ASF, Catasto 1022, Microfilm 2474, fo. 366 ff, 'chartte per mano di ser mo[n]tt[e] di ve[n]ttura nottaio a cha[l]zolai'. E882, fo. 214r, lists an account from 1476 (m.f.) in the name of 'ser Monte di ventura notaio al arte de chalzolai', who is probably the same man listed on fo. 10v, 'ser Monte di

Ventura notaio alla merchatantia', an entry dated 1490. This suggests that he transferred from the guild to the merchants' court at some point.

39. ASF, Notarile Antecosimiano 10586, fo. 136r.

40. K. Park, *Doctors and Medicine in Early Renaissance Florence* (Princeton: Princeton University Press, 1985), 123.

41. *Ibid.*, 22.

42. *Ibid.*, 67.

43. *Ibid.*, 23, 69.

44. *Ibid.*, 67.

45. P.F. Grendler, *Schooling in Renaissance Italy: Literacy and Learning, 1300–1600* (Baltimore: Johns Hopkins University Press, 1989).

46. Park, *op. cit.* (note 40).

47. *Ibid.*, 110, n.76.

48. Ciasca, *op. cit.* (note 30), 746.

49. M. Ficino, *Three Books on Life*, C.V. Kaske and J.R. Clark (trans.), (Binghampton: Medieval and Renaissance Texts and Studies, 1989), 449, n.19, refers to Mengo Bianchelli da Faenza as a 'distinguished physician' who was present at a dinner held at Lorenzo de Medici's house in 1489. He was also a lecturer on medicine at Pavia. F. Raspadori (ed.), *I maestri di medicina ed arti dell'Università di Ferrara, 1391–1950* (Florence: L.S. Olschki, 1991), 12–13, further notes that he was 'lettore allo Studio' at the University of Ferrara during the academic years 1466–72.

50. *De omni genere febrium. Et de morbidis particularibus a capite usque ad pedes.* (Venice: Stefano dei Nicolini da Sabbio, 1536); *De aqua Porretae* (Florence, 1487); *Contro alla peste. Il consiglio di Messer Marsilio Ficino. Il Co'siglio di Maestro Tommaso del Garbo. Una Ricetta duna polvere co'posta da Maestro Mingo da Faenza. Una Ricetta fatta nello Studio di Bolognia et molte altri Remedii* (1523).

51. E882, fo. 119r, 'Fruosino di Cece da Verrazano', 3 January 1493 (m.f.), purchase of 8 oz of 'latt.o daupilati', 'ordino maestro mingho per suora chaterina' and fo. 319v, 28 June 1494, purchase of syrup 'per suora chaterina sua sirochia monacha in santo anbruogio', 'ordino m.o mingho'; fo. 357v, 'Fratti e monaci della badia di firenze', 30 May 1494, purchase of 4 scruples of 'p'le ordino m.o mengho per i.o monacho'.

52. E882, fo. 61r, 'Manfredi inbasciadore di ferrara', 31 October 1493, purchase of 'polvere damatricia', 'ordino m.o mingho perla donna'; 2 November 1493, purchase of 2 drams of 'trefola mangnia', 'p.o m.o mingho'.

53. E882, fo. 329r, 21/06/1494, purchase of 0.5 drams of 'p'le reuberberate daupilate di m.o mingho'; fo. 257v, 10 April 1494, purchase of 8 'p'le del maestro mengho'; fo. 220v, 16 January 1493 (m.f.), purchase of 6 'p'le di m.o mingho'; fo. 350r, 18 August 1494, purchase of 12 'p'le del m.o mengho'. For other clients, see fo. 306v, 'Andrea di pagholo niccholini',

14/04/1494, purchase of 3 oz of 'latt.o ferrato di m.o mingho' and
14/04/1494, purchase of 4 oz of 'latt.o ferrato di m.o mingho'; fo. 346r,
'Rafaello di guliano bastiere a san chasciano', 5 July 1494, purchase of 3 oz
of 'latt.o ferrato di m.o mingho'.

54. E882, fo. 124v, 'Ruffino di [BLANK] oste alaporta alachrocie', 19 October
1493, purchase of a powder, 'per rufino ordino m.o christofono'. The
doctor's boy sometimes delivered medicines to clients, which were probably
also prescribed by his master: E882, fo. 348v, 18 July 1494, 'per fare
bangniuolo ale braccia e ale ghanbe p.o eraghazo di m.o christofano'; fo.
352r, 23 July 1494, 'p.o eraghazo di m.o christofano'.

55. Park, *op. cit.* (note 40), 157.

56. *Ibid.*, 32.

57. *Ibid.*, 29.

58. S.R. Ell, 'Governmental Regulation of Medicine in Late Medieval Venice',
Fifteenth-Century Studies, 2 (1979), 83–9.

59. Although for a later period, the work of Carlo Cipolla deals with much of
the history of public health and plague control in Renaissance Florence, see
C.M. Cipolla, *Cristofano and the Plague: A Study in the History of Public
Health in the Age of Galileo* (London: Collins, 1973); C.M. Cipolla, *Miasmi
ed umori: ecologia e condizioni sanitarie in Toscana nel seicento* (Bologna: Il
Mulino, 1989).

60. L. Colapinto, 'The "Nuovo Receptario" of Florence', *Medicina nei secoli*, n.s.
5 (1993), 39–50.

61. R. Ciasca (ed.), *Statuti dell'arte dei medici e speziali* (Florence: L.S. Olschki,
1922), 46, 180.

62. D. Gentilcore, *Healers and Healing in Early Modern Italy* (Manchester:
Manchester University Press, 1998).

63. E. Welch, *Shopping in the Renaissance: Consumer Cultures in Italy 1400–1600*
(New Haven: Yale University Press, 2005).

64. M. Laughran, 'Medicating without "Scruples": The "Professionalization" of
the Apothecary in Sixteenth-Century Venice', *Pharmacy in History*, 45
(2003), 95–107.

65. K. Park and J. Henderson, '"The First Hospital among Christians": The
Ospedale di Santa Maria Nuova in Early Sixteenth-Century Florence',
Medical History, 35 (1991); J. Henderson, *The Renaissance Hospital: Healing
the Body and Healing the Soul* (New Haven: Yale University Press, 2006).

66. J. Henderson, 'Healing the Body and Saving the Soul: Hospitals in
Renaissance Florence', *Renaissance Studies*, 15, 2 (2001), 188–216; B.J.
Trexler, 'Hospital Patients in Florence: San Paolo, 1567–8', *Bulletin of the
History of Medicine*, 48 (1974), 41–59.

67. M.A. Katritzky, *Women, Medicine and Theatre, 1500–1750: Literary
Mountebanks and Performing Quacks* (Aldershot: Ashgate, 2007). Extensive

discussion of the relationship between mountebanks and apothecaries can be found in D. Gentilcore, 'Apothecaries, "Charlatans", and the Medical Marketplace in Italy, 1400–1750 – Introduction', *Pharmacy in History,* 45 (2003), 91–4; D. Gentilcore, '"For the Protection of Those who have both Shop and Home in this City": Relations between Italian Charlatans and Apothecaries', *Pharmacy in History,* 45 (2003), 108–21; D. Gentilcore, *Medical Charlatanism in Early Modern Italy* (Oxford: Oxford University Press, 2006).

68. K. Park, 'Country Medicine in the City Marketplace: Snakehandlers as Itinerant Healers', *Renaissance Studies,* 15, 2 (2001), 104–20.

69. L. Landucci, *Diario fiorentino dal 1450 al 1516: continuato da un anonimo fino al 1542,* I. Del Badia (ed.), (Florence: Sansoni, 1883), 299–300; see also P. Camporesi, *Bread of Dreams: Food and Fantasy in Early Modern Europe* (Cambridge: Polity, 1989), 22.

70. S. Cavallo and D. Biow, *The Culture of Cleanliness in Renaissance Italy* (Ithaca: Cornell University Press, 2006).

71. Park, *op. cit.* (note 40).

3

Keeping Shop

The Speziale del Giglio was a large, carefully organised, city-based retail outlet. Its owner lived elsewhere in town and in his country 'villa'; he was far from being a small-town or rural apothecary where living space and workspace shared the same building.[1] This division was important. One of the key differences between the mobile mountebank, such as the vendor of 'snake oil' shown in a fifteenth-century illumination, the empiric working from home or even the doctor who made his own pills, and the apothecary, were the physical spaces from which they operated and the social opportunities that this offered (see Image 3.1, overleaf). While travelling vendors made sales and then moved on, preventing redress in case of poor service or quality, the apothecary had to face his clients every day. The expense of maintaining premises was a feature that Guild members stressed in their complaints against pedlars and mountebanks, but the investment also allowed for a dense network of inter-shop relations and exchange and a high degree of specialisation and mutual support. By 1493, the Giglio was well established and could rely heavily on its neighbours, many of whom were also apothecaries – one of the nearby streets was called Via degli Speziali – and gain custom from the local community as well as from those who came from other neighbourhoods.[2]

The first owner of the Speziale del Giglio was Tommaso di Giovanni di Piero Guidi, who set up his business sometime in the 1460s.[3] His name simply means, Thomas, son of John, son of Peter, suggesting a relatively modest background. He had arrived in Florence from Montevarchi, a small town in the countryside and took his last name, Guidi, from the Counts who dominated that region. In 1480 he went to register his family, income and debts in Florence's Catasto, the city's main tax records.[4] Here, he stated that he was forty-three years old and lived in the neighbourhood of San Giovanni, Gonfalone Chiavi, in the parish of Santa Maria Nipotecosa. He was married to Brigida and had three sons and five daughters. Even at this stage, he hadn't lost touch with his birthplace. The family still had a number of smallholdings in Montevarchi, which provided rents of fourteen and seventeen staia of grain annually. He had also bought land near Fiesole and an additional house in Florence which was rented to a stocking-maker for fifteen florins per annum. But, perhaps with a view to reducing his tax

James Shaw and Evelyn Welch

Image 3.1

Historiated Initial 'D' from Historia Naturalis,
depicting a mountebank holding snakes, fifteenth century,
Biblioteca Marciana, Venice, Italy/The Bridgeman Art Library.

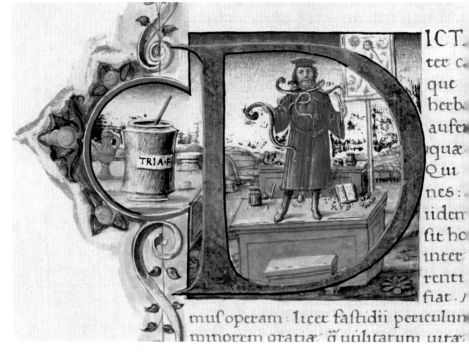

burden, he presented himself as a man of only moderate wealth. The total amount of his possessions was eventually rated at a modest 168 florins.

Florentines were notorious at underestimating their property and pleading poverty when confronted by tax officials.[5] Even so, Tommaso di Giovanni was not a wealthy man and we have no way of knowing how he came to set up his establishment. His matriculation in the Guild of Shoemakers rather than that of the Doctors and Apothecaries may reflect the fact that he had not undertaken an apprenticeship within the city itself. It is possible that his wife's dowry provided the initial sum that allowed the couple to invest in the goods and space required. Luca Landucci gives an indication of the investment needed to establish a business in his diary:

And on the 4th September, 1462, I left Francesco, son of Francesco, the apothecary, at the sign of the Sun, who gave me, the sixth year, the salary of

54

fifty florins, and I joined company with Spinello, son of Lorenzo, the hope of gaining more causing me to give up the gain which was sure. And we opened an apothecary's shop in the *Mercato Vecchio*, at the sign of the King, which had formerly been the shop of a second-hand dealer, which had a very low roof. We raised the roof, and spent a fortune, although I was unwilling to outlay so much. All was done without stint, one cupboard alone costing fifty gold florins.[6]

Shortly afterwards, Landucci fell out with his partner and they separated on 27 July 1463. After working with various other apothecaries, he then bought the shop of the Tornaquinci on 1 September 1466.

Tommaso di Giovanni's itinerary was far more stable. He managed his shop well, was able to make further investments and eventually bought his own country estate. It is not clear when his first wife, Brigida, died but he remarried at some point before October 1501, when he was married to Lucrezia, the daughter of a notary from Pontassieve.[7] By the time of his death, Tommaso di Giovanni could have been described as a well-to-do, if not wealthy, reasonably educated and devout member of the Florentine community. His home was decorated with the heavy wooden furnishings typical of the Tuscan *palazzo*, including a large walnut bed.[8] There were numerous religious images on the walls ranging from the traditional madonna tabernacles to a large image of the Last Supper and a fashionable roundel or *tondo* which was probably also of the Virgin Mary. Tommaso also had four 'heads', probably portrait busts in his bedroom. Three of these were sited above his bed while the fourth was over a doorway. This arrangement was one that would have been familiar to the city's élite and it is interesting to find it in an apothecary's home. Tommaso's ownership of such a large number of devotional artworks may not be unconnected to his close friendship with the Florentine painter, Cosimo Rosselli. Although Rosselli is not highly regarded today, he was considered one of the city's leading artists in the fifteenth century, participating in the painting of the Sistine chapel alongside Botticelli, Perugino and Domenico Ghirlandaio.[9] Rosselli enjoyed a very close relationship with Tommaso, appearing frequently in the Giglio accounts and acting as an executor of the apothecary's will.[10]

As well as sharing an appreciation of Florence's artistic workshop production, Tommaso also had many of his contemporary's literary interests. He owned at least twenty-five books, including at least one in Greek. Some of these are simply described as 'books of medicine', including two editions of Mesue of particular interest to an apothecary, but there are also the works of Dante, Cicero, Horace, Livy, a book on Florentine history, and a 'book of prayers of Fra Ruberto' (the Franciscan preacher Roberto Caracciolo).[11] The substantial amounts of cash found in his desk along with six pieces of unicorn horn and a number of small bags of highly valuable azure pigment suggests that he had had a very successful career in his chosen profession.[12]

Although this was a family business, none of Tommaso's four sons would inherit the shop despite the fact that at least two of the boys, Lorenzo and Marco, worked with their father. Lorenzo travelled to Venice on Giglio business while Marco received payments from clients.[13] By August 1504, when Tommaso drew up his will, both Lorenzo and Marco had died (Marco leaving behind a daughter, named Brigida like his mother). His other son Cristofano had become a Dominican monk at San Marco, the centre of the Savonarolan movement in those years. Tommaso therefore resolved in his will to hand over his business to his daughter Marietta, who in December 1479 had married Lapino Lapini, the son of a mercer.[14] The shop was to be run by Lapino, with the assistance of Giovanni di ser Stefano da Pontassieve, Tommaso's brother-in-law through his second marriage. In addition to the mercery business, Lapino on occasion worked alongside his father-in-law, and when Tommaso died in 1504 he was able to build up the business to even greater profitability becoming a supplier to the ducal court in the 1530s.[15]

In the 1490s, however, the shop was doing reasonably well, if not spectacularly so. This was in part because Tommaso used the business to satisfy his own personal needs rather than for major commercial expansion. Indeed, along with members of his family and staff, he was one of the chief customers of the shop. This had the advantage, of course, of minimising taxable profits but it also suggests that a clear separation between the domestic and the commercial sides of the business was not regarded as essential.

The shop certainly supported a reasonable number of additional employees. Along with his sons and son-in-law, Tommaso employed apprentices or *garzoni*. At least five were mentioned in 1493–4. They were kept busy undertaking deliveries and the hard but essential work of grinding materials with heavy pestles and mortars. One was specifically referred to as a *'pestatore'* or grinder, a figure like that pictured in the fresco in a castle in Issogne, North Italy, of an apothecary where an impoverished beggar is shown grinding ingredients (see Image 3.2 inset).[16] Although not beggars, these young men would typically work at very low wages in return for training, room, board and basic items of clothing. Thus, when local stocking-makers paid for goods with stockings, these were handed out to shop staff whose wages were docked in turn for these supplies.[17]

Interestingly, although apprentices were expected to stay with their master for a period of up to three years, there are suggestions that there was a relatively high turnover in Tommaso's shop. One apprentice only stayed for four months; others seem to have had relatively casual arrangements. But

Image 3.2

Fresco Interior of a Pharmacy,
Italian School, fifteenth century. Castello di Issogne, Val d'Aosta, Italy.

Inset: detail of ingredients.

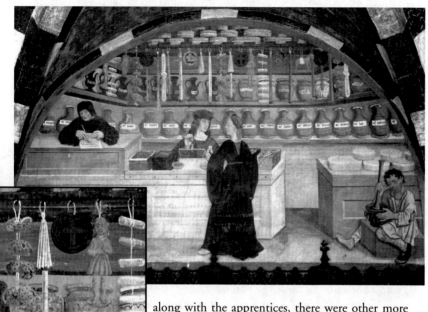

along with the apprentices, there were other more experienced staff members who performed specialist tasks. As the Giglio's meticulous records indicate, the business of book-keeping was crucial. This may have been done by Tommaso himself, but he probably had the help of Duccio di Zanobi Tolosini, who was referred to as 'nostro schrivano' or clerk.[18] There were also 'fattori', or factors, who made deliveries and collected payments and, most importantly, professional debt-collectors. The shop used two such men to bring in payments that were overdue.[19]

There is no record of either of Tommaso's wives or any of his daughters serving in the Giglio although such work would not have been uncommon. Their absence from the accounts may simply be due to the fact that they were not involved in deliveries or payments. Certainly, other fifteenth-century Florentine shopkeepers found it very useful. But in the absence of evidence, we have to assume that from Tommaso's viewpoint, this was essentially a masculine site where he, his sons and son-in-law and his male apprentices prepared a wide range of goods for sale to a much more mixed clientele. However, in 1501–2, his second wife, Lucretia is notable for supplying the shop with small quantities of rose water, which she may have manufactured at home.[20]

Making medicines and the spectacle of shopping

The shop itself could have accommodated the substantial number of staff described above. The 1504 shop inventory describes a 'bottega' or main room and indicates that there was a kitchen for preparing goods and a terrace for drying medicinal and three other main rooms, a much larger interior than most Tuscan shops.[21] The other difference was the fact that exchange and manufacture took place primarily inside the building. In most other shops, the salesman stood at a counter which looked directly out onto the street.[22] While shelves at the back might provide a rich display, the bulk of their premises were devoted to storage. Mezzanine areas and basements were crammed with bulk products while rear rooms might be used as living spaces or to prepare goods. In contrast, the apothecary used a very high proportion of the interior space to provide an area where clients could gather. It is not surprising that when Landucci took over a second-hand dealer's shop in Florence and turned it into an apothecary, he had to raise the roof. The former probably only used the space for storage; Landucci needed to offer his customers a greater degree of comfort. The 1504 inventory of the Speziale al Giglio suggests that this shop was at the higher end of the spectrum in terms of luxurious display. It had the standard image of the Virgin Mary on the wall and its furnishings seem to have been of very high quality. The door and window fittings, writing desks and money box were made in early 1494 by the carpenter and engraver Cervagio Del Tasso,[23] who later worked on the ceiling of the Great Council Chamber in the Palazzo Ducale.[24] Within the shop, the space was dominated by shelves, estimated at over forty-six metres in total,[25] and a large sales counter that was around 5.8 metres long and 1.2 metres wide, a piece of furniture that may have resembled the almost contemporary image in Issogne illustrated above.[26] This structure incorporated a number of other storage devices for dry commodities: a large unit with fifty-five drawers below and shelves above,[27] with a smaller unit of forty-eight drawers below,[28] a smaller cupboard with seven drawers,[29] and two little shelf units for storing small pre-prepared compositions of drugs: one held twenty boxes of pills, and the other thirty-three boxes of pills and trochisks.[30] There were fifty-two estamins, the white fabrics that were used to make sieves, stored in a special box.[31] To the side were additional cupboards with drawers that held ingredients, recipe books and boxes and vials for dispensing goods. In addition, the shop contained a very substantial quantity of vessels, in both ceramic and glass, to store drugs. These included over two hundred *albarelli* jars of different sizes ('half', 'quart' and 'half quart'), probably elegantly decorated, forty-four syrup jars, thirty ceramic oil flasks and fifty-eight glass flasks for distilled waters. Pills were held in small boxes while forty boxes of dried herbs provided stock ingredients for the manufacture of decoctions, fomentations and drugs.[32] On top of the counter was an iron disk to cover cakes, presumably protecting them from dust and insects.[33] There were also wooden containers for plaster.[34] There were also eighteen 'long boxes', perhaps the same as those sold as packaging when customers bought large quantities of sweets such as *confetti*. Finally, there were a large number of coloured glass bottles used to store syrups and electuaries, presumably those supplied to customers to transport liquids.[35]

Financial business and account-keeping was carried out at a separate, smaller writing-desk that contained drawers to hold money and a cupboard of books, containing two receptaries, and copies of the key texts such as Mesue and Serapione.[36] Elsewhere in the shop there was a chest 'full of books' which presumably were referred to less frequently.[37] An inventory taken about the same time of another apothecary shop in Florence also listed over five hundred *albarelli*, sixteen wooden boxes, thirty-two pill boxes; a 'great cupboard with seventy-four drawers' and numerous other cabinets.[38] The presence of a 'writing desk with a doctor's chair' makes it clear that diagnosis and prescribing took place within the shop.[39] The overall impression of wood, painted ceramics and glassware must have resembled some of the illustrations that depict pharmacies from this period, such as the fifteenth-century Italian illuminated Avicenna or the astonishing image of Christ as a pharmacist from a sixteenth-century Parisian manuscript (Images 3.3 and 3.4 overleaf).

But as well as an impressive site of sale and medical advice, the shop was a place of production both in front of clients and out of sight. The Speziale al Giglio was filled with equipment for all types of manufacture. There was the press, a *strettoio pacholo*, used for making oils such as that of almonds.[40] Grinding and mixing were also key processes and the inventory listed three stone and seven bronze mortars of varying weights and sizes, ranging from small versions weighing ten lbs each – ie., just over three kilos – to an immense bronze mortar weighing 130 lbs – ie., forty-four kilos. This was attached to a stone column, ensuring that it became an integral part of the shop's architecture.[41] There were also two special bronze 'mortars for pills' as well as three pairs of scales of various sizes for accurate weighing, iron and brass spatulas to dose materials, and a stove for boiling and heating, along with numerous copper and brass pans and cauldrons.

Mortars were expensive items; in one case, the bronze pestle was suspended above the mortar, suggesting it was immensely heavy.[42] The more elegant versions, bronze basins, two large green pans for making honey

Image 3.3

Page from the Canon of Medicine *by Avicenna (Ibn Sina),*
Biblioteca Estense, Modena, Italy.
The Bridgeman Art Library.

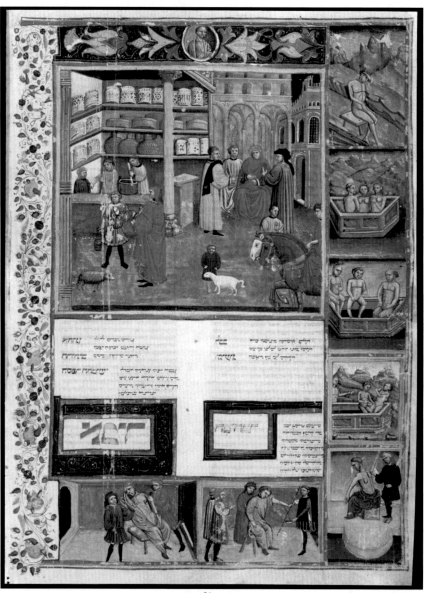

Image 3.4

'*Christ the Pharmacist with Adam and Eve*',
from Chants royaux sur la Conception couronnee du Puy de Rouen,
French School, sixteenth century. Bibliotheque Nationale, Paris, Ms Fr 1537,
Archives Charmet/The Bridgeman Art Library.

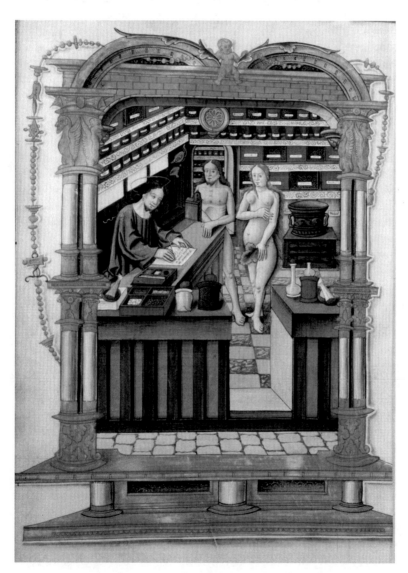

roset,[43] and sixteen smaller pans, copper and brass basins were all on display at the front of the shop. The specialist items needed for the shop's messier business of candle making were kept in the kitchen at the rear. Some of these were extremely heavy – one for wax weighed 120 lbs, a smaller one for vinegar weighed 19 lbs. There were also ten small copper cauldrons – weighing an average of 8 lbs each – and a *caratello* for making verjuice, a vinegar by-product of the grape. The back area also had spatulas, ladles, scales, a *fornello* [small oven] for heating, and two lead alembics with iron bases for distillation.[44] There was also a separate 'kitchen' or workshop containing large numbers of glass flasks with pans for treating white wax and a stove.

Not everything, however, was made in the shop, which had an important wholesale as well as retail function. The most important commodities bought by the shop both for use and redistribution were sugar and spices. The Speziale al Giglio did not obtain such exotic goods directly but relied on a variety of intermediaries. The most important suppliers were Florentine trading companies, such as the banking firm Carlo Ginori & Co.,[45] Francesco Del Pugliese & Co.,[46] and the silk merchants Battista Dini & Co.[47] Alongside these were a number of other companies, often described as bankers, or wool, silk and linen drapers, which also had retail outlets in Florence.[48] Such businesses imported spices (and other groceries) because payment in kind was built into the structure of Mediterranean trade – Florentine cloth exports to the Middle East were often paid for in the form of spices, which could easily travel alongside bulkier cargoes.[49] So, for example, the bankers Giovanni di Ser Francesco & Co., supplied myrobalans, ceruse, capers and incense,[50] and the wool merchants Lorenzo Segni & Co., supplied peppercorns.[51] Most of these suppliers were Florentine, but a number of foreign merchants also imported speciality products, such as a merchant from Genoa who supplied 'Genoese glue',[52] and a number of merchants from Ragusa who supplied wax.[53] No Venetians are listed, which may reflect the disruption of their trade following the opening of the Cape Route – some of the Florentine companies may however have obtained their supplies in Venice.[54]

Purchases from trading companies were generally mediated by brokers.[55] Only a small minority of transactions – about five per cent – were organised in this way, but they were the most valuable purchases of goods in bulk, usually supplied in whole bales or barrels.[56] As well as placing buyers and sellers in contact, the brokers supervised and recorded the formalities of the transaction, such as the weighing of goods. Although Tommaso di Giovanni was not himself a member of the Guild of Doctors and Apothecaries, this did not prevent him from using the services of the official guild brokers.[57] Some of them, like Girolamo Maringhi, were also clients of the Giglio.[58] This would have been a convenient way of paying for his services in kind, but it is also suggestive of a long-established personal and business relationship. Maringhi even acted as shop supplier, trading in damascene sugar candy in his own right.[59] Credit accounts were a convenient means of payment in an economy that was short of cash, and brokers too were involved in the shop's web of personal connections. Another broker, Piero Maringhi, paid for a client's debts to the Giglio by transferring his own credit for brokerage.[60]

In addition to the foreign import trade, the shop also obtained supplies from local producers. A local butcher supplied the shop with lard,[61] and a rope-maker provided pitch.[62] The *bicchieraio* Chimenti d'Agnolo supplied the shop with pharmacy jars.[63] Some of these supply networks extended into the regional state, for example, the shop bought paper from dealers in the production centre of Colle,[64] and charcoal from a furnace at Pontassieve.[65]

This core group of professional merchants and local producers was supplemented by a much broader group of private individuals, often with no given occupation,[66] who took advantage of one-off trading opportunities as they arose. This was particularly important in an economy where cash was short and debts were often settled in kind, since people might often end up with surplus goods to dispose of. Many of these suppliers were carters, whose work in the transport sector exposed them to many business opportunities. They were mostly involved in supplying locally produced raw materials, such as honey, pitch and lead.[67] Approximately two thirds of suppliers were involved in only a single transaction during the three-year sample period, indicating the *ad hoc* nature of supply.[68] Many of these were old clients of the shop.[69] The barber Bernardo di maestro Chimenti, who bought medicines and candles in the 1490s, supplied six barrels of wine in 1502.[70] Luigi Scarlatti, who sold land to the apothecary in 1472, and who was a customer in the 1490s, supplied peppercorns and damascene incense in 1500.[71] Established personal and business ties fed into the supply networks, creating commercial opportunities.

Within this multitude of shopkeepers, businessmen and private citizens dabbling in the wholesale trade on an *ad hoc* basis, a small group of 'regular' suppliers can be identified.[72] They were responsible for relatively small quantities of goods – but on a more frequent basis. Unlike the high-value bulk transactions of the merchant companies, these were petty transactions that did not require mediation by brokers.

These regular suppliers include two rather anomalous figures. Firstly, the apothecary himself supplied both imported and locally produced materials to his associates.[73] Among the former, cassia, pepper, manna, nutmeg, cotton and cloves were particularly important. He also supplied goods from his own household, such as half a barrel of oil, or three flasks of vinegar.[74] In other cases, Tommaso bought goods in his own right that were delivered to the shop and entered as credits in his account, such as three *staia* of almonds,[75] and 'two barrels of sweet oil'.[76] He probably obtained these commodities through private trading, perhaps receiving them as payments in kind, and they could be conveniently disposed of via the shop. Closely related to this supplier, although listed separately with her own account, was the apothecary's second wife, Lucrezia, who, as described above, supplied small quantities of rose-water at irregular intervals. She may have manufactured these herself, since these products were distinct from the ordinary goods from their home – the latter were entered in Tommaso's account.[77]

Secondly, the miller Lorenzo Vochato, tenant of the apothecary's mill,[78] who regularly provided grain, flour, fish, eggs and pigeons. These were probably rent payments in kind, as was standard for agricultural tenancies, Unusually they were not accounted for in monetary terms, probably because the contract specified payment in the form of goods.[79] It is unclear why these goods were paid to the shop instead of to Tommaso personally. Some of the products may have been used in manufacturing (flour was an ingredient in cakes, and eggs might be used to make 'plasters'), but most had to be disposed of.[80] Grain was often used to pay suppliers,[81] as when Salvestro di Donato da Montevarchi was paid fourteen *staia* of grain,[82] or to pay wages to the apothecary and shop staff.[83] It might also be sold in bulk, as when the shop sold 111 *staia* of grain to the local baker Jacopo di Ristoro.[84] Like other Florentine shops, the Giglio participated in transactions that lay outside its core business, dealing in a wide variety of goods that were used for payment in lieu of cash.

The other regular suppliers of the Giglio were apothecary shops. The most important of these was the Porcellino, which made the distilled waters that the Giglio sold.[85] A more varied range of products was supplied by the Pina, including honey, capers, musk, amber and spices, and also manufactures such as syrups and plasters.[86] Of lesser importance was a shop called the Medici, owned unsurprisingly by the Medici family. This was run by Piero de' Rossi & Co., who supplied medicinal simples such as opium.[87] Several other Florentine apothecaries supplied goods on a more occasional basis,[88] indicating that a close network of exchange existed among the operators of the sector. These were often tiny quantities, suggesting that apothecaries were able to turn to each other when stocks ran short. When the Porcellino supplied the Giglio with four lbs of cassia pulp, for example, the debt was paid back in kind two days later.[89] Integration into this network also permitted individual apothecaries to specialise, something that was difficult for provincial traders.[90] Although the inventory of the Giglio lists two alembics that were specifically 'for distilling',[91] the shop actually bought in most of its distilled waters from outside,[92] primarily from the Porcellino, who were specialist distillers[93] – the development of more complex stills in the sixteenth century would probably have permitted a further degree of manufacturing specialisation on an almost industrial scale.[94] The Giglio itself appears to have specialised in funerary equipment, which it hired to other apothecaries,[95] and it also sold its marzipan, pepper bread and drugs to other shops.[96] This raises questions about how representative any one shop can be for the market as a whole.

This network facilitated both the petty exchange of commodities and the bulk distribution of goods. Shops bought large quantities as opportunities arose and disposed of the surplus to operators in the same or related sectors: for example, the Pina regularly supplied the Giglio with bulk commodities, such as whole barrels of capers or honey.[97] Included within this network was the dispensary at the city's great hospital of Santa Maria Nuova. It often disposed of its surplus stock to the apothecaries of the city, as when it supplied rhubarb worth twenty-one florins to the Giglio.[98] In turn, the dispensary often obtained manufactured drugs and other raw materials in bulk from the apothecaries. For example, it bought twelve lbs of currants from the Giglio,[99] and thirty-six flasks of Porretta water from Luca Landucci.[100] This distribution network was not restricted to, or organised by, the Guild, but was a private matter.[101] Tommaso di Giovanni was not registered with the Guild, but he was nevertheless part of this network, along with many Guild operators. The network was particularly dense in the city centre; however, it also extended out to provincial centres – as when the Pina supplied the hospital of Santa Fina in San Gimignano.[102]

Like other Florentine traders and tradesmen, therefore, apothecaries were not simply retailers. Instead, much of their stock was destined for distribution in bulk. This has important consequences for the way that historians can use the inventories of apothecaries, often the only surviving evidence of their activities. Inventories present a 'snapshot' of the stock at a particular moment in time – they must be considered in relation to the *ad hoc* nature of shop supply. The fact that infrequent purchases were made in bulk as opportunities arose means that stocks of many commodities are highly variable. In particular, commodities with a long shelf life are likely to be over-represented, since they could be safely stockpiled. This is evident by comparing the inventory stocks of 1504 to the records of wholesale purchases for the preceding period 1500–2 (see Table 3.1, overleaf).[103] This gives a rough approximation of turnover, identifying commodities that had to be continually replenished, like cassia pulp and distilled waters (both commonly used to manufacture medicines),[104] and those that tended to clog up the shop, like wax or mastic. The inventory therefore overestimates the importance of commodities that had a long shelf life, that were bought occasionally and stockpiled for future use, but which had a very low turnover. They also underestimate the importance of products with a limited

Table 3.1

Wholesale Supplies: Top Fifteen Commodity Groups, 1500–02

Commodity group	Mean annual purchases 1500–2 (soldi)	% of total purchases 1500–2	Inventory 1504 (soldi)	% of total inventory	Approx. turnover (annual supply/ inventory)
Sugar	33,374	34.3%	6,726	7.0%	5.0
Wax	15,839	16.3%	18,672	19.4%	0.8
Spices	11,403	11.7%	4,379	4.5%	2.6
Honey	5,804	6.0%	539	0.6%	10.8
Cassia Pulp	5,231	5.4%	595	0.6%	8.8
Wheat Flour	2,494	2.6%	0	–	–
Cotton	2,417	2.5%	727	0.8%	3.3
Waters	2,125	2.2%	280	0.3%	7.6
Mastic	1,758	1.8%	1,970	2.0%	0.9
Paper	1,421	1.5%	810	0.8%	1.8
Almonds	1,233	1.3%	469	0.5%	2.6
Rhubarb	1,178	1.2%	1,740	1.8%	0.7
Soap	924	1.0%	864	0.9%	1.1
Myrobalans	910	0.9%	879	0.9%	1.0
Glue	845	0.9%	191	0.2%	4.4

shelf life, such as many compound drugs,[105] and especially those that were made on the spot, as was the case for many medicines. Many of the best-selling products were either absent from the inventory, or present in only small quantities.

Some indication of the Giglio's involvement in the bulk distributive trade is given by comparing total annual retail sales (around 88,609 soldi) to average annual wholesale supplies (around 97,000 soldi).[106] The shortfall is all the more striking because the nominal prices that were billed to customers were higher than the sums that the apothecary could realistically expect to recoup. Although these data are taken from different time periods (there is no record of wholesale supplies for 1493–4), for this level of retail sales the associated costs of raw materials cannot have been much higher than around 53,000 soldi for the apothecary to make any profit.[107] Unless the retail trade had picked up dramatically by the early 1500s, a considerable proportion of the supplies (close to half) must have been bought for bulk distribution rather than retail. These kinds of transactions do not appear in the retail records and were accounted for separately, but we do have some evidence of this side of the business: for example, the hospital of Santa Maria Nuova purchased 12 lbs of currants from the Giglio in September 1493, which falls within the sample period, but because this was a bulk transaction the hospital does not appear as a client in the retail records.[108]

Close examination of some of the commodities that are prominent in the inventory supports this hypothesis. Artists' materials amounted to a considerable proportion of stock (seven per cent), but were rarely purchased by the shop, suggesting a low turnover.[109] Retail sales were also very low,[110] and most of the colours in stock, such as verdigris, or orpiment, are almost entirely absent from the retail sample.[111] An explanation is suggested by examining the kind of clients who bought these materials. The few clients who bought colours retail at the Giglio were not professional artists. Instead we find individuals such as a carter and a monk, as well as one monastic institution.[112] In only one case is there a link to an artist, when a company of silk merchants bought 11 lbs of green paint for their shop, which was collected by the painter, Giovanni di Chimenti.[113] Instead, the artists listed as clients of the shop (see the previous chapter) almost always only bought medicines.[114] It was not that the Giglio never sold colours but rather that it tended to sell them in bulk, as when the shop exported 239 lbs of verdigris to Siena. Thus they do not appear in the retail records.[115] Artists' workshops probably bought their materials in large amounts – on this evidence there was not much of a market for small quantities of colour sold retail.

Other commodities reveal similar patterns. There was 810 soldi-worth of paper in stock (less than one per cent of the total), and annual supplies exceeded this (1,421 soldi), suggesting a high turnover, but retail sales were insignificant (approximately 18 soldi). Paper was probably not bought for retail but for redistribution (some was probably also used by the shop). Similarly, there was 864 soldi-worth of soap in stock, which was exceeded by supplies of 924 soldi per annum,[116] but retail sales were insignificant (about twenty soldi). Although some of the soap was probably used in production, the bulk of it must have been for wholesale distribution, probably to barbers. Similar patterns can be found for glue and vitriol, where again the vast majority of stock was for distribution in bulk to other operators (probably tanners and cloth manufacturers in the case of vitriol), rather than retail to the general public. Many of the commodities listed in the fourteenth-century statute were in fact of little importance for the retail trade. Items like paper, soap, artists' materials or string, were occasionally sold retail but were insignificant in terms of the total.[117] Apothecaries like the Giglio specialised their retail activities far more closely.

Conclusion

The inventory gives a strong sense of the capital investment that was made in both the front and back of the shop. In the more public areas, the display reassured customers that their products were being prepared with care. Just over a century later, Tommaso Garzoni would mock this assumption, accusing apothecaries of having:

> [A]mongst them frauds and tricks, not only of ridiculous appearance – like those jugs, those jars and boxes with large capital letters, which tell of a thousand unguents or confections or precious aromatics – but they are empty inside, carrying these ridiculous inscriptions outside, as the jars of master Grillo of Conigliano do – but there are also evil acts of sinister souls, making dangerous medications by switching one thing for another, or mixing poor quality stuff, old and rotting in their goblets, and sometimes they are aware of this, and other times it is due to the shameful ignorance with which they buy goods from Levantine barbarians at a cheap price in order to cobble together a shop as best they can....[118]

While Garzoni's witty attack was delivered in 1585, the concept that fine packaging might mask a poor product was a long-standing one. The wary consumer needed to see for him- or herself what was going into the goods they bought. Importantly, this seems to have been possible at the Giglio. While, as we will see, some items were bought from other suppliers, and distillates, candy-making and wax were created in the back of the shop, the manufacture of specific recipes for an individual patient using the mortar and pestle seem to have taken place in full view of customers. Given the fears of substitutions, inferior ingredients and fraud, this provided an important assurance of quality.

Similarly, even if they were unable to observe the apothecary's activities directly, customers could assume that they had a good understanding of what went on at the back of the shop as well as at the front. With the possible exception of the alembic and oven, the only thing to differentiate the Giglio workshop from a domestic kitchen was the size and weight of the equipment, and the scale of the operation. Otherwise, many of the activities undertaken would have been recognisable and indeed feasible in a Florentine home. Manuscript recipe books from the fourteenth and fifteenth centuries indicate that home remedies and those that made it into the *Ricettario fiorentino* had more in common than might be expected. Eventually compiled and printed, these recipes for everything from how to treat an ulcer to the best way to prevent baldness were composed of ingredients that would be purchased from the apothecary. Thus, while the shop was designed to suggest that the professional way in which prescriptions written by a doctor were made was very different from the potions created by one's wife, mother or maid-servant, the distinctions may not have been so clear cut.[119] To understand the ways in which the shop and its patrons interacted, not only in terms of medical knowledge but also in terms of social connections, we need to identify the actual customers themselves. The Giglio, with its long lists of the men and women who came to buy its products, gives us the means to do so.

Notes

1. J.-P. Bénézet, *Pharmacie et médicament en Méditerranée occidentale: (XIIIe–XVIe siècles)* (Paris: H. Champion, 1999), 259, argues for a hierarchical distinction between small and large operators on this basis.
2. M.L. Bianchi and M.L. Grossi, 'Botteghe, economia e spazio urbano', in F. Franceschi and G. Fossi (eds), *La grande storia dell'artigianato* (Florence: Giunti, 1999), 27–64.
3. R. Ciasca, *L'arte dei medici e speziali nella storia e nel commercio fiorentino dal secolo XII al XV* (Florence: Leo S. Olschki, 1927), 746, quotes Benedetto Dei's list of thirty-two 'Speziarie grosse nella città di Firenze', which is dated 1470. This list includes 'Tommaso di Giovanni, all'insegna del giglio'. Estranei 903, gives the earliest date for the shop business activity as 1464.
4. ASF, Catasto 1022, Microfilm 2474, fo. 366.
5. G.A. Brucker, 'Florentine Voices from the Catasto, 1427–1480', *I Tatti Studies*, 5 (1993), 11–32.
6. L. Landucci, *A Florentine Diary from 1450 to 1516*, A. De Rosen Jervis (trans.), (London: J.M. Dent & Sons, 1927), 3.
7. E541, fo. 24r, 'm.a Luchrezia donna di tomaso di giovanni nostro'. ASF, Notarile Antecosimiano 10586, fo. 136v, describes her as the daughter of Ser Stefano de Pontassieve.
8. E878, fo. 2r, 'chamera di d.o thomaso in sulla sala' lists 'una tabernach0lo e trovi i.o crorsello dinhevo, una nostra donna a ½ tondo chon un fioretto di sopra, uno quadretto entrovi uno sangirolamo dipinto al chornice doro, iiij.o teste dinhevo 3 insulla lettiera e i.o sopra lusio, una piata dipinta intela cho chornicie doro, una lettiera di b[r] 5 in pielarata di nocie agorneone.'
9. A.R. Blumenthal, *et al.*, *Cosimo Rosselli Painter of the Sistine Chapel* (Winter Park Florida: Cornell Fine Arts Museum, 2001).
10. E878, fo. 2r, 'chosimo di lorenzo dipintore' and 'franc.o di giovanni dan*drio*and*ri* [?]' were named as 'asechutori e fidechomessari'.
11. E878, fo. 2v, lists various books: 'lib[r]o di morali disan giachomo, bibbia in forma chorda di choio paghonazo, uno dante, uno pl'mo [?], lib[r]o disposizionedi vangieli, uno lib[r]o de frutti della linxua, lib[r]o in forma d.o chansomere delp chasa, lib[r]o delle preghere di fra rub[er]to, lib[r]o in linxua grecha, uno mesue, lib[r]o di medicina, lib[r]o di medicina, lib[r]o

della storia fiorentina'; ff. 8r–8v lists further books in the study: 'lib[r]o di morali di san giechono, tulio damicizia [i.e. Cicero, 'On Friendship'], lib[r]o della x'polana religione, vergho chiosato, lib[r]o di medicina, lib[r]o di medicina, lib[r]o dorazio, lib[r]o detto pungi linxua, lib[r]o delle deche [i.e. Livy], lib[r]o di santuario, lib[r]o di mesue, lib[r]o... delo spechio duemtenzia.'

12.   E878, ff. 2v–3r, lists on the desk 'uno schatolino truovi 6 pezi di chorno di liochorno', various bags of money totalling around fl 390 and L7461s0d6, and attached to the desk a 'chasone' containing several different sacks of azures.

13.   E882, fo. 113r, 'Ferrando di chastro spangniuolo', 29 October 1491, 'venne da vinegia di suo cho[n] nostre chose quando ando lorenzo nostro a vinegia cho[n] lui'; fo. 96v, 'Giovanbatista di benedetto dighoro', 22 March 1493 (m.f.) and 18 June 1496, 'per marcho di tomaso nostro'.

14.   ASF, Notarile Antecosimiano 10586, ff. 136r–139v, for Tommaso's will.

15.   On this, see Estranei 904–6 and 592–4.

16.   E882, fo. 252v, 'Niccholo di marchionne del m.o ridolfo nostro gharzone' – see also fo. 104v, 21 September 1493, 'porto nichclo nostro fattore' and fo. 354r, 1 August 1494, 'porto nichlo n.o gharzone'. E882, fo. 319r, 'Girolamo di tomme da volterra nostro gharzone' – fo. 352r, 27 July 1494, 'p.o girolamino n.o', may be a reference to this character. For other apprentices listed see, fo. 80r, 'Girolamo d'andrea da san giovanni nostro gharzone'; fo. 131r, 'Lorenzo diachopo di mafio berti nostro gharzone'. E882, fo. 331v, 'Antonio diachopo nostro gharzone pestatore'.

17.   E882, fo. 146r, 'Cristofano di paradiso chalzaiuolo', 23 November 1493; fo. 146v, 'Charlo di bartolomeo chalzaiuolo fratello di franc.o da santo andrea', 3 January 1493 (m.f.), for payments with *calze*, which were then given to members of the shop and placed in their own account as debts.

18.   E882, ff. 246v, 350v, 'Duccio di zanobi tolosini nostro schrivano'.

19.   E882, ff. 138v, 330v, 'Ugenio di tommaso fiaschi nostro rischotitore' – see also fo. 349r, 25 September 1494, 'per noi a ugenio di tomaso fraschi n.o rischotitore'. E882, ff. 253v, 268r, 'Bardo di taddeo di stagio da ghiaccietto nostro rischotitore'.

20.   E541, fo. 24r, transactions dating from 2 October 1501.

21.   J. DeLancey, 'Dragonsblood and Ultramarine: The Apothecary and Artists' Pigments in Renaissance Florence', in M. Fantoni, L.C. Matthew, and S.F. Matthews-Grieco (eds), *The Art Market in Italy: 15th–17th Centuries. Il mercato dell'arte in Italia (secc. XV–XVII)* (Modena: Franco Cosimo Panini, 2003), 141–50: 145.

22.   E. Welch, *Shopping in the Renaissance: Consumer Cultures in Italy 1400–1600* (New Haven: Yale University Press, 2005); D. Clark, 'The Shop Within? An

Analysis of the Architectural Evidence for Medieval Shops', *Architectural History*, 43 (2000), 58–87.

23. E882, fo. 257r, 'Ciervagio di franc.o deltaso lengniaiuolo', 8 January 1493 (m.f.), payment of L26s13, 'sono per piu lavori fatti a tomaso nostro in chasa e in bottegha cioe usci finestre scrittoi e lachasetta de danari'. For details of work on Tommaso's desk, see also fo. 333r, 6 December 1494, which records purchase of nails and metal fittings for Cervagio's work.

24. R. Ciabani, *Le famiglie di Firenze*, 4 vols (Florence: Bonechi, 1992), 355.

25. E878, fo. 19r, 'b[raccia] 80 di schafali in circha'.

26. E878, fo. 19r, 'Uno descho da vendere in bottegha di b[raccia]10 in circha lungho + largho b[raccia] 2 chon armari di fuori + 15 chassette d[is]eni[e]?'. According to M.S. Mazzi and S. Raveggi, *Gli uomini e le cose nelle campagne fiorentine del quattrocento* (Florence: L.S. Olschki, 1983), the Florentine *braccio* was 0.583m.

27. E878, fo. 19r, 'armario dal descho [ad] 55 chasette + schafali di sopra'.

28. E878, fo. 19r, 'armariuzo sotto dt.o armario di 48 chasettine'.

29. E878, fo. 19r, 'Un armaruzo insuldescho di 7 chasettine'.

30. E878, fo. 19r, 'schaffette da pillole in sul descho di xx bossoli di pillole'; 'schafetta chonfitta da pillole + turcissi [c]on 33 bosoli + schatoline da turcissi + pillole'.

31. E878, ff. 18v, 19r, 'Stamingne bianche 52' and a 'chassa da stamingne'.

32. E878, fo. 19r, 'Schatole da erbe seche'.

33. E878, fo. 19v, 'tondo di ferro dachoprire le torte'.

34. E878, fo. 19r, 'bichonzuoli da giesso'. According to G. Nardelli, *Farmacie e farmacisti in Umbria: dagli statuti degli speziali all'ordine* (Perugia: Umbrafarm, 1998), 184, a *bigonzuolo* was a 'recipiente in legno tondeggiante'.

35. E878, fo. 19v, '74 mezine tragialle +altri cholori dalatovari + sciloppi inchucina'.

36. Ciasca, *op. cit.* (note 3), 342–3.

37. E878, fo. 20r, 'chassone pieno di libri'.

38. ASF, Notarile antecosimiano 14293, fo. 25r, inventory of 23 September 1500.

39. ASF, Notarile antecosimiano 14293, fo. 25v.

40. Bénézet, *op. cit.* (note 1), 290.

41. A. Martini, *Manuale di metrologia ossia misure, pesi e monete in uso attulamente ed anticamente presso tutti i popoli* (Turin: Loescher, 1883) gives the Florentine pound as the equivalent of 339.54g.

42. E878, fo. 19r, 'Mortaro grande cholpestone di bronzo peso'.

43. E878, fo. 19r, 'Pentole verde grande da mele rosato'.

44. E878, fo. 19v, 'champane di pionbo dastilare [su]lfondo di ferro'.

45. E541, ff. 17v, 18v, 22r, 29v, 'Charlo di lionardo ginori e chonpangni', for a total value of 31,898 soldi, amounting to about 11% of the total value of supplies in the three year period. Most of this was specifically described as being for 'Madeira sugar'. The company also supplied incense and soap. On Ginori, see D. Franklin, 'Rosso Fiorentino's Betrothal of the Virgin: Patronage and Interpretation', *Journal of the Warburg and Courtauld Institutes*, 55 (1992), 180–99: 180.

46. E541, ff. 6r, 9v, 'Francesco di Piero delpugliese e chonpangni', for a total value of 19,088 soldi, all of it described as 'Portuguese sugar'.

47. E541, ff. 28r, 29v, 'Batista di franc.o dini e chonpangni setaiuoli', for a total value of 11,543 soldi. Together, these three suppliers (Ginori, Del Pugliese, Dini) accounted for 62,529 soldi, 22% of the total spending over the three-year period (290,242 soldi).

48. Some examples – E541, fo. 34r, 'Lorenzo di bernardo sengni e chonpangni lanaiuoli'; ff. 12v, 14v, 'Guliano di guolo setaiuolo'; ff. 22r, 27r, 'Franc.o di guliano di giovencho de medici e chonp.a lanaiuoli'; fo. 20v, 'Franc.o di filippo delpugliese e chonpagni lanaiuoli'; ff. 12r, 13v, 'Zanobi di franc.o di bartolo e chonpangni linariuoli'; ff. 24v, 27v, 33r, 'Giovanni di ser franc.o da anbra e chonpangni banchieri'.

49. Ciasca, *op. cit.* (note 3), 447–50.

50. E541, ff. 24v, 27v, 33r, 'Giovanni di ser franc.o da anbra e chonpangni banchieri'.

51. E541, fo. 34r, 'Lorenzo di bernardo sengni e chonpangni lanaiuoli'.

52. E541, fo. 4v, 'Davitti lomellino da gienova', 6 February 1499 (m.f.), purchase of 1 balla of 'Cholla gienovese'.

53. E541, ff. 7r, 19v, 'Giorgio di ghoccio da raghugia' (for wax); fo. 36v, 'Valenzino di lorenzo da raghugia' (for pepper); fo. 35v, 'Nicholo di nicholo da raghugia' (for wax); fo. 28v, 'Girolamo di nichol darghugia [sic]' (for wax).

54. Ciasca, *op. cit.* (note 3), 495, suggests that by the end of the century most supplies were probably imported to Florence via Pisa.

55. On the guild brokers and Maringhi in particular, see A. Astorri, 'Il "Libro delle Senserie" di Girolamo di Agostino Maringhi (1483–1485)', *Archivio storico italiano*, 146, 3 (1988), 389–408.

56. Only 38 out of 758 wholesale transactions (5%) were mediated by brokers, but these were the most valuable transactions, amounting to 93,908 soldi out of 290,242 soldi (32%). The primary factor in these cases appears to have been the size of the transaction. The *Porcellino*, which regularly sold small quantities of goods to the Giglio without using a broker, nevertheless used an official guild broker to sell a large quantity of sugar – see E541, fo. 36r, 15 November 1502, sale of 439 lbs of Portuguese sugar from the *Porcellino* to the Giglio, brokered by Girolamo Maringhi.

57. These included Cosimo del Falcone, Girolamo Maringhi, Cosimo Petrucci, Antonio Corbizzi, Piero Maringhi.
58. 'Girolamo daghostino maringhi' was both a client and supplier of the Giglio – see E882, fo. 14v, and E541, fo. 30r. Astorri, *op. cit.* (note 55), states that in 1483, Maringhi formed a brokerage company with Zanobi di Davizo. The latter was also a Giglio client and supplier – see E882, ff. 270r, 294v, 'Zanobi di davizo sensale' and E541, fo. 5v, 'Zanobi di... sensale'.
59. E541, fo. 30r, 26 April 1502, 20 lbs of 'chandi domaschini'.
60. E882, fo. 204r, 'Chimenti di piero battiloro chon guliano ghondi', 24 December 1493, 'per lui da piero maringhi e quali ritenne tomaso n.o a detto piero di piu senserie fatte'.
61. E541, fo. 5r, 'Niccholo di brunetto beccharo', 17 February 1499 (m.f.), for 47 lbs of lard.
62. E541, fo. 18v, 'Piero di zanobi funaiuolo', 30 March 1501, for 252 lbs of 'pecie nera'.
63. E541, fo. 7r, 'Chimenti dangniolo bichieraio', for an unspecified quantity of 'alberegli'.
64. E541, fo. 16v, 'Bastiano di franc.o dimorozo dacholle' and ff. 10r, 13v, 'Benedetto di bastiano moro[l]i dacholle' were the biggest suppliers of paper (and they were probably related). Also important were fo. 34r, 'Iachopo di ghaleotto chovoni', fo. 3v, 'Ghoro diachopo dacholle', and fo. 28v, 'Ant.o di ghoro da cholle'. On the Colle paper industry see D. Herlihy and C. Klapisch-Zuber, *Tuscans and their Families: A Study of the Florentine Catasto of 1427* (New Haven: Yale University Press, 1985), 126.
65. E541, fo. 36r, 'Vicho fornaciaio al ponte a sieve', 22 November 1502, for 560 lbs of 'charboni molli'.
66. 92 out of 126 suppliers (73.0%) had no given occupation.
67. E541, fo. 10r, 'Franc.o di simone da artimino vetturale' (for honey); ff. 11r, 11v, 13v, 'Franc.o delciba vetturale dasandonnino' (for honey); fo. 12r, 'Pippo dant.o Vetturale' (for pitch); ff. 31r, 24v, 'Giovanni di benozzo vetturale' (for honey); fo. 7r, 'Niccholo di scharino vetturale' (for lead).
68. 83 out of 126 suppliers (65.9%) were involved in only a single transaction in the sample period.
69. Although positive identifications cannot always be made, at least 13 out of 126 suppliers (about 10%) were listed as clients in the retail register E882, and possibly as many as 30.
70. E882, ff. 22r, 44r, 48v, 54v, 'Bernardo di m.o chimenti barbiere'; E541, fo. 35r, 30 September 1502.
71. E882, ff. 76v, 240r, 'Luigi dant.o scharlatti'; E541, fo. 7v, 3 June 1500 and 13 June 1500, for 30 lbs of peppercorns and 7 lbs of damascene incense.
72. There are only 6 out of 126 'regular' suppliers (about 5% of the total), defined as those involved in ten or more transactions over the three-year

sample period. Purchases from these 'regular' suppliers amounted to only 37,257 soldi out of a total of 291,521 soldi in the sample period (13%).

73. E541, ff. 3r, 10v, 21r, 33r, 'Tommaso di Giovanni di Piero nostro prop[r]io' provided 11,235 soldi-worth of goods in the sample period, 4% of the total.

74. E541, fo. 3r, 27 March 1499, 'un mezo barile dolio avemo di chasa sua'; 14 July 1500, '3 fiaschi d'acieto venne dichasa'.

75. E541, fo. 3r, 15 February 1499 (m.f.), 'per istaia tre di mandorle nostrali avemo per lui da Giovanni da bernardo di betto e per lui da lucha suo nipote'; 17 February 1499 (m.f.) 'per otto schatole piene avemo per lui da bertolino vetturele'; 16 June 1500, 'per v schatole piene a vemo per lui da bortolino vetterale'. The phrase *per lui* ('for him') indicates that these goods were to be credited to his account, not that he would consume them.

76. E541, fo. 3r, 12 May 1500, L10s18 'sono per due barili dolio dolcie avemo per lui da messer franc.o ghualterotti anostro ghabella posto messer franc.o abidato'. This man is also listed in E882, fo. 313v, 'messer Franc.o di lorenzo ghualterotti'.

77. E541, fo. 24v, 'm.a Luchrezia donna di tomaso di giovanni nostro', lists four flasks in October 1501, one flask in July 1502, and one flask in August 1502.

78. E541, ff. 4v, 15r, 16r, 20r, 32v, 38v, 'Lorenzo di … vochato ilmoro mungniaio almulino di tommaso nostro', supplied 8,080 soldi-worth of goods in the sample period, 3% of the total. The mill was not mentioned in Tommaso's *Catasto* entry of 1480, and must have been added to his holdings subsequently, or owned by the shop.

79. E541, fo.38r, 'Saldamo chonto chon lorenzo sopradetto ogi questo di p.o di novembre 1503 choma ppare al quaderno de medici s.o c72 resto debitore di tomaso di staia 46 di ghrano e barili 4 di vino e paia 70 di pipioni e lib 70 ½ di pesci e 273 vuova dachordo cholui e ttutto quello che lui dara da qui inanzi si porra nella faccia al dirinpetto c39'. In order to assess the relative importance of these supplies in monetary terms, we have applied general price estimates for the period.

80. It is unclear what happened to perishable produce such as pigeons and fish – were these perhaps consumed by the shop staff?

81. On grain as an alternative to currency, see E882, fo. 73v, 7 September 1493 and 30 August 1494.

82. E541, fo. 11r, 'Salvestro di donato damonte varchi', 2 September 1500, for an unspecified quantity of opium.

83. E882, fo. 34r, 'Tommaxo di Giovanni di piero nostro', 29 November 1493, 'pagho laportatura di 16 fascidighrano', ie. Tommaso paid the delivery.

84. E882, fo. 218r, 'Jachopo di ristoro fornaio a san bra[n]chazio', 9 November 1493, sale of 111 staia of grain, for an agreed price of s17 per staio.

85. E541, ff. 2v, 8v, 13r, 23r, 29r, 31v, 34v, 36r, 38r, 'Iachopo di bernardo e chonpangni speziali al porcellino', for a total value of 11,155 soldi. See also Bénézet, *op. cit.* (note 1), 298–9.

86. E541, ff. 2v, 12r, 17r, 24r, 37v, 'Franc.o e ser piero di pagholo pinadori e chonpangni speziali ala pina', for a total value of 4,009 soldi.

87. E541, ff. 3r, 19r, 23v, 'Piero di giovanni derossi & chonpangni speziali a medici', for a total value of 2,339 soldi. The same shop appears with different owners in E882, fo. 167v, 'Michele di bernaba e chonpangni speziali a medici', and shows how their account was 'reckoned' in 1500, leaving the new owner with a credit of L9s10, 'fatto chreditore di questo saldo piero di giovanni de rossi'. Ciasca, *op. cit.* (note 3), 746, quotes Benedetto Dei's 1470 list of *speziarie grosse*, which includes 'Giovanni di Ser Martino a' Medici, di Mercato'. A. Astorri, 'Appunti sull'esercizio dello speziale a Firenze nel quattrocento', *Archivio storico italiano*, 147 (1989), 31–62: 58, refers to a shop located in the Mercato Vecchio called 'i Medici' and owned by the Medici family.

88. 8 out of 126 suppliers (6.3%) were described as apothecaries, making it the most common occupation listed among suppliers.

89. E882, fo. 107r, 'Bernardo e Nicholo e chonpangni speziali al porciellino', 3 April 1494 and 1 April 1494.

90. Astorri, *op. cit.* (note 87), 61, suggests that the retail of medicines was a specialist sector of the market.

91. Described in the inventories as 'champane di pionbo dastilare sulfondo di ferro'.

92. E541, shows spending of 2,518.5 soldi on 1371 lbs 10 oz of waters in 1500.

93. Smaller suppliers of distilled waters include E541, ff. 11r, 16r, 'Marchion monacho in badia di firenze'; fo. 24v, 'm.a Luchrezia donna di tomaso di giovanni nostro'; ff. 3v, 6r, 25v, 'Bernardo di serafino delbiada' (who also supplied verjuice).

94. R. Palmer, 'Pharmacy in the Republic of Venice in the Sixteenth Century', in A. Wear, R.K. French, and I.M. Lonie (eds), *The Medical Renaissance of the Sixteenth Century* (Cambridge: Cambridge University Press, 1985), 115. See for example Mattioli's *Del modo di distillare le acque da tutte le piante* (1565), available as appendix to Mattioli's *I discorsi di M. Pietro Andrea Matthioli Sanese, Medico Cesareo, nei sei libri di Pedacio Dioscoride Anazarbeo della materia medicinale* (Venice, 1585).

95. E882, fo. 107v, 'Giovanbatista e chonpangni speziali al chanto alerondine', 18 March 1493 (m.f.) to 14 April 1493; fo. 109v, 'Niccholo e baldino trosci e chonpangni speziali ala cholonna' 9 January 1493 (m.f.), 25 August 1494, 4 August 1492; fo. 169r, 'Morello di giovanni e chonpangni speziali ala luna', 10 January 1497 (m.f.); fo. 187r, 'Piero di [BLANK] lorenzi speziale al diamante', 6 March 1494 (m.f.), 27 May 1497; fo. 208v, 'Bernardo di

giovanni mini e chonpangni speziali alla chrocie', 17 May 1494; fo. 221r, 'Giovanni di bartolomeo baroncini e chonpangni speziali', 18 May 1497; fo. 249v, 'Domenicho di franc.o e chonpangni speziali al sole', 16 January 1493 (m.f.) to 16 May 1494.

96. E882, ff. 99r, 323r, 'Ugholino di bartolomeo di chanbio e chonpangni speziali'.

97. E541, fo. 2v, 'Franc.o e ser piero di pagholo pinadori e chonpangni speziali ala pina', 3 January 1499 (m.f.), 26 August 1500, 210 lbs of capers and 350 lbs of honey.

98. E541, fo. 35r, 'L'ospedale di santa maria nuova', 3 November 1502.

99. ASF, Santa Maria Nuova 5079, fo. 52r, 23 Sep 1493, L2s8 for 12 lbs of currants from 'tomaso del giglio speziale'.

100. ASF, Santa Maria Nuova 5079, fo. 52r, 23 Sep 1493, L6s6 for 36 flasks of mineral water 'aqua di poretta' from 'lucha landucci speziale'. The water came from a famous local spring and was believed to be particularly effective in curing eye problems – see G. Chellini, *Le ricordanze di Giovanni Chellini da San Miniato, medico, mercante e umanista (1425–1457)*, M.T. Sillano (ed.), (Milan: F. Angeli, 1984), 30, n.26.

101. J.E. Shaw, *The Justice of Venice: Authorities and Liberties in the Urban Economy, 1550–1700* (Oxford: Oxford University Press, 2006), 80–1, for the mechanisms to enforce the fair distribution of wholesale supply applied by many Venetian guilds. This does not appear to have applied in Florence in the 1490s.

102. G. Borghini, *et al.*, *Una farmacia preindustriale in Valdelsa : la spezieria e lo spedale di Santa Fina nella città di San Gimignano secc. XIV–XVIII* (San Gimignano: Città di San Gimignano, 1981), 124–6.

103. Although the accounts contain entries spanning the period 27 March 1499 to 21 February 1504 (m.f.), they are only complete and comprehensive for the three-year period 1500 to 1502 (the limited records for 1503 consist almost entirely of supplies from Lorenzo the miller).

104. Average annual cost of distilled waters (2,125 soldi) in 1500–2 was nearly eight times as high as the stock in 1504 (280 soldi). Average annual cost of cassia pulp (5,231 soldi) in 1500-02 was nearly nine times as high as the stock in 1504 (595 soldi).

105. For information on the limited shelf life of simples and pre-prepared drugs, see the *Ricettario fiorentino*, doctrine 11.

106. Annual average expenditure was 96,747 soldi in the sample period 1500-02.

107. After allowing for returns (see Chapter 5), total retail sales in the sample year cannot have been more than around 83,238 soldi. If we apply a typical discount on payment of 20% (see Chapter 4 on payment), and then assume a minimum 20% profit margin (from which the costs of rent, labour, fuel etc. would also have to be deducted), then we can estimate that the cost of

supplies destined exclusively for the retail market cannot have amounted to much more than 53,272 soldi. This sort of profit margin would have given the apothecary a maximum income of 13,318 soldi, ie. *c.*100 florins per annum, assuming that costs of rent, labour and fuel were zero.

108. ASF, Santa Maria Nuova 5079, fo. 52r, 23 Sep 1493, L2s8 for 12 lbs of currants from 'tomaso del giglio speziale'.

109. The only artists' materials purchased during the sample period were a large quantity of verdigris (mean spending 756 soldi per annum), and a much smaller quantity of sinoper (mean spending 50 soldi per annum). Verdigris appears to be an exception to the pattern of low turnover, since there was only 42 soldi worth in stock in 1504. E878, fo. 15r, lists 6 lbs of 'Verderame pesto'. On supplies of verdigris, see E541, fo. 15r, 'Anbrogio dant.o dipor[c]i da milano', 30 December 1500, 2,238 soldi for 373 lbs of verdigris. The apothecary also occasionally bought smaller quantities (*c.*½ lb), presumably to meet a shortfall in his own stocks – see E541, 'Franc.o e ser piero di pagholo pinadori e chonpangni speziali ala pina', fo. 2v, 23 January 1500 (m.f.); 17r, 3 February 1500 (m.f.); fo. 24r, 19 March 1501 (m.f.). See also E541, fo. 6r, 'Sandro di Stefano dapogimele', 15 April 1500, for 150 soldi worth of sinoper.

110. Retail sales in the sample year amounted to 603 soldi. This consisted of two major sales of azure (360 soldi), one sale of 'green' (165 soldi) and several small sales of sinoper (78 soldi).

111. Orpiment does not appear in either the wholesale purchases 1500–2 or the retail records 1493–4. E882, fo. 46r, 'Bartolomeo di nicholaio dallaquila', 19 August 1493, for the only appearance of verdigris in the retail sample, s1d8 of 'alume di rocho arso e verderame', which was probably for medicinal application.

112. E882, fo. 103v, 'Benedetto di piero da san donnino vetturale', 20 September 1493, L18 for 4 lbs of azures; fo. 117v, 'Fratti di san franc.o daladoccia', 24 September 1494, s19 for 1 oz of 'gialolino', ½ oz of 'verdazzurro' and ½ oz of 'azurro fine'; fo. 172r, 'fratte Lorenzo chorsi frate deloservanza di san franc.o', 7 November 1494, L8s9 for 169 lbs of 'sanopia macinata'.

113. E882, fo. 259v, 'Boninsengnia di niccholo boninsengni e chonpangni setaiuoli', 22 February 1493 (m.f.), L8s5 for 11 lbs of 'verdetto fine', 'porto giovanni di chimenti dipintore inpinti per dipingiere la bottegha', for an agreed price of s15 per lb. This artist was probably the client listed in E882, ff. 79r, 184r, 'Giovanni di chimenti rosselgli dipintore'.

114. The only exceptions in the sample are E882, fo. 161r, 'Chosimo di lorenzo rosselgli dipintore', 18 June 1494, s2 for ½ lb of 'olio di linseme'; fo. 261v, 'Bernardo di stefano rosselgli dipintore', 10 April 1494, s10 for 20 lbs of 'giesso volterrano'.

115. DeLancey, *op. cit.* (note 21), 146. For payments related to these activities, see Estranei 572, ff. 3v, 43v, 44v, 45v, 46v, 48v.

116. Soap was not manufactured on the premises but obtained wholesale. E541, ff. 18v, 26r, 36v, 'Piero di zanobi funaiuolo', was the biggest single supplier, supplying 1,227 lbs of soap in the sample period (44% of the total).

117. E882, fo. 268v, 'Girolamo di pagholo federighi', 13 August 1494, for the only sale of string in the sample period, one 'ghomitolo' of 'spagho sottile', for a price that cannot have been much more than 1 soldo.

118. T. Garzoni, *La piazza universale di tutte le professioni del mondo*, P. Cherchi and B. Collina (eds), 2 vols (Turin: Einaudi, 1996), Vol. 2, 1063, 'Ci sono anco fra loro di molte fraudi e inganni non solamente di apparenza ridicolosa – come quei bussolotti, quegli albarelli, e quelle scatole che con lettere maiuscole e grosse, e alludono talora a mille unguenti o confezioni o aromati preziosi, e nondimeno sono vacui di dentro, portando lo soprascritto ridicoloso di fuori come fanno i bussoli di maestro Grillo da Conigliano – ma di malizia sinistra di animo, componendo alle volte medecine mortifere col ministrare una cosa per una altra o col meschiar nei calici dalle bevande robba marcia, vecchia, stentita e fracida quanto dir si possa, la quale alle volte conoscono, e alle volte ancora con disconcia ignoranza hanno comprata da barbari levantini a buon mercato per levar su bottega alla meglio che succeda … E resteranno i protomedici avvertiti che tocca più a loro che a me a dannare i speciali, facendo essi le visite alla teriaca, al mitridate e al resto delle medicine c'hanno in bottega'. See also M. Laughran, 'Medicating without "Scruples": The "Professionalization" of the Apothecary in Sixteenth-Century Venice', *Pharmacy in History*, 45 (2003), 95–107: 103; and E. Welch, 'Space and Spectacle in the Renaissance Pharmacy', *Medicina e Storia*, 15 (2008), 127–58.

119. S. Pennell, 'Perfecting Practice? Women, Manuscript Recipes and Knowledge in Early Modern England', in V.E. Burke and J. Gibson (eds), *Early Modern Women's Manuscript Writing* (Aldershot: Ashgate, 2004), 237–58.

PART TWO

CUSTOMERS AND CREDIT

4

People and their Purchases

The Giglio account books are essentially long lists of names, purchases and debts. Transforming this basic economic and legal information into the people they once represented means looking at how and why they were recorded in this way. How did new clients open accounts and obtain credit? What could they then buy? Can we say something about the social groups that they came from? Can we literally 'people' the spaces that we described in Chapter 3?

This type of investigation assumes that the names written in these books represent the majority of customers. Certainly, anyone could walk into the shop and buy goods immediately using cash – when they did so it was carefully recorded. But this was very inconvenient in an economy where hard currency was in short supply.[1] Although a minority of clients used cash, most did their shopping on credit. This was the norm in almost every sector of the Florentine economy, where wealth circulated on paper to a significant extent.[2] But this was particularly important in the medical sector – treatment was often an urgent and expensive requirement that lay outside the ordinary household budget.[3]

The Giglio records make it clear that shop credit was not available to all. It was a function of wealth, status and, most importantly, some form of personal contact with the apothecary. In the early modern city, this meant *knowing* people, having the right connections: this might be a direct personal connection, or a more indirect *knowing about* people, either through mutual social ties or their wider reputation. It was only through knowing people, their families, or third parties willing to vouch for them, that the apothecary could make the decision to open a credit account for them.[4] Lacking any independent mechanism to assess creditworthiness, the apothecary was obliged to base this decision on information gathered at a personal level. Business decisions were not taken in isolation from social factors but were inextricably bound up with the ways in which the apothecary knew people and established relationships with them. It is worth stressing that such relationships were not strictly economic but intrinsically social in nature.[5]

Something of this process is apparent from the ways in which the apothecary recorded his clients. Rather than systematically recording the key details such as name, patronymic, surname, place of residence and occupation, clients were listed in an *ad hoc* fashion. What was recorded could be quite limited, serving only as a reminder of who the person was. The personal data that the historian would ideally like to have is therefore missing or incomplete in many cases, making it difficult to identify clients; in other instances, we get fascinating additional information about clients – the painter Piero di Jacopo was identified by his patronymic and his occupation, but for the apothecary it was also important to note that he was the brother of Antonio del Pollaiuolo.[6] What the apothecary chose to record about clients therefore tells us something about *how* he knew them. He probably recorded only the bare minimum for people he already knew well, but set down full details when the opening of the account marked the start of a new relationship.

Clients were often identified in terms of relationships to other people that the apothecary already knew. Members of the apothecary's existing personal network were key intermediaries in his formation of new relationships. Sometimes we learn more about these third parties than we do about the client themselves. One client, for whom we have only the first name, 'Nanni', was further identified as 'the brother of Scorinci the baker'.[7] In another case, the apothecary did not even record the client's name, identifying him only as the 'worker of Niccolò Sernigi'.[8] The apothecary was more concerned to record people's *connections* than their personal details. Another client, 'Andrea', was identified only as the brother of Bartolomeo Scala,[9] the Chancellor of Florence – the key to his obtaining credit was his relationship to one of the shop's most important customers.[10] Similarly, Mona Chiara was identified only as the *orditore* (threader of looms) of the wool-manufacturer Dionigi di Chimenti, and her debts were subsequently transferred to his account.[11]

People were identified by the connections through which the apothecary made an assessment of credit, a point which is well illustrated by the use of patronymics. While the apothecary usually followed the standard Florentine practice of identifying men primarily through reference to their father, he sometimes recorded other relatives, presumably because these were the connections that seemed most relevant. In such cases, a blank space was left for the expected patronymic. For example, 'Giovanni di [BLANK] nephew of Piero Zuccheri', was identified through his uncle, rather than his father.[12] Many clients were identified in relation to their marital kin, such as the goldsmith Francesco, noted primarily as the brother-in-law of the doctor Ugolino Mazinghi.[13] Less frequently, clients were identified through a father-in-law,[14] and in one exceptional case, a son-in-law.[15] As for women, the apothecary usually followed the standard Florentine practice of referring to husbands (living or dead), but they might also be identified as sisters, mothers, aunts, 'relatives', daughters, and servants of men that the apothecary knew.[16] Clients might also be identified by household, as in the case of the otherwise unidentified 'Mona Cosa' who 'lives with' the silk manufacturer Francesco di Bettino.[17] Less frequently, clients might be identified through ties of friendship, as with Mona Veronica, described only as the 'friend of Cibaldo',[18] or Mona Antonia of Bergamo, described as 'the soldier's woman'.[19] Although such forms of identification are in some ways unhelpful, being too vague to allow cross-referencing with other sources, what is more interesting here is not the detail of these relationships so much as the fact that the information was included. This tells us something about *how* the apothecary knew people – in terms of their relationships to others, whether by blood, marriage, business, household or friendship.

One consequence of the process by which new client relations were formed was a high level of interconnectivity amongst the shop's many clients. The clientele can be envisaged as an expanding network of personal relationships, in which one client led to another. This was a two-way process of information flows that allowed potential clients to know the shop and also allowed the apothecary to know something about the clients, helping to establish trust on both sides. A connection to an existing client gave the apothecary some indication of the family's ability to pay and reputation. The result was a marked clustering of clients who were connected in various ways. A good example is the Bracci family, a group of clients descended from a common ancestor, most of whom were members of the Guild of Oil- and Sausage-traders.[20] In addition to two of the sons of Ser Tomme,[21] five of the grandsons also had accounts,[22] as did a number of the women of the family, including Mona Alessandra and the maidservant Ginevra.[23] Another cluster can be identified around Andrea di Berto Lapi.[24] Account holders from his family included his wife Piera,[25] three cousins, and two of his cousin's nephews.[26] In addition to this extended family, the cluster also included a group of five Spaniards who resided in Andrea's house,[27] and two of the servants dedicated to their service,[28] each with their own account. Since it was difficult for foreigners to obtain credit, the connection to the Lapi household may have been essential for these Spanish clients.

These examples are based solely on the limited data present in the account records, and many of these personal connections must have gone unrecorded, even if they played a role in the apothecary's decision to grant credit. For example, the ties that linked Bartolomeo Scala to other account-holders, including his son-in-law Niccolò di Antonio da Filicaia, his wife's nephew Lorenzo di Tommaso Benci, or his banker Bernardo Rinieri, are not mentioned in the shop accounts, although they were probably known to the apothecary.[29] It is a difficult task to tease out these sorts of connections but supplementary evidence reveals something of the possibilities. For another example, the apothecary's tax declaration describes his purchase of land at

Fiesole in 1472, and a number of the people involved in this transaction subsequently appeared in the shop books. These include the vendor Luigi Scarlatti,[30] and the notary Ser Andrea Mini,[31] while the money used for the purchase was transferred from shares in a house belonging to the family of another client, Bartolomeo de' Medici.[32] None of these connections are described in the accounts but the case shows how major transactions of this sort could establish permanent ties of trust (perhaps underpinned by credit), and create long-term relationships with clients. Both Luigi Scarlatti and Ser Andrea Mini continued to be active as clients in the 1490s, over twenty years after the purchase of land had taken place. Luigi Scarlatti also supplied pepper and incense to the shop in 1500.[33] Similarly, the tax declaration refers to Benedetto di Goro, a stocking-maker who was renting the apothecary's other house in Florence in 1480, and he too is listed in the shop accounts.[34] The clustering apparent from the limited information recorded in client descriptions is just a tiny proportion of the ties that knit the shop clientele together.

The importance of social ties is also evident when clients had to provide a surety, somebody who guaranteed their debt in the event that they were unable to pay. This allowed people who did not know the apothecary, or whose economic status was questionable to make purchases without paying immediately. Sureties were usually members of the same family, or people from the same household, trade or neighbourhood.[35] Employers sometimes provided such guarantees for their servants and workers. The painter Alesso Baldovinetti provided surety for Luca, one of his workers.[36] Similarly, the factor at the convent of Sant'Ambrogio acted as surety for one of the gardeners there.[37] Despite the ease of setting up such guarantees – the name of the surety, presumably present to give their consent, was simply written into the ledger when the account was opened – it is striking that the apothecary only insisted on this in a small minority of cases.[38] Over ninety per cent of clients were offered credit simply on the basis of personal trust and the standard protections offered by the law.[39] Those who were required to provide sureties were often people with no defined occupation,[40] and in particular, women.[41] Conversely, having a defined trade – particularly if organised in a guild – implied a certain solidity of income and status, and was one of the keys by which male members of middling artisan class were able to obtain credit.[42]

It was particularly important for sureties to have established ties to the apothecary: the apothecary already knew them and their credit history, and if they were clients then any bad debts could be easily transferred to their account:[43] for example, the Badia of Florence, one of the shop's biggest clients, was surety for at least three other Giglio clients.[44] Davide and his brother Giovanni, bakers, whose family had a long-standing relationship with the Giglio going back to their father, were able to act as surety for four other Giglio clients.[45] The majority of sureties (sixty per cent) were existing clients of the shop,[46] and those who weren't often had close ties to somebody who was.[47] Particularly effective in this respect were direct ties to the apothecary and his shop staff. The apothecary's son-in-law,[48] his son,[49] the clerk,[50] the apprentices,[51] and a factor,[52] all acted as sureties for clients.[53] With direct personal ties to the apothecary, they played an important role in vouching for and guaranteeing the debts of people who could not otherwise obtain credit.

The vertical nature of the relationship between clients and surety meant that women are mostly found on one side of the relationship. Few women acted as sureties in their own right because they were usually the dependents of men and lacked financial autonomy.[54] Nevertheless, there was no legal impediment to women doing so. The wealthy widow Mona Maddalena acted as surety for her son-in-law, Domenico di Bono Rinucci, allowing him and other members of his family to obtain credit.[55] In another case, we find one married woman acting as surety for another, even though their husbands were alive,[56] and in one exceptional reversal of standard gender and working relationships, a female servant called Mona Rosa acted as surety for a male client of rank, Ser Alessandro di Matteo Strozzi.[57] Although the reasons for this are unclear, the case underlines the variety of personal arrangements that might be produced by death, bankruptcy and other shifts of fortune.

Many clients are identified by reference to place, but these generally indicate place of origin rather than residence. In addition, where customers are described as being 'of Venice', 'of Urbino', 'of Genoa' or 'of Bergamo', it is unclear whether they had migrated to Florence on a temporary or permanent basis or whether they were actually native Florentines who had inherited the reference to place, as with the surname 'Da Romena'.[58] Nevertheless, there is some evidence to suggest that the shop drew clients from some of the peripheral towns and villages of the Florentine regional state,[59] especially in the immediate environs, such as Fiesole, Signa, Calcinaia, Settignano, Sesto and San Donnino. Centres of particular importance that lay a little further away included San Casciano, Impruneta, Incisa and Panzano. The Giglio also supplied a number of apothecaries based in regional centres such as Pisa and Pistoia.[60] Particularly prominent was the apothecary's home town of Montevarchi in the Upper Arno valley. This confirms the importance of personal ties to the apothecary, established before he migrated to Florence, or formed subsequently through his ongoing connection to that town (especially his landholdings), and to the immigrant community living in Florence.[61] These included Jacopo di Martino Menchi, from whom the apothecary had bought property in Montevarchi, and other members of this family.[62] Also important was the Franciscan monastery at

Montevarchi, and a number of its personnel.[63] The ties remained active back to the home town: Bastiano di Giovanni, who acted as factor for the apothecary, presumably overseeing his landholdings in Montevarchi, continued to send money and goods to that town.[64]

The accounts provide very little indication of the geographical distribution of clients within the city. The electoral and tax records can provide some idea of the distribution of clients, although this approach can only be used for families who can be readily identified by surname. Many of the leading families were based in the San Giovanni quarter, although this simply reflected the general residential pattern of the patrician élite. There is a slight concentration of clients from the immediate surrounding area in the parish of Santa Maria Nipotecosa, including local shopkeepers and priests. There is no detectable concentration of clients in the apothecary's own residential neighbourhood in the quarter of Chiavi, even though some prominent figures came from this area, such as the descendants of Paolo di Piero of the Albizzi clan,[65] based in and around the nearby Borgo Albizzi, who were major clients of the shop.[66] Overall, the shop appears to have drawn its clients from across the city rather than any particular neighbourhood. Rather than considering geographical proximity, it is more helpful to consider the clientele as a *network* of people connected by various ties. With its central location, the shop was a space where people from all across the city could meet and network, transcending the limits of neighbourhood sociability to make contact with others from Florence and beyond. Rather than being concentrated in any particular district, clients clustered around certain leading families, such as the Albizzi, Niccolini, Capponi and Strozzi families. This meant that coming into the shop inevitably carried political overtones, an issue which will be discussed below.

Clustering also occurred in terms of the particular institutions that were frequented by the apothecary. This is particularly true for the commercial court of the *Mercanzia*, where the apothecary often went to take actions against debtors. Over time, many of the permanent staff of the *Mercanzia* had been Giglio clients, most importantly the chancellor,[67] but also four of the notaries, and a *donzello* (one of the minor officials).[68] In particular, one of the *procuratori* (the lawyers attached to the court) was the notary Ser Giovanni di Maso, and along with his son Tommaso; he regularly worked for the Giglio in pursuing claims against debtors.[69] The apothecary also pursued claims for debt at the tribunal of the Podestà, and the Giglio clients included the notary Ser Benedetto dalla Scarperia, who acted as their *procuratore* here,[70] five other notaries and another *procuratore*.[71] Similarly, there were Giglio clients at the customs office, the *dogana*, where the apothecary paid duties on imported merchandise.[72] This close relationship between institutions that Tommaso di Giovanni frequented and the officials who used his shop may be explained as a form of barter. It could have been a convenient way of paying for such men's services in a cash-poor economy, allowing them to take payment in the form of apothecary goods. But it is also easy to imagine that long-term personal connections with key bureaucratic officials at these courts and offices resulted in favourable treatment.

In addition, a number of clients were members of the Guild of Doctors and Apothecaries.[73] Among the most influential were Stagio di Lorenzo Barducci, one of Tommaso's wealthy neighbours, and one of his biggest private clients.[74] He and his son Giovanni – also a client – may have been particularly important contacts due to their influence in the Guild and more widely.[75] Stagio's close relationship with the Guild can be seen by the fact that Guild officials even delivered goods from the shop to his house at times.[76] In addition to the Barducci, six of the forty men (ie. fifteen per cent) who served as Guild consuls across the two-year period 1493–4 were Giglio clients,[77] and at least six more were closely related to Giglio clients.[78] These connections may have been important in shielding Tommaso di Giovanni from prosecution as an unlicenced trader who was not registered with the Guild. Many of the leading members of the Guild, elected as its consuls, were aware of Tommaso's activities, but did nothing to prosecute him, perhaps because so many of them were his customers. Not all of these men necessarily practised the trade, since many of those who registered in the guilds did so solely in order to conduct a political career. This may explain why the Guild's trading monopoly was so poorly enforced, since its governing body had little direct interest in policing the trade. In addition, in a guild where so many different trades were represented, it was difficult for any individual group to assert its interests.

Further key sites were the areas at or just outside the city gates, especially the Porta alla Croce to the east,[79] and the Porta San Piero Gattolini – now known as the Porta Romana – to the south, where there were concentrations of shops.[80] Particularly prominent clients were a number of businesses such as barbers, innkeepers and blacksmiths, which provided essential restorative services for travellers: wine, food, and a bed; a shave, bloodletting and haircut; shoeing horses. At Porta alla Croce, clients included the barber Simone di Domenico,[81] the blacksmith Antonio,[82] and Ruffino, described as 'shopkeeper and innkeeper'.[83] At Porta San Piero Gattolini, they included the barbers Lorenzo di Guido[84] and Lione d'Antonio,[85] the shopkeeper Luca di Paradiso,[86] and the blacksmith Piero.[87] These premises, strategically located at the city–country interface, where travellers met, exchanged news and made deals, may also have been key spaces for the formation of new relationships.

The city's religious institutions also provided foci for social interaction around which clusters of clients formed. At the Badia of Florence, a major corporate client in its own right,[88] these included several monks,[89] as well as the chamberlain Don Vettorino.[90] Similarly, the Benedictine convent of Sant'Ambrogio, which grew rapidly in this period, was among the shop's biggest clients, along with the sacristy attached to the church.[91] The network of clients clustered around Sant'Ambrogio included the factor Antonio di Tommaso,[92] the prior Messer Francesco di Stefano,[93] and a number of priests and chaplains.[94] The accounts also list a number of the local traders with connections to the convent, including a gardener and a baker.[95] Overall the accounts suggest that a number of physical locations outside the shop itself – the tribunal, the customs house, various churches, and the city gates – were key places in the formation of the client network, probably because they were frequented by the apothecary himself.

Religious institutions may have been particularly important for bringing the apothecary into contact with Florentine artists. Cosimo Rosselli, an important client of Giglio and the executor of the apothecary's will, painted the frescoes in the Cappella del Miracolo at Sant'Ambrogio in 1486.[96] Other Giglio clients who worked on Sant'Ambrogio included the sculptor Mino da Fiesole and the carpenter Chimenti del Tasso – whose brother Cervagio carried out woodwork for the Giglio.[97] Cosimo Rosselli also did work at a number of other religious institutions listed on the Giglio books, such as the convent of the Murate, the church of Cestello, and the confraternity of San Bernardino.[98] Like Sant'Ambrogio, the Cistercian church of Cestello was one of the shop's major corporate customers. Bartolomeo Scala, one of the most important clients, played an important role in financing the development of the monastery, which lay opposite his house, hiring the architect Giuliano da Sangallo – also a Giglio client.[99] Many of the artists who worked on this church were Giglio clients, including Cosimo Rosselli,[100] Sandro Botticelli,[101] and Domenico Ghirlandaio,[102] and they in turn were linked to many other artists who were clients.[103] As a supplier of artists' materials, the Giglio had a vital role to play in artistic production, with many of the leading artists of the city in the late fifteenth century listed on its books.[104] Bernardo Rosselli is recorded as buying colours there in 1476, for example.[105] While there is no evidence to suggest that the Giglio was fully responsible for bringing these figures together (indeed the project may have brought all these artists to the shop), it does demonstrate that the Giglio tapped into the key networks of artistic production and patronage that formed around religious sites and reinforced these in turn.

Florence was also a city of faction, and certain semi-public spaces served as important meeting places for political discussion and networking. Along with barber shops, apothecary shops were notorious for this, though seemingly at a rather higher social level.[106] A number of the 'new men' associated with the Medici were shop clients, in particular the chancellor Bartolomeo Scala and his brother Andrea (the sons of a miller from Colle),[107] and Filippo di Piero Da Gagliano (who managed banking and financial matters for Lorenzo de' Medici).[108] The clientele included many prominent Florentines from among the pro-Medici faction, such as Messer Bernardo Buongirolami, Pierfilippo Pandolfini and Piero di Giovanni Capponi.[109] Strikingly, of the six ambassadors who went on the Florentine diplomatic mission to Rome in 1492, whose number included Piero de' Medici, three were Giglio clients: Tommaso Minerbetti, Messer Puccio d'Antonio Pucci, and Pierfilippo Pandolfini.[110] Eleven further clients (ie. sixteen per cent of the total) were members of the council of seventy in 1489, a sign that they were closely trusted Medici allies, including Lapo Niccolini, Braccio Martelli, Piero Capponi and Tanai de' Nerli.[111] Similarly, Piero Soderini, who was favoured by Piero de' Medici and who would be elected Gonfaloniere for life in 1502, was also a Giglio client.[112]

The presence of Bartolomeo Scala, an able political survivor, also raises interesting possibilities of connections to the Savonarolan faction after the fall of the Medici in 1494.[113] More than eleven per cent of the over five hundred leading citizens who signed a petition in favour of Savonarola in 1497 were listed as Giglio clients,[114] including prominent leaders of the movement such as Andrea Cambini,[115] Francesco Gualterotti,[116] and Ulivieri Guadagni.[117] Jacopo di Paolo Niccolini, who handed down some of Savonarola's speeches, was also a Giglio client.[118] Other possible sympathisers, such as Sandro Botticelli and his brother Antonio, were also among the shop clients.[119] Whether these connections are coincidental, reflecting simply a broad section of the elite of Florentine society, or whether the shop was itself a space for the formation and negotiation of faction and political opinion remains an intriguing possibility. Certainly, shops were important meeting places for political socialisation and it is significant that Manfredo Manfredi, the Ferrarese ambassador sympathetic to the Savonarolans, was one of the most important clients.[120] Did his patronage of the Giglio reflect a desire to gather news and measure the strength of factions? The best one can say without further evidence of Manfredi's activities is that the shop was patronised by a broad section of the political élite, from which factions were to emerge in the era of political upheaval to come.

This discussion of guilds, workshops and faction has emphasised a world of men, and in fact women constituted only a tiny proportion of clients – just over five per cent.[121] Around a fifth of these were corporate institutions like the convent of Sant'Ambrogio,[122] and almost half of the remainder were widows.[123] This partly reflects the high incidence of widows in a city where men tended to marry much later than women, but also the greater financial independence that came to many women following widowhood.[124] Mona Agnola, the widow of ser Domenico Pugi, had her own account at the shop, and also came there in person.[125] With control of their sexuality no longer so tightly bound up with male honour, especially if they were old or had no parental household to return to, widows were freer to move about town than were wives or unmarried daughters, even though this might represent a necessity forced on them by difficult circumstances rather than a positive choice. While he was alive, Domenico di Bono Rinucci often bought items for his wife Lucrezia,[126] but immediately after his death she commenced her own account.[127] Similarly, Maddalena Minerbetti opened her own account only after her husband Tommaso died.[128] But there was nothing to stop married women having accounts at the shop at the same time as their husbands,[129] as in the cases of Mona Piera, wife of Andrea Lapi;[130] Alessandra, wife of Niccolò Rinucci;[131] and Girolama, the wife of Puccio Pucci. The only women who can be positively identified as unmarried were mostly servants of low social status, and a smaller number of nuns.[132] This was related to the tight controls placed on women's movements in Renaissance Florence, particularly for unmarried girls.

Even though there was therefore no impediment to women having their own account, few women did so in practice. Nevertheless, this assumption seriously underestimates their participation as consumers. Shopping accounts were extremely flexible and could be used by other members of the household and family, both men and women. In one transaction, the account-holder, a blacksmith called Biagio di Stefano, was not involved at any point: his surety came to the shop to order goods, which were for delivery to his wife, and these were then transported by one of his workers.[133] No limits were placed on this sharing of accounts, though further authorisation might be necessary if third parties were not known to the apothecary. When the Abbot of Santa Trinità ordered wax for delivery by a worker, the apothecary noted that the transaction had been personally authorised by the account-holder, Giovanni de' Libri.[134] In a context of frequent litigation over debt, such information was carefully recorded in order to authenticate transactions. If clients attempted to deny liability for goods, it would be helpful to know if they had come to the shop in person, who had carried the goods away, or to whom the goods had been delivered.

'Remote shopping', by means of servants, workers or relatives,[135] was particularly important in the medical sector where clients were often confined to bed: for example, Domenico di Tone had many of his medicines brought to him by his maidservant Nanna.[136] It was also important where clients lived at a distance, or if they had farms and villas in the countryside. One client used his son-in-law as a proxy to collect goods from the shop for delivery to his villa at Panzano.[137] Similarly, Michele di Bernardo Niccolini arranged for a blacksmith called Sandro to deliver pudding pipe from the shop to his country villa.[138] Pills were even sent as far as the Levant.[139] Local deliveries might also be carried out by shop staff, sometimes even the apothecary himself. On the account of Girolamo di Paolo Federighi, one of the shop's most important clients, the apothecary delivered a purge of rhubarb to Mona Costanza, 'to be tempered at home', suggesting that he may have carried out the final adjustments to the purge at the client's house.[140] He also delivered sugar candy and syrup to the family of Bartolomeo Settecieli, wool manufacturers.[141] Such deliveries were probably carried out as a personal favour, since no additional delivery cost was incurred. This information was carefully recorded, not to charge clients for the service, but to substantiate claims in the event of a dispute.

This sort of shopping by proxy allowed women to participate in the market from home, without having to go there in person or carry goods. Many women received goods as the wives, daughters and other relatives of male account-holders. This was particularly important for the women who were closed up in the city's convents, many of them patrician daughters.[142] It was extremely unusual for nuns to have their own accounts – one exception was Sister Agnola of the *Polverine*, who opened an account just to buy a single purge – delivered to her by another nun.[143] This perhaps reflected the greater freedom of movement accorded to this community of reformed prostitutes, given that they had little left to lose in terms of moral honour. Most nuns were obliged to rely on the support of their convents and families. Some of the shop's biggest clients were convents (especially Sant'Ambrogio), which collectively bought large quantities of goods on behalf of the nuns.[144] The accounts also list many examples of families buying goods for delivery to sisters and daughters in the convents, as when Bernardo Monti sent syrups and medicines to his sister, a nun at San Martino.[145] This means of accessing goods was particularly important for female workers, nursemaids and servants, who would otherwise have been unable to obtain credit.[146] It is not clear from Giglio evidence how such debts were resolved within the household, but the sums were probably docked from the servant's wages rather than being offered out of charity.[147]

Women were not merely the passive recipients of deliveries commissioned by male account-holders but could also use the accounts of male relatives in an active fashion. This can be seen in the case of Mona Caterina, a woman with her own business – she was a shopkeeper at San Niccolò – but whose account was in the name of the husband, 'Magi'. The fact that the entry describes Magi as 'the husband of Mona Caterina' implies that the account was opened in his name simply to provide formal cover for her shopping.[148] Caterina was, in practice, the principal client, and the goods are specifically described as for her in the account. Similarly, the account of Jacopo di Bartolomeo Galli was opened specifically 'on behalf of his mother', and she used it to buy goods for herself and other women of the household.[149] Andrea Lapi was prepared to allow his servant to use his shop account to buy her own medicines, perhaps because he knew that she would be denied credit, or because she was sick in bed and unable to go out.[150] In almost all of these cases it was also the women of the household who came to the shop to collect the goods.[151] As a result, goods might be ordered by a woman, collected from the shop by women, and destined for women's use, even though the account-holder was male. Apparently insignificant as account-holders, women become more visible as consumers when we look at the detail of the transactions.

Furthermore, despite the controls placed on the mobility of patrician women in particular, the shop was not an exclusively male space. Many of the servants sent to buy items by wealthier families were female. To give just a few examples, Giovanbattista di Benedetto sent his maidservant to collect honey roset,[152] while Bernardo di Pierfrancesco had his servant Sandra collect cinnamon and coriander.[153] In addition to servants, respectable women of middling rank, almost always married or widowed, could also be found in the shop, buying goods and handling money.[154] Lucrezia Mannini came to the shop to buy her own medicines on several occasions, using her son's account.[155] Similarly, Raffaella Chomi came to the shop to buy pills using her son's account,[156] returning several months later with cash to settle the bill.[157] Another client's aunt came to the shop to buy medicines on his behalf.[158] The Gianfigliazzi brothers, Antonio and Francesco, sent their mother Mona Bartolomea to the shop with saffron and almonds.[159] The blacksmith Paolo di Meo sent his wife with cash to pay the bill.[160] Aside from serving girls, the only unmarried women coming to the shop were *fanciulle*, prepubescent girls. The stocking-maker Cristofano di Paradiso sent his daughter Caterina to the shop to buy soap.[161] Similarly, the stocking-makers Antonio and Francesco di Giano had their niece Ginevra carry goods for them on occasion.[162] One young girl, the daughter of a notary, also delivered rhubarb pills to her brother.[163]

The practice of sharing accounts means that the names of account-holders only partially reflect the nature of the customer base. Although each individual member of a family or household sometimes had their own account, they often shared an account registered in the name of a single family member. It was more useful to understand consumer demand as being *mediated* by the account-holders: each client was a conduit connecting the shop to an extended network of dependents, kin and associates. Rather than a free market, the difficulty of obtaining credit constrained the market to operate through personal networks of patronage. The account-holders, those within the circle of shop credit, mediated access to the shop's products among their networks of clients and dependents. This was especially important for women and other dependents such as children, servants and workers, but it also applied to relatives, members of the household, and friends. The accounts reveal something of the way that commodities circulated in broader social networks beyond the immediate transaction between the client and the apothecary.

Shop staff in particular provided key nodes in this network of consumption, mediating the flow of goods to their personal social networks. The apothecary, his immediate relatives and shop employees numbered among the principal clients of the shop. However, not all of the goods debited to their accounts were for their own consumption. They were also often distributed to friends and relatives, who in this way contracted personal debts with the employee rather than the shop. For example, Lapino Lapini, the apothecary's son-in-law, supplied candles, pepper and pepper bread to one of his tenants,[164] and pepper, spices and saffron to his bailiff.[165] The apothecary's sons similarly supplied goods to relatives and others.[166] Lorenzo, for example, supplied spices to the stocking-maker Cristofano di Paradiso,[167] and he in turn often sent goods to Lorenzo, suggesting particularly close relations between these two.[168] Even lowly employees like the apprentice Niccolò supplied pills, sweets and sugar to his sister-in-law,[169] purges to his sister,[170] and sugar roset and cassia pods to his brother-in-law's nursemaid in Val d'Elsa.[171] The apothecary himself used his personal account to supply others, sometimes recorded as debts but sometimes as gifts that incurred less formal kinds of obligation.[172] In this way, people could deal with shop staff as intermediaries, contracting debts and obligations with them, rather than with the shop.

Consumption

The tightly woven network of figures that patronised the Speziale al Giglio came into the shop for many reasons, to collect an order, pay a debt, perhaps even simply to hear the latest gossip and news. In fact, only a surprisingly small number came in to actually buy something. More than two thousand names were recorded in the account-books, but many of these were old debts or inactive accounts. There was much more limited group of 515 'active clients' who made purchases in the year between July 1493 and July 1494.[173] This group spent nearly 89,000 soldi that year, a mean average of just over 170 soldi per client (just over a florin each).[174] Although this is strictly speaking a nominal figure, it provides a useful starting point for gauging consumption levels and consumer behaviour.

The vast majority of clients bought relatively little throughout the year, only making purchases very occasionally, probably in response to illness. As

Table 4.1

Distribution of Purchasing at the Giglio, 1493–4

Annual purchasing (soldi)	Cumulative frequency (number of clients)	Cumulative proportion (% of all clients)	Cumulative purchasing (soldi)	Cumulative proportion (% of all purchasing)
10	98	19%	596	1%
≤20	162	31%	1,531	2%
30	211	41%	2,754	3%
≤40	244	47%	3,902	4%
50	276	54%	5,351	6%
≤60	295	57%	6,415	7%
70	312	61%	7,490	8%
≤80	324	63%	8,386	9%
90	336	65%	9,401	11%
≤100	349	68%	10,646	12%
110	359	70%	11,685	13%
≤120	367	71%	12,603	14%
130	374	73%	13,486	15%
≤140	380	74%	14,294	16%
150	393	76%	16,185	18%
≤160	398	77%	16,958	19%
170	406	79%	18,283	21%
≤180	413	80%	19,493	22%
190	415	81%	19,868	22%
≤200	420	82%	20,841	24%
250	433	84%	23,753	27%
≤500	474	92%	38,943	44%
1000	502	97%	59,932	68%
≤5000	513	100%	77,194	87%
6000	515	100%	88,609	100%

a result, consumption varied widely, from one soldo at the bottom end to a tiny minority of clients whose expenditure exceeded five thousand soldi. Because consumption was so polarised, the median average of 45 soldi per year gives a much more realistic idea of 'typical' consumption. If we arbitrarily choose the level of 150 soldi per annum, less than the mean average, seventy-six per cent of clients fell within this group.[175]

Table 4.2

Top Ten Clients, Sample Year

Name	Total Transactions	Consumption (soldi)	Proportion[176]
Sacristy of Sant'Ambrogio	23	5,890	6.6%
Badia of Florence	270	5,525	6.2%
Giovanni di Lapo di Lorenzo Niccolini	24	3,088	3.5%
Convent of Sant'Ambrogio	212	2,137	2.4%
Jacopo di Ristoro, baker at San Brachazio	1	1,887	2.1%
Antonio and Francesco di Giano, stocking-makers	195	1,617	1.8%
Bartolomeo di Ser Francesco da Anbra	59	1,352	1.5%
Ser Zanobi di Jacopo Borgianni	59	1,332	1.5%
Bernardo di Piero Del Palagio	142	1,315	1.5%
Antonio di Giovanni Del Caccia	40	1,298	1.5%

As this indicates, over half the clients bought less than fifty soldi-worth of goods per annum – this made them insignificant in business terms, at only six per cent of total consumption. Many only came to the shop once during the sample period and bought only a tiny quantity of goods. Far more important for the business was the 'long tail' formed by a minority of clients (twenty-four per cent) whose individual consumption exceeded 150 soldi per annum, accounting for eighty-two per cent of total consumption.[177] Even within this latter group there was considerable polarisation: the far extremity of the tail was constituted by a handful of thirteen clients who bought more than a thousand soldi-worth of goods, and who accounted for almost a third of total consumption. The business was dominated by a relatively small group of regular, high-consuming clients, but it also served a much larger mass of occasional and petty clients who may have been vital elements in the maintenance of a broad social network, even if they counted for little in financial terms.

Table 4.2 focuses on the top-end clients who accounted for the bulk of the shop's business. This is dominated by religious corporations.[178] The shop's biggest customer was the Sacristy of Sant'Ambrogio, which ordered close to 6,000 soldi worth of wax, candles, tapers and torches.[179] Closely related to this institution, but accounted for separately, was the Convent of

Sant'Ambrogio, which purchased over 2,000 soldi-worth of medicines and spices for the nuns during the sample year.[180] The second most important customer was the Badia of Florence, which bought goods to the value of over 5,500 soldi, including medicines, sweets and spices.[181] Sometimes the spices were described as being 'for the kitchen', while the medicines were usually for various individuals, such as Don Stefano, the Abbot, and usually transported 'by the nurse'.[182] They bought no wax or candles, apart from a few wicks for the sacristy.[183] In contrast to the prevailing image of self-sufficient institutions reliant on their own herb gardens, monasteries and convents were enthusiastic consumers of shop-bought drugs. They enjoyed significant shop credit thanks to their extensive landholdings and institutional continuity.

Individual clients rarely approached this sort of level of consumption, with the important exception of Giovanni di Lapo Niccolini, who bought 3,000 soldi-worth of candles for his father's funeral over a four day period.[184] The baker Jacopo di Ristoro is an anomalous case – his purchase of 111 *staia* of grain in a single bulk transaction does not represent the sort of goods normally on sale and was probably entered in the retail records by mistake.[185] A better example of the kind of individual clients who made up the bulk of the big consumers are the stocking-makers Antonio and Francesco di Giano.[186] They were regular clients who came to the shop frequently and carried out a high number of transactions over the year (195 in total).

But if we can identify these clients, can their consumption patterns be linked to available data on their social status? This is a problematic exercise for a number of reasons. Firstly, the Giglio retailed a wide range of different commodities, for which the consumption patterns varied significantly, as will be explored in detail in Chapters 6 to 8. Some clients, like the Sacristy of Sant'Ambrogio, or Giovanni Niccolini, used the shop rarely, but were leading consumers because of the type of commodities they bought: expensive wax products. Other clients, like the Badia of Florence, or the stocking-makers Antonio and Francesco di Giano, were regular customers who were primarily interested in lower value products, such as medicines, confectionery and spices.

A related problem is that demand for many apothecary goods was highly variable, rather than a constant requirement such as bread or wine. Demand for medicines was closely linked to health – some clients bought medicines only in response to an irregular pattern of acute disease, while others had a more constant demand related to a chronic condition. Demand for wax products also varied dramatically in relation to the pattern of deaths (leading to funerals) within a family. The irregular nature of demand for apothecary products helps to explain why credit practices were so strongly established here, because household budgets might be stretched by the need to respond to unplanned events. All this makes it more difficult to establish links between wealth and consumption, because the demand for apothecary goods varied according to particular circumstances. The accounts contain many examples of wealthy patricians bearing illustrious surnames who bought little or nothing at the shop over the sample year – but this is probably an indication of a limited requirement for the apothecary's goods at that particular time, rather than an inability to afford them.

Secondly, in the absence of tax records for the 1490s, we are forced to use approximate guides to social level contained in the client descriptions, such as the possession of occupational titles, surnames, the need to provide a surety, or gender.[187] Yet, as we have seen, these data are problematic because the apothecary did not record information about clients in a systematic way, but on an *ad hoc* basis according to what he thought was relevant. Even though every client had a father, the apothecary did not always record this information; similarly, he did not always record surnames or occupations, even if clients had them. To give some examples: the account of Giovanmatteo di Marco Nelli contains no indication that he is a mercer,[188] the account of Bernardo di Stoldo Rinieri fails to mention that he was a banker,[189] and that of Francesco di Paolo Mini fails to record that he was an apothecary.[190] Conversely, the account of Manfredo Manfredi, the Ambassador of Ferrara, records his occupation but not his surname.[191] Occupational bynames are further complicated by the possibility that they might be inherited as surnames, rather than describing the present occupation. The data present in the records is therefore partial; in particular, the *absence* of any particular piece of information does not allow us to draw definitive conclusions about an individual. Furthermore, this focus on individuals can be misleading, because, as this chapter has shown, accounts were not just linked to individual clients who can be neatly classified, but were access points to broader social networks.

The data are therefore problematic, but some tentative conclusions can be reached in the aggregate. One indicator of the social status is the fact that just under half of all clients were identified by surname, approximately the same proportion as found for the Florentine populace in general.[192] A number of members of the patrician elite can be identified, such as Alamanno Rinuccini,[193] the famous critic of the Medici regime. The proportion of clients identified by occupation (thirty-six per cent) is by contrast lower than expected, suggesting that the working population was under-represented.[194] The most commonly recorded occupations were other apothecaries (6.5 per cent), reflecting a significant trade among the operators in the sector, both within the city and out to regional centres. Below this a wide span of skilled trades and shopkeepers are represented, including in particular stocking-makers (4.5 per cent), painters (3.9 per cent), carpenters

Table 4.3

Purchasing Patterns by Client Type

Client Type	No. of Clients	% of Clients	Mean Purchasing (soldi)	Median Purchasing (soldi)	Total Purchasing (soldi)	% of Total Purchasing
All	**515**	**100%**	**172.1**	**45.0**	**88,609**	**100%**
Corporate	**19**	**4%**	**843.1**	**35.7**	**16,018**	**18%**
Individual	**496**	**96%**	**146.4**	**45.2**	**72,591**	**82%**

(3.6 per cent), shoemakers (3.2 per cent), notaries (2.5 per cent), goldsmiths (2.5 per cent), linen drapers (2.5 per cent), and second-hand dealers (2.5 per cent). The particularly high proportion of shoemakers and stocking-makers may reflect the solid personal and commercial links between the shop and this guild, of which the apothecary was a member. Also notable are religious functions such as priests and chaplains (4.7 per cent), or friars (2.3 per cent). More lowly occupations such as servants (1.1 per cent), and labourers (2.5 per cent), or low-end artisan trades such as cobblers, builders, spinners and shearers, are present, but are under-represented relative to their importance in the wider population.[195] No group was entirely excluded, with the exception of the agricultural labourers that made up the bulk of the rural population outside the city walls. Overall then, the clients span a broad social range of the urban population, from maidservants, unskilled labourers and fishermen to the upper levels of the patrician elite, but the distribution is weighted towards the middling strata of skilled artisans and shopkeepers and the upper levels of society.

These figures can be broken down by client type to draw out connections between social factors and consumption patterns. Firstly, corporate clients (see Table 4.3) must be handled separately.[196] These included a number of consumers who were extremely important for the shop's business – hence the very high mean and disproportionate contribution to total consumption – such as the Badia, but there were also a number of poor corporations which bought very little – hence the surprisingly low median – including the Observant Franciscans at San Michele alla Doccia whose purchases amounted to only four soldi,[197] or the Confraternity of San Giovanni Scalzo, who spent five soldi.[198] Not all corporations were wealthy, and some were even obliged to provide sureties in order to get credit, including some confraternities, churches and minor communes like Favuglia.[199]

Turning to individual clients, Table 4.4 demonstrates that clients *without* given occupations and *with* surnames tended to spend more.[200] This suggests

Table 4.4

Consumption Patterns by Client Type

Client Type	No. of Clients	% of Clients	Mean Purchasing (soldi)	Median Purchasing (soldi)	Total Purchasing (soldi)	% of Total Purchasing
All	**496**	**100%**	**146.4**	**45.2**	**72,591**	**100%**
Individual						
Surname	252	51%	168.3	58.3	42,400	58%
No Surname	244	49%	123.7	33.3	30,192	42%
No Occ. Title	312	63%	160.1	48.6	49,955	69%
Occ. Title	184	37%	123.0	35.3	22,636	31%
Female	21	4%	184.7	47.7	3,879	5%
Male	475	96%	144.7	45.0	68,712	95%
No Surety	454	92%	149.2	45.5	67,723	93%
Surety	42	8%	115.9	43.5	4,869	7%

that the shop's biggest consumers were mostly members of the patrician élite. Clients identified by occupational titles, most of whom were master artisans, were a minority of clients (thirty-seven per cent of the total), and also tended to consume less than average (thirty-one per cent of total consumption). While there were exceptional figures like the stocking-makers Antonio and Francesco di Giano, most artisans were small-scale consumers, below 150 soldi per annum. Certain occupations, such as friars, spent even less than that on average.[201]

Perhaps surprisingly, the mean consumption of the minority of female clients was higher than that of men. Women with their own accounts were exceptional, and although some of these were poor servants, they were outweighed by a number of patrician ladies with high levels of consumption, such as Francesca Mormorai[202] and Silvaggia Strozzi[203] (both widowed), and Girolama Farnese – whose younger brother Alessandro went on to become Pope Paul III.[204] However, these were exceptional cases and the median consumption of women was equivalent to that of men.

Finally, the mean expenditure of clients who were obliged to provide sureties was lower than the average. This is because their lower credit fixed a ceiling on their consumption.[205] Although a surety meant that they were able to enjoy credit equivalent to that of most of the clientele – as the median figures show – they were unable to run up debts like those of the 'tail' of big consumers, and so the mean average is lower.

The presence of surnames, occupational titles and sureties therefore provide an approximate means of identifying the wealth of clients. Although unreliable as a guide to individual wealth, the aggregate data permit the identification of a group of people who bought goods more often, and spent more money. In the following chapters, these identifiers will be used to examine what *sort* of products tended to be bought by the rich and which by the poor.[206] In this way we will identify which products were, in comparative terms, 'popular' items within the reach of all, and which were 'elite' products limited to a wealthy minority.[207]

Clients can be further characterised in three broad groups according to their pattern of expenditure over time. A first group were the 'crisis' clients who came to the shop at times of need, their accounts lasting only as long as their sickness. At the bottom end of this group were the poorest clients (including carters, labourers and servants), whose consumption was limited to the cheapest varieties of medicines. Zanobi, a carter from Signa, is exemplary. In July 1493, he bought a cheap purge with pudding pipe for his brother for eight soldi.[208] Later that year, his brother Andrea used the account to buy a purge in 'date' form, again for a few soldi.[209] That was the last purchase until April 1496, when Zanobi bought some oils and syrup, bargaining over the price.[210] Comparable behaviour can be seen with Ginevra, a maidservant, whose only purchases in the sample period consisted of a cheap purge, some honey and some stomach ointment.[211] Similarly, a manual labourer came to the shop on two occasions to buy items for his sick wife: first a cheap purge, and a few days later syrup, honey and confectionery to build up her strength.[212] Although the poor might have been able to afford this kind of spending in the short term, it would have been unsustainable for the chronically sick. At times of economic difficulty, such people might be excluded from the market altogether, unless they could rely on the help of a generous master or patron, and their best option would probably have been to resort to the city hospital.

The upper end of this group of 'crisis' clients included many artisans who had the credit to buy the very best medicines, but who only used the shop at times of need. People of middling rank had access to even the most expensive products. Lorenzo, a butcher, bought expensive purges, accompanied by syrups, pills, unctions, clysters and sweets, and even a fabulously costly confection of chicken in a gilded box. Yet his account was only open for sixteen days, probably as long as his sickness lasted.[213] Similarly, a fisherman from Signa bought an epithem containing precious musk and amber, along with comfits, pennets, *manuschristi* and *cotognato*, but his purchases in the sample year were concentrated in three short bursts, presumably linked to sickness.[214] Again, these were 'crisis' clients; they were prepared to buy the very best over a short period of time, but they did not habitually shop at the apothecary's and limited their purchases to medicinal products. If they bought sweets, this was only as part of their medical treatment. Perhaps such levels of expenditure could not always have been sustained but they were often only necessary for a short period linked to a specific illness. The generous level of credit that the shop offered to middling folk of this sort allowed them access to its most expensive products, the same sorts of things that were bought by the elite. Lorenzo the butcher, who spent over 350 soldi in sixteen days, is comparable to an elite patrician widow like Lucrezia Rinucci, who spent nearly 650 soldi in twenty-five days. Both bought a similar range of costly purges, epithems, electuaries, plasters, clysters and syrups.[215] The most expensive purge in the sample, costing over twelve lire, was bought by a client who used the shop for only a five-day period in the whole sample year and then closed his account.[216] They differed from the bottom end of poor clients (carters and servants) in terms of the quantity of their spending and the kinds of products they bought, rather than in the kind of consumer behaviour they exhibited.

These 'crisis' clients can be distinguished from a small minority of 'habitual' clients who came to the shop on a regular basis, not just when they needed medicines, but also to buy luxury products such as sweets and spices. 'Indacho Raghugieo' (probably a merchant from Ragusa) bought some of the most expensive purges in the sample, in one case costing eleven lire. Along with medical items such as gilded trochisks, pills of rhubarb, syrups, clysters and epithems, he also bought confectionery, marzipan, capers and candles. He bought something from the shop almost every day over a two-month period, items that were not always connected to sickness.[217] Another regular long-term client was Manfredo Manfredi, the Ambassador of Ferrara, who bought items two or three times a month, but more often at times of special need. Although he could afford expensive purges, he generally spent little on medicines. What stands out about his spending is his regular purchase of items that were hardly ever bought by the poorer clientele. These included various sorts of confectionary, such as comfits (some of them gilded), aniseed, sugar candy, *pinochiati*, pennets and marzipan; spices, such as saffron, cloves, cumin, coriander, cinnamon and pepper; and miscellaneous items, such as torches, almonds, currants, soap, and candles.[218] Manfredi was a member of the political elite, but similar behaviour is evidenced by people like Antonio and Francesco di Giano, described as 'stocking-makers'.[219] They could afford the most expensive medicines when necessary, and also habitually bought large quantities of sugar, sweets and spices. What marked the 'élite' consumer was not so much access to medicines as to the delights of confectionery and spice, and not just on special occasions or linked to sickness but on an habitual basis. These were the people most significant for the business, along with its corporate clients, but they were also those who were least likely to pay promptly.

Overall, these data suggest a considerable range of consumption patterns. The bulk of clients came to the shop infrequently and bought very little.[220] The majority of artisan masters, priests, notaries, friars, carters and maidservants fall into this category. However, because demand for apothecary products was highly irregular, even wealthier clients might consume little if there was no particular need. The clients who used the shop on a regular basis, and whose high consumption made them essential for its business, were mostly drawn from a more elevated social group – the patrician families who were distinguished in the accounts by their possession of illustrious surnames and lack of occupational titles. It is important to emphasise again, however, that these are aggregate tendencies – the clients do not fall neatly into clearly defined groups but present a variable pattern according to specific individual circumstances, needs and connections. The most important result of this analysis is the central role played in the shop's economic activity by a relatively small number of key clients, most of whom were patricians, flanked by a mass of petty and occasional clients. Although the clientele was therefore fairly broad in terms of social participation, most of them were insignificant for the business in purely financial terms.

Conclusion

Analysis of account-holders reveals a clientele that consisted mostly of wealthy patrician families, but with a sizeable group drawn from the middling artisan and shopkeeper population. There was only a small minority of account-holders from the lowest trades such as porters, servants and manual workers. However, the client base was wider than the sample of account-holders suggests. Women are an exemplary case. Although constituting only a tiny minority of account-holders, this severely underestimates their participation in the market. They were often the recipients of goods bought on somebody else's account; they used accounts registered in the names of males in an active manner; and they might come to the shop to select, transport or pay for goods, although their freedom to do so was related to marital and social status. The focus on account-holders also misrepresents the nature of the shop space, which was frequented by a much broader group of people. Clients were often distanced from the actual transaction by the use of proxies, people who chose and transported the goods.[221] Wealthy patricians might find themselves waiting alongside maidservants and carters, old widowed mothers and young children, artisan masters and manual workers.

The Giglio had a large client base, with high numbers of people listed on the books, but many of these were extinct or dormant accounts and relatively few of those listed were active as clients during the sample year. Within this group, the majority were petty and occasional consumers who had very little significance for the business, as measured in purely financial terms. The provision of such services may however have paid off in terms of the broad personal connections that they offered. The apothecary was tapped into a wide network of operators, many from the political elite, many of whom owed him money, and who therefore constituted a reserve of contacts and favours on which he might draw. Only a relative minority of clients (little more than one hundred) were of any real significance as consumers, and these tended to be members of the patrician elite, many of them readily identifiable through their prestigious surnames. This pattern of polarised consumption and the credit practices that were particularly prevalent in this market sector can both ultimately be related to the irregular nature of demand for apothecary products. Most clients were 'crisis' consumers who only came to the shop when strictly necessary, spending intensely in short bouts that are strictly delimited in time; 'habitual' clients were a rarity and many of them large corporate institutions.

This chapter has emphasised that the ways in which clients obtained credit and used their accounts can only properly be understood in the context of a network of personal relationships. Participation in the market was mediated by the social factors that conditioned access to credit and the use of accounts. A person (or family) who lacked the necessary credit to open a shop account might be able to participate in the market through connections of family, work or institutional affiliation to an existing account-holder. Even dependents such as workers, apprentices and servants could benefit from medicines purchased by their masters. Each account-holder was potentially a conduit for the flow of material goods to their own circle of kin, dependants, and friends, either indirectly by making them the recipients of goods, or directly by permitting them to use the account. In any case, such participation was at the discretion of the account-holder – their decision to share their credit was a form of favour. A further example of how patronage intersected with economic life is in the way that people could offer to stand surety for those whose credit was insufficient by itself. Particularly important in this respect were the apothecary and the close circle of relatives and employees who staffed the shop, including even the lowly apprentices. They were key nodes in this network of consumption and credit, vouching for the credit of new clients, acting as their sureties, or using their own accounts to provide people with goods.

Access to credit was therefore a function of hierarchical ties of obligation, dependency and patronage. Although the fifteenth century has been seen as a period of emergent individualism in Florence, social and economic behaviour were strongly conditioned by these sorts of social bonds.[222] The retail of goods to all (for cash) was of limited import relative to the bulk of the shop's trade, which was mediated by access to credit and therefore conditioned by contact with the apothecary, his close circle or with existing account-holders already within the shop's credit network.

This explains the pronounced clustering that can be identified among the clientele, even with the limitations of the evidence. Clients formed groups based around links to existing account-holders, and most importantly through the personal connections of the apothecary himself, finding new clients through his personal business and property transactions. Many of the key sites frequented by the apothecary stand out as particularly important for the formation of client relationships – the Mercanzia, the Podestà, the customs house, the guilds, the city gates, religious institutions. Such networks were far more significant than geographical proximity in determining the client base of the shop, which benefited from its central location to attract a clientele from across the city, penetrating into the surrounding territory to a more limited extent. The apothecary stands out as being extremely well-connected, with links to many influential figures in guild and communal government, and most of the leading artists' workshops. These networks of contacts were bound together by forms of social and economic credit to which we turn in the next chapter.

Notes

1. C. Muldrew, '"Hard Food for Midas": Cash and its Social Value in Early Modern England', *Past & Present*, 170, 1 (2001), 78–120.
2. R.A. Goldthwaite, *The Building of Renaissance Florence: An Economic and Social History* (Baltimore: Johns Hopkins University Press, 1980), 306–16.
3. J.E. Shaw, *The Justice of Venice: Authorities and Liberties in the Urban Economy, 1550–1700* (Oxford: Oxford University Press, 2006), 151.
4. I. Naso, *Una bottega di panni alla fine del trecento: Giovanni Canale di Pinerolo e il suo libro di conti* (Genoa: Università di Genova, 1985), 55.
5. This is a finding that is confirmed in M. O'Malley and E. Welch (eds), *The Material Renaissance* (Manchester: Manchester University Press, 2007). See particularly the chapter by Guido Guerzoni, 'The Social World of Price Formation: Prices and Consumption in Sixteenth-century Ferrara', *idem*, 85–105.
6. E882, fo. 218v, 'Piero diachopo dipintore fratello dant.o del polaiuolo'.
7. E882, fo. 24r, 'Nanni fratello dischorinci fornaio'.
8. E882, fo. 41v, '[BLANK] lavoratore di nicholo sernigi'.
9. E882, fo. 35r, 'Andrea di [BLANK] fratello di messer bartolomeo schala'.
10. E882, ff. 49r, 338r, 'messer Bartolomeo di [BLANK] schala'.

11. E882, fo. 43v. 'M.a Chiara di [BLANK] orditore de dionigi lanaiuolo', 8 July
    1491, her debt of s16d8 was 'posto a chonto di dionigi di chimenti
    lanaiuolo'; see also fo. 7r, 'Dionigi di chimenti lanaiuolo', for a debt of s16d8
    'quali ci promisse per m.a chiara orditore'.
12. E882, fo. 149r, 'Giovanni di [BLANK] nipote di piero zucheri'.
13. E882, fo. 88v, 'Franc.o di [BLANK] orafo chongniato di m.o ugholino
    mazinghi'; see fo. 71r, 'm.o Ugholino di messer paradiso mazinghi medicho'.
14. There are only three cases: E882, fo. 25v, 'Andrea dalla serra gienero di
    nencio di guliano da singnia'; fo. 92v, 'Biagio di [BLANK] della roccha gienero
    dicabaldo righattiere'; fo. 198r, 'Michele di [BLANK] ghardi gienero di papino
    delfrale'.
15. The only case is E882, fo. 85v, 'm.o Lucha di [BLANK] suociero di ser
    Giovanni da falghano'.
16. E882, fo. 99v, 's[uor]a Girolama sirochia di giovanni chartolaio'; fo. 168v,
    'm.a Adola donna fu di [BLANK] e sirochia di ruberto delglialbizi'; fo. 202v,
    'm.a Lucia di lionardo tavolaccino madre di donant.o delgli angnioli'; fo.
    245r, 'm.a Lisabetta madre di tomasino viviani'; fo. 35v, 'Chaterina di
    [BLANK] zia dineri ghualzelgli'; fo. 279v, 'm.a Dianora di giovanni parente di
    frate franc.o in san franc.o'; fo. 289v, 'm.a Lisabetta figliuola che fu di ser
    guliano bardini' (despite the fact that this woman was married, the
    apothecary identified her in relation to her dead father, rather than her
    husband; he also knew her brother: fo. 15r, 'Pierfranc.o di ser Guliano
    bardini'); fo. 228v, 'Lacheccha di giovanni serva di fantino deluivaio'.
17. E882, fo. 135r, 'm.a Chosa di [BLANK] sta chon franc.o di bettino setaiuolo';
    fo. 168r, 'Giovanmaria di ser ant.o da chotongniano sta cho nicholo del
    necha'.
18. E882, fo. 162r, 'm.a Veronicha di [BLANK] amicha di cibaldo'; fo. 113v,
    'Lorenzo di [BLANK] tanalgli chalzaiuolo amicho di m.o ant.o da san
    giovanni'; fo. 301v, 'Niccholo dant.o amicho di domenicho chardaiuolo'.
19. E882, fo. 216r, 'm.a Antonia da berghamo cioe quella del soldato'.
20. E882, fo. 22v, 'Aghostino di Giovanni di ser tomme bracci'; fo. 124v,
    'Jachopo di giovanni di ser tome bracci'; fo. 263v, 'Tommaso di marcho di
    ser tomme'. They were all involved in the guild of Oliandoli e Pizzicagnoli –
    see Tratte 1724, 64742, 64477, 108546, 108547, 108549, 108550.
21. E882, fo. 26r, 'Marcho di sertomme bracci'; fo. 153v, 'Giovanni di ser tome'.
22. On Giovanni's side these included E882, fo. 22v, 'Aghostino di Giovanni di
    ser tomme bracci'; fo. 124v, 'Jachopo di giovanni di ser tome bracci'. On
    Marco's side these included fo. 199v, 'Nicchodo di marcho di ser tomme
    bracci'; fo. 263v, 'Tommaso di marcho di ser tomme'; fo. 33v, 'Chostantino
    di marcho di ser tomme bracci'.
23. E882, fo. 184v, 'm.a Alessandra in chasa giovanni di ser tomme'; fo. 152v,
    'Ginevra serva di ghostantino [*sic*] di marcho di ser tome bracci'.

24. E882, ff. 53v, 181r, 'Andrea di Berto di michele lapi'. Tratte 400926, lists an Andrea di Berto di Michele di Salvestro Lapi, born 1447.
25. E882, fo. 257v, 'm.a Piera donna dandrea di berto lapi'.
26. E882, fo. 158r, 'Antonio di silvestro lapi'; fo. 190v, 'Giovanni di salvestro lapi'; fo. 165v, 'Piero di salvestro lapi'; fo. 16v, 'Guliano e Nicholaio Fratelgli e Filgliuoli di Girolamo di Salvestro Lapi'; fo. 177r, 'Niccholaio di girolamo lapi'.
27. E882, fo. 46r, 'Chancia spangniuolo in chasa andrea lapi'; fo. 250r, 'Diegho salamancha spangniuolo in chasa andrea di berto lapi'; ff. 83r, 120r, 262r, 323r, 'Giovanni Salamancha spangniuolo in chasa andrea di berto lapi'; fo. 88r, 'Martino di polo spangniuolo in chasa andrea di berto lapi'; ff. 51v, 122r, 306r, 'messer Ghirighoro ghovascho spangniuolo in chasa andrea lapi'.
28. E882, ff. 113r, 245v, 'Anna serva delgli spangniuoli in chasa andrea lapi'; ff. 13v, 62v, 322r, 'Jachopo di [BLANK] familglio degli spangniuoli in chasa andrea lapi'.
29. E882, ff. 49r, 338r, 'messer Bartolomeo di [BLANK] schala'; ff. 121v, 308v, 'Niccholaio dant.o da filichaia'; ff. 112v, 118r, 167r, 334v, 'Lorenzo di tomaso benci'; fo. 179v, 'Bernardo di stoldo rinieri'. See A. Brown, *Bartolomeo Scala, 1430–1497, Chancellor of Florence: The Humanist as Bureaucrat* (Princeton: Princeton University Press, 1979), 245–7; R.A. Goldthwaite, 'Local Banking in Renaissance Florence', *Journal of European Economic History*, 14, 1 (1985), 5–55: 45 n.58.
30. E882, ff. 76v, 240r, 'Luigi dant.o scharlatti'; ASF, Catasto 1022, fo. 366, 'luigi dannttonio di scharlato'.
31. E882, ff. 167r, 266r, 'ser Andrea di ser giovanni mini'; ASF, Catasto 1022, fo. 366, 'ser anndre[a] di ser giovanni mini'.
32. E882, fo. 301v, 'Michele di bartolomeo de medici'; ASF, Catasto 1022, fo. 366, 'chonpramolo di dinari avemo insulachasa de figluoli di barttolomeo de medici'.
33. E541, fo. 7v, 'Luigi d'Ant.o scharlatti', 3 June 1500 and 13 June 1500.
34. E882, fo. 191v, 'Benedetto di ghoro chalzaiuolo'; ASF, Catasto 1022, fo. 366, 'benedetto di ghoro chalzaiuolo'.
35. E882, fo. 142r, 'ser Raffaello di ser gherardo gherardini', with surety 'ser Giovanni suo fratello' – see fo. 122r, 'ser Giovanni di ser gherardo gherardini'; fo. 317r, 'Lionardo di ser gherardo gherardini', with sureties 'ser Giovanni di ser gherardo e ser rafaello suo fratelgli'; fo. 193v, 'Domenicho di [BLANK] fratello di chincho ferretti', identified by reference to his brother, who was also his surety; fo. 109r, 'Piero di giovanni chapponi', with surety 'Giovanni suo filgliuolo' – see ff. 299r, 312v, 'Giovanni di piero chapponi'; fo. 25v, 'Andrea dalla serra gienero di nencio di guliano da singnia', identified through reference to his father-in-law, who was also his surety.

36. E882, fo. 110v, 'Lucha di domenicho lavora[n]te dalesso baldo vinetti', whose surety was his master 'alesso baldovinetti'; fo. 152v, 'Ginevra serva di ghostantino [sic] di marcho di ser tome bracci e per lei promisse detto ghostantino', whose surety was her master – see fo. 33v, 'ghostantino di marcho di ser tome bracci'; fo. 142v, 'Niccholo lavorante di salvestro sarto', whose surety was his master; fo. 107r, 'Giovanni di stefano lavoratore di nicholo sernigi', whose surety was his master – see ff. 206v, 341r, 'Niccholo di giovanni sernigi'; fo. 107r, 'Giovanni di stefano lavoratore di nicholo sernigi', with surety 'Niccholo di giovanni sernigi'; fo. 41v, '[BLANK] lavoratore di nicholo sernigi'. Other clients who got their employers to act as sureties include a chaplain and a debt-collector, see fo. 202r, 'frate Lorenzo di [BLANK] chappellano di ser nerotto a santa maria achanpi' – his surety was 'ser Nerotto'; fo. 126r, 'Andrea dugholino rischotitore di zanobi di franc.o di bartolo', and for his employer see fo. 39v.

37. E882, fo. 17v, 'Ceo di [christ]ofano ortolano da santo anbruogio', whose surety was a client – see fo. 39r 'Ant.o di Tomaso fattore delle monache di santo ambruogio'; fo. 170v, 'Jachopo di [BLANK] vetturale ala badia a monte schalari' with surety 'dontubia monacho in detta Badia'.

38. There is much evidence that apothecaries required clients to provide pledges as a condition of granting credit elsewhere – see A. Giuffrida, 'La bottega dello speziale nelle città siciliane del '400', in *Atti del colloquio internazionale di archeologia medievale, Palermo-Erice, 20–22 settembre 1974* (Palermo, 1976), 28; R.K. Marshall, *The Local Merchants of Prato: Small Entrepreneurs in the Late Medieval Economy* (Baltimore: Johns Hopkins University Press, 1999), 75; Naso, *op. cit.* (note 4), 57, n.14; J.-P. Bénézet, *Pharmacie et médicament en Méditerranée occidentale: (XIIIe–XVIe siècles)* (Paris: H. Champion, 1999), 350. R. Ciasca, *L'arte dei medici e speziali nella storia e nel commercio fiorentino dal secolo XII al XV* (Florence: L.S. Olschki, 1927), 307, states that Florentine doctors and apothecaries typically required pledges, but this was not the case at the Giglio.

39. Only 185 out of 2,247 clients (8.2%) provided sureties and only 44 out of 515 active clients (8.5%) provided sureties.

40. Excluding corporate clients, only 9 out of 42 clients (21.4%) providing sureties had occupational titles, compared to 175 out of 454 clients (38.5%) without sureties who had occupational titles.

41. Excluding corporate clients, 4 out of 42 clients (9.5%) providing sureties were female. This was over twice the rate for clients without sureties – only 17 out of 454 clients (3.7%) without sureties were female.

42. Excluding corporate clients, only 9 out of 184 active clients (4.9%) with occupations had to provide sureties. The precise trades involved (*bastiere, chalzaiuolo, manischalcho, maziere, ortolano, oste, scharpellatore, serva, stamaiuolo*) were mostly trades not linked to guild organisations.

43. In 21 out of 40 cases where debts were transferred from one customer account to another, a formal legal relationship of suretyship was in place.

44. E882, fo. 199r, 'Filippo di samuello', fo. 175r, 'm.a Margherita diromigi barbiere', fo. 174v, 'Andrea di [BLANK] dattorri', all listed the Badia as their surety.

45. E882, fo. 51v, 'Davitte di landino fornaio' was surety for three clients listed on fo. 99r, 'Ghuasparre di Geremia da palazuolo', 'Vergilio di [BLANK]', 'Vicho di [BLANK] da palazuolo'. He also had close ties to other clients, including his business partner ff. 58v, 89v, 'Nanni di [BLANK] fornaio chon davitte di landino' and his brother-in-law fo. 286r, 'Baccio di ventura chongniato di davitte di landino'. See also fo. 247v, 'Giovanni di [BLANK] santini di mugiello', whose surety was 'Giovanni di landino fornaio'. The brothers are listed together on fo. 9v, 'Filgliuoli erede di landino fornaio', and their father is probably ff. 161v, 291r, 'Landino di vanno fornaio'.

46. 111 out of 185 sureties (60%) were clients of the Giglio.

47. E882, ff. 44r, 46v, 'Franc.o di giovanni di nofri dalterrio', whose surety was his cousin Filippo di Jacopo. Filippo's brother was also a client, see ff. 245v, 258r, 319r, 'Domenicho diachopo di nofri dalterrio'.

48. E882, fo. 116r, 'Lapino dangniolo lapini nostro' was surety for fo. 50v, 'Stefano di baldanza da lugliano'. Lapino also covered the debts of other men, including his *balio* and a carter – see fo. 116r, 26 September 1492, 'ci promisse per zanobi dangniolo suo balio', 17 July 1492, 'ci promisse per ant.o di vettorio vetturale da chalcinaia'.

49. E882, fo. 5r, 'Lorenzo di Tommasso di Giovanni nostro' was surety for fo. 94v, 'Bernardo di [BLANK] salviati'.

50. E882, ff. 246v, 350v, 'Duccio di zanobi tolosini nostro schrivano'. Tratte 405863 lists him as Duccio di Zanobi di Luigi Tolosini, born 3 July 1453. Tratte 35064, he was elected Prior in 1518, although ineligible. He was surety for fo. 353v, 'Jachopo di simone baroncielgli'.

51. E882, fo. 80r, 'Girolamo d'andrea da san giovanni nostro gharzone' was surety for the client listed on fo. 98v, 'Ristoro di [BLANK] lavoratore di ser lorenzo', and also another man 'e quali ci promisse per girolamo darezo'; fo. 252v, 'Niccholo di marchionne del m.o ridolfo nostro gharzone' was surety for the client listed on fo. 354v, 'Giovanni di christofano chongniato di nicholo di marchionne n.o gharzone'.

52. E882, fo. 95r, 'Girolamo di maestro piero della barba nostro fattore', was surety for his aunt, fo. 115r, 'm.a Fiametta donna fu di m.o pagholo dela barba'.

53. E882, fo. 192v, 'Antonio di maso dicuccio da san chasciano', a former employee (his account records sums 'per piu ttempo servitto ala bottegha'), was surety for the client listed on fo. 181v, 'Santi randelgli'.

54. E. Muir, '"In Some Neighbours We Trust": The Exclusion of Women from the Public in Renaissance Italy', in D.E. Bornstein and D. Peterson (eds), *Florence and Beyond: Culture, Society and Politics in Renaissance Italy: Essays in Honour of John M. Najemy* (Toronto: Centre for Reformation and Renaissance Studies, 2008), 271–90.

55. E882, ff. 32v, 335v, 343v, 346r, 348r, 'Domenicho di bono rinucci', whose surety was the client listed on fo. 199r, 'm.a Madalena donna fu di ser domenicho pugi suo suocera'. Other members of Domenico's family were also clients, including his brother, sister-in-law and widow – fo. 179r, 'Niccholo di bono rinucci'; fo. 180r, 'm.a Alessandra donna di niccholo di bono rinucci'; ff. 348v, 352r, 355r, 'Luchrezia donna fu di domenicho di bono rinucci'.

56. E882, fo. 165r, 'm.a Alessandra di bernardo baroncelgli', whose surety was the client listed on fo. 206v, 'm.a Gismonda donna di bartolomeo lapi'.

57. E882, fo. 226v, 'ser Alessandro di matteo strozi e per lui promisse m.a rosa serva di ser anselmo'.

58. E882, fo. 354r, 'Tommaso di ser marcho daromena'; fo. 188r, 'ser Benedetto di niccholo daromena'.

59. E882, fo. 163r, 'Simone di matteo sta a ghrieve'; fo. 176r, 'Franc.o dant.o sta a monte ritondo'; fo. 57v, 'Biagio di piero becchaio a sesto'; fo. 217r, 'Marcho di michele scharpelatore a settingniano'.

60. E882, fo. 226r, 'Franc.o di taddeo cioci speziale in pistoia'; fo. 230r, 'Giovanni di niccholaio lenzi e chonpangni speziali in pistoia'; fo. 324r, 'Guliano di piero speziale in terra nuova'; fo. 76r, 'Giovanni dandrea di papi speziale a sam miniato al tedescho' (near Pisa). On city apothecaries as centres of regional distribution, see I. Ait, *Tra scienza e mercato: gli speziali a Roma nel tardo medioevo* (Rome: Istituto Nazionale di Studi Romani, 1996), 89.

61. E882, fo. 230v, 'Balduccio di [BLANK] da monte varchi'; fo. 205v, 'Bastiano di giovanni da monte varchi nostro fattore'; fo. 27r, 'Franc.o di ghuasparre da Montevarchi'; fo. 273v, 'Franc.o di rosino da monte varchi'; fo. 225r, 'Franc.o di ser iachopo da monte varchi'; fo. 141v, 'Fratti di monte varchi'; fo. 24v, 'Giovanni di ghuasparre damonte varchi'; fo. 241v, 'Jachopo di martino menchi da monte varchi'; fo. 290v, 'Luolo di piero di luolo da monte varchi'; fo. 201v, 'm.a Chaterina da monte varchi serva di tomaso di salvestro spini'; fo. 226r, 'm.o Mariotto di [BLANK] da monte varchi de fratti di san franc.o'; fo. 303r, 'messer Giovanni di filippo priore di monte varchi'; fo. 301v, 'Nanni di bartolo di ferro vetturale da monte varchi'; fo. 168v, 'Piero di ser christofano da monte varchi'; fo. 222v, 'ser Lodovicho di christofano menchi da monte varchi'; fo. 182r, 'Ulivieri di bindo da monte varchi'; fo. 340v, 'Vicho di [BLANK] cialdaio da monte varchi'.

62. E882, fo. 241v, 'Jachopo di martino menchi da monte varchi'; ASF, Catasto 1022, fo. 366, 'chonpramolo da iachopo di martino menchi da monte varchi'. See also fo. 222v, 'ser Lodovicho di christofano menchi da monte varchi'.

63. E882, fo. 141v, 'Fratti di monte varchi'; fo. 226r, 'm.o Mariotto di [BLANK] da monte varchi de fratti di san franc.o'; fo. 303r, 'messer Giovanni di filippo priore di monte varchi'; fo. 301v, 'Nanni di bartolo di ferro vetturale da monte varchi'.

64. E882, fo. 205v, 'Bastiano di giovanni da monte varchi nostro fattore', 25 October 1494, purchase of saffron 'disse per mandare a monte varchi', 23 February 1494 (m.f.), debit of one florin 'disse per mandare a monte varchi'.

65. ASF, Catasto 1022, fo. 188, 'Pagholo di piero di lucha degli albizi', described as 'vechio e infermo'. Tratte 415970, 204583, 90880, show that he was born in 1418, elected Prior in 1462, and had died by 1491.

66. E882, fo. 40v, 'Filgliuoli e rede di pagholo di piero delglialbizzi'. Most of the items bought on this account were for Marsilio di Paolo, born 11 Apr 1476 (tratte 413953), and therefore only 18 at the time. See also fo. 103v, 'Raffaello di pagholo dipiero delglialbizi', whose account was later transferred to that of the other heirs. Raffaello was the eldest brother, born in 1459 and elected Gonfalone di Compagnia in 1493 (tratte 417436, 98798).

67. E882, fo. 179v, 'ser Antonio di ser batista chancieliere ala merchatantia'.

68. E882, fo. 156r, 'Adamo di [BLANK] donzello ala merchatantia'; fo. 83v, 'Giovanni di maso notaio ala merchatantia', whose son was also a client – see fo. 89v, 'ser Franc.o di ser Giovanni di maso notaio ala merchatantia'; fo. 10v, 'ser Monte di Ventura notaio alla merchatantia'; ff. 91r, 183v, 'ser Vivaldo di chonte notaio ala merchatantia'.

69. E882, fo. 83v, 'Giovanni di maso notaio ala merchatantia'. He appears on fo. 12r, 7 November 1493; fo. 38r, 15 June 1497; fo. 78r, 31 October 1493; fo. 260r, 31 October 1495, and also fo. 58r, where he is referred to as 'ser Giovanni di maso n.o prochuratore'. Fo. 129r, 8 August 1496, records L1s6, 'per piu spese fatte ala merchatantia per ser giovanni di maso che detto di sebe la sentenzia'. Fo. 128v, 'Luchant.o di piero di tomaso di ser iachopo' lists Giovanni as the surety. His son Tommaso appears on ff. 129r, 194r.

70. E882, fo. 149r, 'ser Benedetto di [BLANK] dalascharperia'. He appears in the account of a number of clients pursued for debt at the Podestà, see fo. 7r, 1 August 1496; fo. 6r, 1 August 1496; fo. 59v, 1 August 1496; fo. 131r, 1 August 1496; fo. 174r, 1 August 1496; fo. 196v, 1 August 1496; fo. 202r, 1 August 1496; fo. 250v, 1 August 1496; fo. 264r, 1 August 1496.

71. E882, fo. 298v, 'ser Bernardo di domenicho notaio al podesta'; fo. 195r, 'ser Giovanmattio di franc.o di ser iac.o notaio al palagio del podesta'; fo. 317v, 'ser Jachopo di martino notaio al palagio del podesta'; fo. 88r, 'ser Niccholo di ser michele di ghiudotto del chanpana notaio al palagio delpodesta'; fo.

86v, 'ser Tommaxo del mazo notaio al palagio del podesta'; fo. 212r, 'ser Girolamo dant.o del chalzolaio proquratore al palagio del podesta'.

72. E882, fo. 264v, 'Bartolomeo del zacheria veditore in doghana'; fo. 12r, 'Franc.o di Lucha sta in doghana'; fo. 159v, 'ser Lorenzo di [BLANK] notaio in doghana'.

73. For clients explicitly described as doctors, see E882, ff. 54r, 232v, 'm.o Bartolomeo di [BLANK] da pisa medicho'; fo. 172v, 'm.o Raffaello di charlo medicho'; fo. 71r, 'm.o Ugholino di messer paradiso mazinghi medicho'.

74. E882, ff. 31r, 118v, 'Stagio di lorenzo barducci'. ASF, Catasto 1022, fo. 315, shows he was aged 57 in 1480. Tratte 202741, 305712, 310630, 105190, 105194, 105200 show that he was elected Prior in 1459 and 1470, Gonfalone di Compagnia in 1488, and Consul of the Guild of Apothecaries and Doctors across the period 1468 to 1489. He was registered as an apothecary back in 1433. R. Ciasca (ed.), *Statuti dell'arte dei medici e speziali* (Florence: L.S. Olschki, 1922), 510, states that Barducci was one of the reformers of the Guild statutes in 1482.

75. E882, ff. 47v, 198v, 'Giovanni di stagio barducci'. ASF, Catasto 1022, fo. 317, shows he was aged 22 in 1480. Tratte 58099, 58116, 312437, 300298, 300588, 58114 for his political career based in the Guild of Apothecaries and Doctors.

76. E882, fo. 118v, 18 May 1495, L2s6d4 for various spices and 1 lb 10 oz of sugar, 'porto ant.o che sta alarte delgli speziali'.

77. E882, fo. 133r, 'Giovanni di girolamo bonsi', elected consul 16 December 1492 (tratte 54248); ff. 47v, 198v, 'Giovanni di stagio barducci', elected Consul 17 April 1493 (tratte 58116); ff. 139r, 173v, 'Lionardo di franc.o mini', elected Consul 16 August 1493 (Tratte 68139); fo. 207v, 'Filippo di tommaso pucci', elected Consul 16 December 1493 (Tratte 37971); fo. 18v, 'Particino di guliano particini', elected Consul 28 April 1494 (Tratte 91311); fo. 280v, 'Bernardo di franc.o lapaccini', elected Consul 18 April 1494 (Tratte 22250). None of these men are identified in the Giglio accounts as apothecaries or doctors.

78. E882, fo. 128r, 'Lodovicho dant.o masi' may be related to Carlo di Antonio di Ser Tommaso Masi, elected Consul 16 December 1492 (tratte 27343); fo. 145v, 'Puccio di franc.o pucci', related to Piero di Francesco di Puccio Pucci, elected Consul 16 December 1492 (tratte 94505); fo. 32v, 'Aniballe di domenicho ditano petrucci' related to Agostino di Annibale di Domenico Petrucci, elected Consul 17 April 1493 (tratte 1533); fo. 280v, 'Bernardo di franc.o lapaccini' and fo. 159v, 'm.a Chostanza donna fu di franc.o lapaccini' related to Giovanni di Francesco di Zanobi Lapaccini, elected Consul 17 April 1493 (tratte 53906); fo. 279v, 's[uor]a Maddalena di matteo charnesechi' with surety 'Matteo di manetto charnesecchi', who was elected Consul 16 August 1493 (Tratte 79059); fo. 2r, 'Ghaleotto di [BLANK] cei'

111

and E541, fo. 33v, 'Giovanbatista di ghaleotto ciei', probably related to Salvestro di Galeotto di Francesco Cei, elected Consul 16 December 1493 (Tratte 101478).

79. E882, fo. 265r, 'Franc.o dant.o dal borgho abita ameza strada fuori della porta ala [croce]'.

80. A. Astorri, 'Appunti sull'esercizio dello speziale a Firenze nel quattrocento', *Archivio storico italiano*, 147 (1989), 31–62: 55.

81. E882, ff. 88r, 262v, 293v, 'Simone di domenicho delfora barbiere della porta alla chrocie'.

82. E882, fo. 69v, 'Antonio di [BLANK] fabro alla porta alla + [croce]'.

83. E882, ff. 124v, 169v, 326r, 'Ruffino di [BLANK] oste e botteghaio fuori della porta ala chrocie'. He may have been a *fornaio* – ASF, Catasto 1148, fo. 182r, lists a 'Rufino di Giovanni di rannuccio fornaio', owning 'Una casa co' i.o casolare p.o i' detto p'p'lo alato alla porta alla + fuori della porta detta del quale chasolare ebi afatto una casa co' i.o forno di sotto a detta chasa...'. The same source lists a son, Bartolomeo, a name which also appears in the Giglio account.

84. E882, fo. 89r, 'Lorenzo di ghuido barbiere fuori dela porta a san piero ghattolini'.

85. E882, fo. 274r, 'Lione dant.o di ghuido barbiere ala porta a san piero ghattolini'.

86. E882, fo. 131v, 'Lucha di paradiso botteghaio fuori della porta a sanpiero ghattolini'.

87. E882, fo. 166r, 'Piero di [BLANK] fabro ala porta a san piero ghattolini'.

88. E882, ff. 34v, 79v, 220v, 257v, 309r, 329r, 342v, 350r, 'Frati e monaci della badia di firenze'.

89. E882, fo. 67v, 'Andrea monacho in badia di firenze'; fo. 136v, 'don Domenicho monacho in badia di firenze'; fo. 157r, 'don Ghraziano monacho in badia di firenze'; fo. 167r, 'don Franc.o da ghaeta monacho nela badia di firenze'; fo. 294r, 'don Masino monacho in badia di firenze'.

90. E882, fo. 92r, 'don Vettorino chamarlingho di badia di firenze'.

91. E882, ff. 75r, 84r, 130v, 204r, 237r, 311r, 321r, 344r, 'Munistero e donne di santo anbruogio'; fo. 102r, 'La saghrestia di santo anbruogio'; S.T. Strocchia, 'Sisters in Spirit: The Nuns of S. Ambrogio and their Consorority in Early Sixteenth-Century Florence', *Sixteenth Century Journal*, 33, 3 (2002), 735–67: 749.

92. E882, fo. 39r, 'Antonio di tomaxo delle monache di santo anbruogio'.

93. E882, ff. 136r, 287v, 'messer Franc.o di stefano della torre priore di santo anbruogio'.

94. E882, ff. 139v, 235r, 244v, 'ser Bernaba di christofano prete e chapellano in santo anbruogio'; fo. 164r, 'ser Lotto prete e chapellano i[n] santo

anbruogio'; fo. 325r, 'ser Portagio di franc.o del tasso chappelano in santo anbruogio'.

95. E882, fo. 17v, 'Ceo di [christ]ofano ortolano da santo anbruogio'; fo. 262r, 'Jachopo di ristoro fornaio a santo anbruogio'.

96. A. Thomas, 'The Workshop as the Space of Collaborative Artistic Production', in R.J. Crum and J.T. Paoletti (eds), *Renaissance Florence: A Social History* (Cambridge: Cambridge University Press, 2006), 424; E882, ff. 111r, 161r, 'Chosimo di lorenzo rosselgli dipintore'.

97. E. Borsook, 'Cult and Imagery at Sant'Ambrogio in Florence', *Mitteilungen des Kunsthistorischen Institutes in Florenz*, 25 (1981), 147–202: 176–8; H.P. Horne, 'A Newly-Discovered Altarpiece by Alesso Baldovinetti', *Burlington Magazine* 8, 31 (1905), 51–9: 51–2; Strocchia, *op. cit.* (note 91), 745. E882, fo. 274r, 'Mino di [BLANK] schultore'; fo. 260v, 'Chimenti di franc.o del tasso lengniaiuolo' (the nephew); fo. 81r, 'Chimenti di domenicho del tasso lengniaiuolo' (the uncle).

98. E882, fo. 290r, 'Munistero e donne delle murate'; ff. 93r, 95v, 'fratti e monaci di settimo eccestello'; fo. 219v, 'La chonpangnia di san bernardino in santa chrocie'.

99. Brown, *op. cit.* (note 29), 130, 233; E882, fo. 133r, 'Guliano di [BLANK] da san ghallo'.

100. E882, ff. 111r, 161r, 'Chosimo di lorenzo rosselgli dipintore'. Many artists linked to Cosimo Rosselli were also Giglio clients – see fo. 234r, 'Neri di bicci dipintore' (his former master); ff. 47v, 261v, 310r, 'Bernardo di stefano rosselgli dipintore' (his cousin); ff. 79r, 184r, 'Giovanni di chimenti rosselgli dipintore' (his nephew); fo. 24v, 'Piero di Lorenzo dipintore' (possibly his pupil, better known as Piero di Cosimo); fo. 11r, 'Como di [BLANK] chongniato di chosimo dipintore' (probably his brother-in-law – Rosselli is the only Cosimo listed as a painter in the accounts).

101. E882, fo. 181r, 'Alessandro di mariano detto sandro di botticiello dipintore'. He had previously worked with fo. 221r, 'Jachopo darchangiolo dipintore' (better known as Jacopo del Sellaio). Jacopo del Sellaio also appears in a joint account with his business partner Filippo di Giuliano on fo. 216v, 'Filippo di guliano eiachopo darchangiolo dipintori'.

102. E882, fo. 127v, 'Domenicho di tomaso di qurado dipintore'.

103. Thomas, *op. cit.* (note 96), 425.

104. In addition to those listed above nn. 99, 100, 101, 102, other artists mentioned in the books include E882, fo. 99v, 'Davide di Tommaso Ghirlandaio'; fo. 218v, 'Piero diachopo dipintore fratello dant.o del polaiuolo', better known as Piero Pollaiuolo; fo. 226r, 'Piero del massaio dipintore'; fo. 231r, 'Domenicho di michelino dipintore'; fo. 144r, 'Nanni ghrosso dipintore'; ff. 79r, 184r, 'Giovanni di chimenti rosselgli dipintore'; ff. 257r, 259r, 'Ciervagio di franc.o del tasso lengniaiuolo'. Cases where the

identification is unclear include ff. 188v, 284r, 'Chimenti e baldo di piero dant.o dipintori', and fo. 71v, 'Benedetto di Giovanni schultore'.

105. ASF Rosselli del Turco p.II, N.2, cc.12r, 18r, records small quantities of colours bought retail by Bernardo di Stefano Rosselli at the Giglio in 1476 – for his account see E882, ff. 47v, 261v, 310r. See also A. Thomas, *The Painter's Practice in Renaissance Tuscany* (Cambridge: Cambridge University Press, 1995), 175.

106. F. De Vivo, *Information and Communication in Venice: Rethinking Early Modern Politics* (Oxford: Oxford University Press, 2007), 98–106.

107. E882, ff. 49r, 338r, 'messer Bartolomeo di [BLANK] schala' and his brother fo. 35r, 'Andrea di [BLANK] fratello di messer bartolomeo schala'.

108. E882, fo. 187v, 'Filippo di piero da ghalgliano'. See A. Brown, 'Lorenzo de' Medici's New Men and their Mores: The Changing Lifestyle of Quattrocento Florence', *Renaissance Studies*, 16, 2 (2002), 113–42: 115, 122–3, 134.

109. E882, fo. 243v, 'messer Bernardo di messer giovanni buongirolami', fo. 166v, for his brother [?] 'Girolamo di messer giovanni buongirolami', fo. 196v, for his son [?] 'messer Giovanni di messer bernardo buongirolami'; fo. 40r, 'Pierofilippo di [BLANK] pandolfini'; fo. 109r, 'Piero di giovanni chapponi', ff. 157v, 190r, for his brothers 'messer Ant.o di giovanni chapponi', 'Gherardo di giovanni chapponi', and ff. 109r, 299r, 312v, for his sons 'Giovanni di piero chapponi', 'Bernardo di piero di giovanni chapponi'.

110. E882, fo. 40r, 'Pierofilippo di [BLANK] pandolfini'; fo. 255v, 'Tommaso di piero minerbetti' and fo. 279r for his wife 'm.a Maddalena donna di tomaxo Minerbetti'; ff. 110r, 115v, 117r, 'Madonna Girolama donna di messer puccio dant.o pucci' was the widow of Puccio Pucci.

111. N. Rubinstein, *The Government of Florence under the Medici (1434 to 1494)* [1966], 2nd edn (Oxford: Clarendon, 1997), 361–2, lists the Council of 70 in 1489. Of these the following are listed in E882, ff. 50r, 288v, 'Lapo di Lorenzo Niccolini', ff. 65r, 93r, for his son 'Giovanni di lapo di lorenzo niccholini' and ff. 5v, 21r, 38v, 125r, for his brothers; fo. 40r, 'Pierofilippo di [BLANK] pandolfini'; ff. 49r, 338r, 'messer Bartolomeo di [BLANK] schala'; ff. 77v, 236r, 'Domenicho di messer charlo pandolfini'; fo. 87v, 'Braccio di M. Domenico Martelli'; ff. 154r, 246v, 'Angolo di Francesco di Lorenzo Miniati'; fo. 154r, 'Piero di gino chapponi'; fo. 164r, 'Maso [BLANK] degli alessandri'; fo. 186r, 'Jachopo di messer alessandro delgli alesandri'; fo. 194v, 'Nicchol [sic] dandrevuolo sacchetti'; fo. 299r, 'Tanai di franc.o denerli'.

112. E882, fo. 107v, 'Piero di messer tomaso soderini'.

113. On Scala's ambivalent attitude to the new regime see Brown, *op. cit.* (note 29), 124-30.

114. L. Polizzotto, *'The Elect Nation': The Savonarolan Movement in Florence, 1494–1545* (Oxford: Clarendon, 1994), 446–60. At least 57 of 503 names listed can be identified as Giglio clients in E882.

115. E882, fo. 251v, 'Andrea dant.o chanbini'.

116. E882, fo. 313v, 'messer Franc.o di lorenzo ghualterotti'.

117. E882, fo. 190v, 'Ulivieri di simone ghuadangni'.

118. E882, fo. 242r, 'Jachopo di pagholo di lapo niccholini'; his father (d.1482)
      was listed fo. 215v, 'Pagholo di lapo niccholini'.

119. E882, fo. 181r, 'Alessandro di mariano detto sandro di botticiello dipintore',
      and his brother fo. 126r, 'Antonio di mariano filipepi'.

120. E882, ff. 61r, 339r, 'messer Manfredi inbasciadore di ferrara'.

121. 26 women out of 515 active clients in the sample period (5.0%), or 114
      women out of 2,247 clients (5.1%).

122. 5 out of 26 active female clients (19.2%) were convents.

123. 10 out of 21 active female individual clients (47.6%) can be identified as
      widows with certainty. The status of the other married women is unclear. 46
      out of 99 of all female individual clients were widows (46.5%).

124. This was higher than the 25% of all women who were widows in 1427– see
      D. Herlihy and C. Klapisch-Zuber, *Tuscans and their Families: A Study of the
      Florentine Catasto of 1427* (New Haven: Yale University Press, 1985), 124;
      C. Klapisch-Zuber, 'The "Cruel Mother": Maternity, Widowhood, and
      Dowry in Florence in the Fourteenth and Fifteenth Centuries', in C.
      Klapisch-Zuber (ed.), *Women, Family, and Ritual in Renaissance Italy*
      (Chicago: University of Chicago Press, 1985), 117–31: 120.

125. E882, fo. 98v, 'm.a Angniola donna fu di ser domenicho pugi', 9 June 1494,
      purchase of 3 oz of julep violet and an ampoule, 'porto lei detta'. Fo. 327r,
      'm.a Angniola di saghramoro', also bought her own medicines.

126. E882, ff. 32v, 335v, 343v, 346r, 'Domenicho di bono rinucci', last
      transactions on 15 July 1494.

127. E882, ff. 352r, 348v, 355r, 'm.a Luchrezia donna fu di domenicho di bono
      rinucci', first transactions from 16 July 1494.

128. E882, fo. 255v, 'Tommaso di piero minerbetti', active in buying items (often
      for his wife) in February 1493 (m.f.), and settled the bill on 1 March 1493
      (m.f.). Fo. 279r, his wife 'm.a Maddalena donna di tomaxo minerbetti', had
      her own account starting shortly after this, 15 March 1493 (m.f.).

129. 40 out of 114 of all female clients (35.1%) were identified as married
      women, with the title 'Mona' (and in one case 'Madonna'), and no
      indication that their husband was dead at the moment the account was
      opened.

130. E882, fo. 257v, 'm.a Piera donna dandrea di berto lapi', who purchased
      items in February and March 1494 (m.f.). Fo. 53v, her husband 'Andrea di
      Berto di michele lapi' had his own account at the shop, which lists
      transactions from 16 Aug 1493 up to 16 October 1495. We can be certain
      that he was her husband because, on 5 October 1495, he bought syrup and
      sugar 'per m.a piera'.

131. E882, fo. 179r, 'Niccholo di bono rinucci'; fo. 180r, 'm.a Alessandra donna di niccholo di bono rinucci'.
132. Excluding corporate clients, 3 out of the 21 active female clients (14.3%) were servants. 9 out of 99 of all female clients (9.1%) were servants, some unmarried. 5 out of 99 female clients (5.1%) were nuns.
133. E882, fo. 305r, 'Biagio di stefano manischalcho', 10 May 1494, 'tolse michele di chante per la donna e porta elavoratore'.
134. E882, fo. 319r, 'Giovanni di maffeo de libri', 6 May 1494, 'porto lorenzo di lolo sta cho le monache di faenza e tolse labate di santa trinita chome disse detto giovanni'.
135. E882, fo. 96v, 17 March 1494 (m.f.), 'porto la serva'; fo. 141r, 24 September 1494, 'porto la sandra sua serva'. See E. Welch, *Shopping in the Renaissance: Consumer Cultures in Italy 1400–1600* (New Haven: Yale University Press, 2005), 217–18.
136. E882, ff. 58v, 261r, 319r, 354r, 'Domenicho di tone'.
137. E882, fo. 73v, 'Franc.o di Benedetto di cianpolo da panzano', 11 October 1495, 'tolse e porto giovanni mancini per mandargli a panzano'. For the relation between them, see entry for 3 December 1494, 'tolse giovanni mancini suo gienero disse per mandagliene in villa'.
138. E882, fo. 323v, 'Michele di bernardo niccholini', 26 May 1494, 'tolse sandro fabro per mandarli in villa'; P.L. Rubin, *Images and Identity in Fifteenth-Century Florence* (New Haven: Yale University Press, 2007), 245–6, discusses the marriage of Michele Niccolini to Oretta Pucci in 1471.
139. E882, fo. 40v, 'Filgliuoli e rede di pagholo di piero delglialbizzi', 2 July 1494, 1¼ oz of 'p'le magistrali' 'disse per mandare a piero suo fratello inlevante'. This elder brother was Piero di Paolo di Piero, b. 25 March 1461 (tratte 417008).
140. E882, fo. 23v, 'Girolamo di pagholo federighi', 14 February 1493 (m.f.), 'una medicina per m.a ghostanza', 'porto tomaso n.o astenperare achasa'.
141. E882, fo. 349r, 'Bartolomeo di tomaso settecielgli e fratelgli lanaiuoli in samartino', 18 July 1494, 8 August 1494. See also fo. 19v, 'Tomme dardingho dasanchasciano', 14 September 1496, for a delivery of syrup 'per la donna di berto di tomme porto tomaso'; fo. 348v, 'Piero di messer tomaso salvetti', 15 July 1494 and 17 July 1494, the apothecary's son Lorenzo delivered items for a sick child.
142. Welch, *op. cit.* (note 135), 216–17.
143. E882, fo. 327r, 's[uor]a Angniola delle polverine', was the only nun with her own account who bought anything during the sample year. This account was immediately settled in cash and struck through. She subsequently opened a second account – see fo. 333v. She spent a total of only 41.3 soldi in the sample year.

144. E882, ff. 75r, 84r, 130v, 204r, 237r, 311r, 321r, 344r, 'Munistero e donne di santo anbruogio'; ff. 68v, 311v, 'Munistero e donne di san nicholo dela via del chochomero'.

145. E882, fo. 45v, 5 August 1493, purchase of syrup 'per una sua sirochia monacha in samartino fuori dela porta al prato'; fo. 119r, 'Fruosino di Cece da Verrazano' often sent medicines to his sister, a nun at Sant'Ambrogio, as on 4 October 1493; fo. 104r, 'Bartolomeo delvantaggio', 26 March 1494, ½ oz of 'channella fine sodo', 'per la monacha delle murate'.

146. E882, fo. 188r, 'Giovanni dalessandro rondinelgli', 21 May 1494, medicine 'per m.a salvestra sua lavoratore'; fo. 307r, 'Antonio e franc.o di giano chalzaiuoli', 28 April 1494, 'disse per la balia'; fo. 122v, 'Michele di bernardo niccholini', 7 January 1493 (m.f.), 1 oz of 'loccho sano e dieiris' and an alberello 'per la serva'; fo. 183v, 'Piero dandrea mazzi', 24 May 1494, a purge 'per la serva'.

147. D. Romano, 'Aspects of Patronage in Fifteenth- and Sixteenth-Century Venice', *Renaissance Quarterly*, 46 (1993), 712–33: 716–17.

148. E882, fo. 285r, 'Magi di [BLANK] marito di mona chaterina botteghaia a san nicholo dirinpetto ala fonte'.

149. E882, fo. 308v, 'Jachopo di bartolomeo ghalli per chonto della madre': 14 April 1494 and 21 April 1494, 'per m.a checcha'; 4 August 1494 to 1 September 1494, 'per la serva'; 25 September 1494, 'per la madre'.

150. E882, fo. 53v, 'Andrea di Berto di michele lapi'. These items were subsequently paid for separately from the rest of the account, suggesting that Andrea was unwilling to advance her much credit.

151. E882, fo. 308v, 'Jachopo di bartolomeo ghalli per chonto della madre', lists mostly women as providing porterage: 'm.a ghostanza', 'm.a biagia', 'm.a brigida'.

152. E882, fo. 96v, 17 March 1494 (m.f.), 'porto la serva'.

153. E882, fo. 141r, 24 September 1494, 'porto la sandra sua serva'. See also fo. 106r, 'Piero di franc.o di bettino setaiuolo', 9 April 1494, the wife of a silk manufacturer sent her nursemaid to the shop, 'porto la balia per la donna'.

154. Most of these women were identified with the title 'Mona', implying that they were, or had been, married. Among the many examples are E882, fo. 83r, 2 October 1493, 'porto m.a chaterina ghardadona'; fo. 115r, 2 October 1493, 'porto m.a margherita'; fo. 90r, 22 May 1495, 'porto m.a uliva'; fo. 96v, 23 December 1493, 'porto m.a mea'; fo. 96v, 10 January 1493, 'porto m.a nanna'; fo. 106r, 29 March 1494, 'porto mona tomasa'. For a clear case where the husband was still alive see fo. 124r, 'Giovanni d'ant.o buricchi pigionale alatorre', 3 June 1494, 'porto la molglie'.

155. E882, fo. 82r, 28 September 1493, 'tolse e porto m.a luchrezia sua madre dachordo [soldi] 7', and entries for 7 December 1493, 1 December 1493.

156. E882, fo. 317r, 6 May 1494, 'porto m.a rafaella sua madre'.

157. E882, fo. 317r, 27 October 1494, payment of L7, 'per lui da m.a rafaella sua madre recho ella detta'.
158. E882, fo. 108r, 24 September 1493, 'per lui', 'porto la zia'.
159. E882, fo. 11r, 'Antonio e franc.o di niccholo gianfilgliazi', 23 December 1493, payment in the form of 3 oz of 'zaferano e mandorle' 'recho m.a bartolomea loro madre dachordo' for an agreed price of L4.
160. E882, fo. 13v, 'Pagholo dimeo fabro atterrenzano', 20 July 1493, payment of L1s3d8, 'recho la donna sua'.
161. E882, fo. 146r, 'Cristofano di paradiso chalzaiuolo', 23 September 1495, 6 oz of 'sapone ghaetano', 'p.o la chaterina sua figliuola'.
162. E882, fo. 307r, 'Ant.o e franc.o di giano chalzaiuoli', 25 April 1494, 'porto la ginevra sua nipote'; 1 May 1494, 'tolse giovanni dala volta e porto la ginevra'.
163. E882, fo. 266r, 'ser Andrea di ser giovanni mini', 4 April 1494, 'pel figliuolo p.o la sua fanculla'.
164. E882, fo. 116r, 'Lapino dangniolo lapini nostro', 30 October 1493, 'demo per lui a ant.o di bernardo dalantella suo pigionale'.
165. E882, fo. 116r, 2 November 1493, 'demo per lui al balio'; for this man see entry for 26 September 1492 'ci promisse per zanobi dangniolo suo balio'.
166. E882, fo. 5r, 'Lorenzo di Tommasso di Giovanni nostro', 12 November 1493, for spices 'dette ala suociera'; fo. 147v, 'Marcho di tomaxo di giovanni nostro', 2 April 1494, for spices 'per lui a fratte bernaba in san bernaba'.
167. E882, fo. 5r, 17 May 1494, 'per lui a christofano di paradiso'. For this client, see fo. 146r, 'Cristofano di paradiso chalzaiuolo'.
168. E882, fo. 5r, 3 March 1494 (m.f.), 5 March 1494 (m.f.), purchases of marzipan 'porto chris[t]ofano di paradiso'. Even customers like Cristofano, who had his own account, sometimes obtained supplies through the shop staff. On this see also entry for 17 June 1494, 'per lui a lorenzo di bernardetto', for delivery of white wax candle on Lorenzo's account to a client who had his own account – see fo. 86r, 'Lorenzo di bernardetto de medici'. Similarly, fo. 147v, 'Marcho di tomaxo di giovanni nostro', 6 September 1494, 'per lui a piero pitozi peschatore', the apothecary's son Marco supplied almonds to a fisherman who had his own account – see ff. 14v, 345v, 'Piero di Lionardo pitozi peschatore da singnia'.
169. E882, fo. 252v, 'Niccholo di marchionne del m.o ridolfo nostro gharzone', 4 March 1493 (m.f.), and 5 March 1493 (m.f.), 'per la chongniata sua'.
170. E882, fo. 252v, 4 August 1494, and 9 August 1494, 'per la sirochia'.
171. E882, fo. 252v, 18 June 1494, 'per mandare in valdelsa ala balia del chongniato'.
172. E882, fo. 34r, 'Tommaso di giovanni di piero nostro', 25 January 1493 (m.f.), for marzipan, 'mando a nich012 sernigi', whose account is listed on ff. 206v, 341r, 'Niccholo di giovanni di sernigi'. See also fo. 34r, 27 January

1493 (m.f.), fo. 255r, 26 March 1494, and 27 March 1494, for yellow torches, *zibibbo*, marzipan and aniseeds sent to the convent of the Murate; fo. 255r, 29 April 1494, 9 May 1494, for red wine and sugar sent to a nun called Sister Orsola.

173. E882, 516 out of 2,247 clients (23%) bought something from the shop during the sample year. However, one of these spent an indeterminate sum and must be discounted from the analysis, leaving 515 active clients for whom spending data exists. By comparison, Bénézet, *op. cit.* (note 38), 210, shop accounts from fifteenth-century Arles reveal *c.*60 clients.

174. Total spending of 88,609 soldi, divided by 515 active clients, giving a mean average of 172 soldi per client.

175. 75% of all clients fell within the upper quartile of the distribution at up to 145 soldi. 79% of all clients fell within the mean average at up to 172 soldi.

176. As a proportion of total retail spending during sample period of 88,609 soldi.

177. Clients spending over 150 soldi in the sample year account for a total of 72,424 soldi.

178. Marshall, *op. cit.* (note 38), 42, found that one monastery (San Domenico) was responsible for 86% of the business of the apothecary Benedetto di Tacco.

179. E882, fo. 102r, 'La saghrestia di santo anbruogio'.

180. E882, ff. 75r, 84r, 130v, 204r, 237r, 311r, 321r, 344r, 'Munistero e donne di santo anbruogio'.

181. E882, ff. 34v, 79v, 220v, 257v, 309r, 329r, 342v, 350r, 'Frati e monaci della badia di firenze'.

182. E882, fo. 350r, 30 August 1494, 'porto lanfermiere'.

183. E882, fo. 220v, 8 January 1493 (m.f.), 'lucingnioli sottili', 'per la saghrestia'.

184. E882, ff. 65r, 93r, 'Giovanni di lapo di lorenzo niccholini'.

185. E882, fo. 218r, 'Jachopo di ristoro fornaio a san brachazio'.

186. E882, ff. 44v, 307r, 318v, 326v, 337v, 'Antonio e franc.o di giano chalzaiuoli'.

187. A. Spicciani, 'Aspetti finanziari dell'assistenza e struttura cetuale dei poveri vergognosi fiorentini al tempo del Savonarola (1487–1498)', in *Studi di storia economica toscana nel medioevo e nel rinascimento: In memoria di Federigo Melis* (Pisa: Pacini, 1987); J. Henderson, *Piety and Charity in Late Medieval Florence* (Oxford: Clarendon, 1994), 394–5; J. Kirshner and A. Molho, 'The Dowry Fund and the Marriage Market in Early Quattrocento Florence', *Journal of Modern History*, 50 (1978), 403–38: 414, also used possession of surname as approximate guide to social rank.

188. E882, fo. 322v, 'Giova'matteo di marcho nelli'. He is listed as a mercer, in a company with his brother, on fo. 103v, 'Benedetto di piero da san donnino

vetturale', 6 August 1494, 'per lui da giovannmatteo e guseppe nelli e chonpangni merciai'.

189. E882, fo. 179v, 'Bernardo di stoldo rinieri'. On his banking firm, see Brown, *op. cit.* (note 29), 222; Goldthwaite, *op. cit.* (note 29), 45, n.58.

190. E882, fo. 276r, 'Franc.o di pagholo di ser giovanni mini', is described as an apothecary in the 1480 Catasto – see Astorri, *op. cit.* (note 80), 40.

191. E882, ff. 61r, 339r, 'messer Manfredi inbasciadore di ferrara'.

192. Excluding 51 corporate clients, there are 2,196 individual clients remaining. 1,022 out of 2,196 (ie. 47%) of these individual clients are identified by surname. A. Molho, 'Names, Memory, Public Identity, in Late Medieval Florence', in G. Ciappelli and P.L. Rubin (eds), *Art, Memory, and Family in Renaissance Florence* (Cambridge: Cambridge University Press, 2000), 240, quotes Catasto data from 1480 showing that 48.3% of persons or households were identified by surname.

193. E882, ff. 315v, 332v, 'Alamanno di filippo rinuccini'.

194. Excluding 51 corporate clients, there are 2,196 individual clients remaining. 785 out of 2,196 (i.e. 36%) of these individual clients are identified by their occupation. This figure is lower than expected, confirming that the clientele was drawn disproportionately from the elite with no declared occupation (64% of clients). Herlihy and Klapisch-Zuber, *op. cit.* (note 124), 127, show that 43.9% of the population had no declared occupation in the Catasto records.

195. Out of 785 clients listed with occupations, we find for example the following totals: *speziale* (51), *chalzaiuolo* (35), *dipintore* (31), *lengniaiuolo* (28), *chalzolaio* (25), *notaio* (20), *orafo* (20), *linaiuolo* (20), *righattiere* (20), *prete* or *chapellano* (37), *frate* (18), *serva* (9), *lavoratore* (20), *zocholaio* (2), *muratore* (13), *filatoiaio* (5), *cimatore* (11).

196. 51 out of 2,247 of all clients were corporate (2.3%).

197. E882, fo. 117v, 'Fratti di san franc.o daladoccia', total spending 4 soldi. On this monastery, see D. Rosenthal, 'The Spaces of Plebeian Ritual and the Boundaries of Transgression', in R.J. Crum and J.T. Paoletti (eds), *Renaissance Florence: A Social History* (Cambridge: Cambridge University Press, 2006), 165.

198. E882, fo. 354v. 'La chonpangnia e vuomini di san giovanni schalzo', total spending 5 soldi.

199. E882, fo. 270v, 'La chonpangnia di santa maria alarciana' with surety 'Maso di nofri di valdifantona'; fo. 252r, 'Pieviere e vuomini di san martino aviminiccio di mugiello' with surety 'Giovanni diachopo masini setaiuolo in bottegha di tomaso alamanni'; fo. 187r, 'Chomune e vuomini [sic] delanpolecchio' with surety 'messer ghuaspare abate di san baronto'; fo. 339v, 'Chomune e vuomini di favuglia', and fo. 339v, 'Chomune e vuomini di

tremuleto', both with surety 'Tanai di veri de medici', whose account is on fo. 2r.

200. Clients with surnames and clients with occupational titles formed two fairly distinct groups with relatively little crossover. Excluding corporate clients, 219 out of 496 clients (44%) had surnames but no occupational title, while 151 clients (30%) had occupational titles but no surnames. Only 33 clients (7%) possessed both occupational titles *and* surnames. This suggests that the apothecary either identified people by reference to family, or by reference to trade, but not both.

201. Average annual spending of the few friars (4) listed as active clients was only 19.6 soldi.

202. E882, ff. 238v, 342r, 'm.a Franc.a donna fu di luigi mormorai e giovanbatista suo figliuolo', total spending 842 soldi.

203. E882, ff. 104v, 254v, 'm.a Silvaggia donna fu di filippo strozzi', total spending 782 soldi.

204. E882, ff. 110r, 115v, 117r, 'Madonna Girolama donna di messer puccio dant.o pucci', total spending 841 soldi. Rubin, *op. cit.* (note 138), 248, on the marriage of Puccio Pucci to Geronima Farnese in 1483, with a huge dowry of 2,700 ducats.

205. The 471 active clients without sureties spent 83,294 soldi, an average of 176.8 soldi per annum. The 44 active clients with sureties spent 5,334 soldi, an average 121.2 soldi per annum. Average debt for clients with sureties was 77 soldi, while for clients without sureties it was 264 soldi.

206. 42,400 out of 72,591 soldi were spent by clients with surnames (58.5%), excluding corporate clients.

207. An alternative to what might seem a rather crude dependence on surnames and occupational titles might be to use total spending as an approximate guide to wealth, see for example Kirshner and Molho, *op. cit.* (note 187), 414. However, because of the irregular nature of spending on apothecary goods, where, for example, a healthy rich man might spend very little until falling sick, it is much more useful to establish factors that are independent from consumption.

208. E882, fo. 17r, 20 July 1493, 'Zanobi di Stefano Vetturale da singnia de dare ad[i] detto p[er] una m[edicin]a p[er] Giovanni suo frattello… [dr] vi di polpa di chasia [dr] i di sugho rosato [dr] i di diefinichon st[emperat]a in aqua di fumost[ern]o e [una] [am]p[oll]a porto e detto… s8 d4'.

209. E882, fo. 17r, 'E adi 29 d'ottobre s2 p[er] resto d'un datt[er]o tolse e porto a[n]drea suo fratello… s2'.

210. E882, fo. 17r, 'E ad[i] 2 d'ap[r]ile 1496 p[er] dua p[r]ese di s[ciropp]o chon zuc[cher]o [e] aque st[illat]a e p[er] olio di spigho e di chosto in tutto da[c]chordo s11 d8'.

211. E882, fo. 152v, 'Ginevra [ser]va di ghostantino di marcho di [ser] to'me bracci e p[er] lei promisse detto ghostantino per questo e quello figli dissi de dare ad[i] xiiii.o d'ottobre p[er] una m[edicin]a p[er] lei in che ent[ran]o [oz] i di diechattolichon fatto datt[er]o chon zuc[cher]o porto ella detta... s10', 'E ad[i] 16 detto p[er] [oz] ii di rosata novella e [oz] ½ d'unzione da stomacho... e ii alb[erell]i... s10 d8'.

212. E882, fo. 31v, 'Lorenzo di Giovanni dant.o lavoratore di maso delglialesandri': 27 July 1493, a purge for s13d8; 1 August 1493, 4 oz of savonia, 2 oz of 's.o di bisanti', 2 oz of 'rosato cholato', plus receptacles, for s14.

213. E882, fo. 56r, 'Lorenzo di Salvetto becchaio a Sanfriano': 25 August 1493, a complex purge costing L8½; 20 August 1493, 4 oz of 'churiandoli inpizichata'; fo. 49v, 12 August 1493, 22.5 oz of confectioned chicken and a gilded box for 4 lire. His total spending was almost 18 lire across the period 10 August 1493 to 25 August 1493, just over 20 soldi per day.

214. E882, fo. 345v, 'Piero di lionardo petozi peschatore da singnia', 5 July 1494, a cordial epithem for L1s7; see also fo. 14v, 29 January 1493 (m.f.), 2 August 1493, 26 August 1493, and fo. 345v, 5 July 1494.

215. E882, ff. 348v, 352r, 355r, 'm.a Luchrezia donna fu di domenicho di bono rinucci', total spending across period 16 July 1494 to 9 August 1494 was s641.5, ie. around s26 per day. For a similar case of intensive spending by a wealthy widow linked to sickness, see ff. 110r, 115v, 117r, 'Madonna Girolama donna di messer puccio dant.o pucci'.

216. E882, fo. 309v, 'Nero di Francesco del Nero', 14 April 1494, a medicine containing 1.5 oz of manna and 1 dr of rhubarb for 243 soldi. His total spending was s252.33, across the period from 14 April 1494 to 18 April 1494, or s50.47 per day.

217. E882, ff. 45r, 53r, 67v, 'Indacho raghugieo'. His total spending across the period 4 August 1493 to 5 October 1493 was s1070.67, or s16.99 per day.

218. E882, ff. 61r, 339r, 'messer Manfredi inbasciadore di ferrara'. His total spending across the period from 4 March 1495 (m.f.) to 21 March 1495 (m.f.) was s94.33, or s5.24 per day.

219. E882, ff. 44v, 307r, 318v, 326v, 337v, 'Antonio e franc.o di giano chalzaiuoli'.

220. Naso, *op. cit.* (note 4), 55, found in her study of a draper's shop in Pinerolo, which had around *c*.150 clients in the period 1398–9, that most of the clients (60%) performed only a single transaction in the whole year.

221. Welch, *op. cit.* (note 135), 243.

222. F.W. Kent, *Household and Lineage in Renaissance Florence: The Family Life of the Capponi, Ginori, and Rucellai* (Princeton: Princeton University Press, 1977); Goldthwaite, *op. cit.* (note 2).

5

Recovering Debts

The previous chapter suggested that the apothecary at the Giglio encouraged and benefited from an integrated social and economic system of close family, neighbourhood and professional ties. As Craig Muldrew has suggested, the trust embedded in these networks made credit possible in the marketplace. Why then, did so many of the Giglio's clients effectively default on all or part of their debts? The carefully maintained account books survived, not as a testimony to the success of this system but to the constant fear of its failure.

When 'Falconiere' the carter came to the Giglio to buy a wax taper in March 1493, he bargained with the apothecary, finally agreeing a price of six soldi and eight denari, which he immediately paid in cash. The transaction was carefully recorded and then the account was 'struck through' with a line from top right to bottom left, because the debt was already settled. This happened again and again across the period April–May 1494 – each time, Falconiere paid in cash, and each time a new account was started and then struck through. In total, there are four separate accounts in his name in the sample period, each one closed almost as soon as it was opened.[1]

This behaviour was very unusual. Only a small minority of customers paid for their goods immediately and in cash. These were primarily people of humble status, often carters like Falconiere. They were men and women whose limited wealth, connections or reputation made it impossible for them to obtain credit. Denied access to credit, they had to find cash, something that could be difficult in an economy where coins were in short supply. We can observe them struggling with the coinage: coins of large denomination might be difficult to dispose of, for example. Unable to get credit, they might have to open an account by paying a large coin in advance, in effect themselves becoming creditors of the shop. The carter Jacopo for example opened his account by paying a florin in advance, which he then got back in the form of supplies.[2] He probably lacked the small coin to pay for each item separately, so this was a useful way for him to dispose of this unwieldy florin. In other cases, poor clients quickly reached their credit limit and could only obtain further goods if they agreed to settle their debts. When a carter called Domenico bought a purge in 1494,[3] he was only granted credit on condition of paying back old debts dating back to 1485,[4] and he duly settled his account about two weeks later.[5]

For most clients, by contrast, the timing, form and extent of payment was an entirely separate question from the purchase and consumption of goods. For example, the shop's biggest customer in the sample year, the Sacristy of Sant'Ambrogio, paid nothing towards its account during this period. The extent of this is clear from comparing the figures recorded for consumption (88,609 soldi) with those recorded for payment (58,011 soldi) in the sample year, only about two thirds of the total. Comparing these figures is potentially problematic: payments made during the sample year relate to consumption that took place not just that year but all previous years as well. There is also evidence to suggest that the apothecary was not always so careful about recording payments.[6] Despite these limitations, the imbalance of incomings relative to consumption is striking. The consequence of this shortfall was that the shop had built up a huge quantity of debt over the nearly thirty years since it had begun trading.

Adding up all the old debts that were transferred into the register during the sample period, some of which date back to 1465, the total was around 490,000 soldi.[7] This figure does not include the shop's biggest debtor by far – Tommaso di Giovanni, the apothecary himself.[8] His debt of over 125,000 soldi made up twenty per cent of the total, but this should properly be interpreted as representing his income from the shop over a period of many years.[9] This was not a 'debt' that he ever intended to repay to the shop – his account was struck through as 'settled' despite never making any payments. It consisted partly of goods and partly of cash, some of which was paid out directly to his personal creditors. Similarly, substantial sums were advanced to the apothecary's son-in-law Lapino, his son Marco, and his apprentice Girolamo d'Andrea. Again, this took the form of both goods and cash; Lapino in particular was a regular consumer of spices, even having them sent out to his villa.[10] Even the *pestatore* who did the heavy work of grinding spices in the mortars was paid in sweets, spices and soap, as well as coin.[11] It is difficult to determine here whether such consumption should be considered as advances or back payments for the wages of staff. On balance it appears that a more realistic figure for the shop's consumer debt can be obtained by excluding the income and wages of shop staff from the total.

As in the case of consumption, debt was not evenly distributed. The mean average level of debt for all clients was 286 soldi, but because of the remarkably skewed distribution, the median of 46 soldi provides a much more realistic idea of a typical client's debt. For most ordinary clients, only petty credit was available at the apothecary shop. The bulk of the enormous 'mountain' of old debt was actually due from a small minority of clients – a group of around fifty clients owed around half of all the debt.

Although well below the level of Tommaso di Giovanni, the next leading debtors at the shop were corporate institutions, mostly religious institutions whose landholdings guaranteed the debt. The Badia of Florence for example, which was the second-biggest customer in the sample year, had debts of over 23,000 soldi in May 1493.[12] Since it consumed goods to the value of over 5,500 soldi during the sample year,[13] and paid just over 1,300 soldi during the same period (a single cash payment of ten florins),[14] the debt had risen to 27,455 soldi by January 1495.[15] That the Badia enjoyed such extensive credit may have been related to the position of the Abbey as a major landlord in the city of Florence.[16] Other major corporate debtors included the monastery of San Donato a Scopeto, with debts totalling over fourteen thousand soldi,[17] and the Guild of Shoemakers, with debts of over ten thousand soldi.[18] Although it is surprising to find a guild among the shop's leading debtors, since their assets were relatively limited, this was a consequence of the special relationship the apothecary had with this guild, of which he was a member. Although not coming close to these levels, certain private individuals were also able to obtain significant levels of credit. Antonio and Francesco di Giano, stocking-makers, had debts of over 4,600 soldi in May 1493.[19] During the sample year they were among the shop's biggest private clients, spending over eighty lire and making payment of only thirteen lire.[20] As we shall see, some of these major debtors were related to the shop's business activity, as in the case of Bartolomeo di Niccolò & Co., glassware-makers, with debts over four thousand soldi and who supplied the shops with drinking glasses.[21]

Only a small proportion of this debt consisted of cash loans. The apothecary did occasionally lend small amounts but these appear to be limited to personal favours, rather than something available to a wider clientele. During the sample year, around 3,512 soldi-worth of cash was distributed to a select group of eighteen clients (about three per cent of those active in the sample year).[22] Of these, more than half were from the immediate circle of shop staff – the apothecary himself, his immediate family, and various employees, all identified by the label 'nostro' in the accounts. So, for example, one of the apprentices took a florin 'to give to his mother'.[23] This group received most of the major advances from one florin upwards, accounting for around three quarters of the total.[24] The vast majority went to the apothecary himself and his eldest son Lorenzo, who accounted for over forty per cent of the total.[25] These should really be considered as 'income' rather than loans.

Very few other clients were ever lent cash, and then only for relatively small sums. One of the biggest borrowers was Maestro Giovanni, probably a merchant from Ragusa, who borrowed small sums of cash for various purposes: to redeem his cloak (probably from a pawnbroker),[26] to pay for the services of porters, as well as a florin as a 'loan'.[27] The recording of these details suggests that these were exceptional loans made as a personal favour (no interest was charged) and which needed to be justified by reference to specific circumstances. One client was given money to buy ingredients for his medicine elsewhere because the shop did not have them in stock, but this sort of cash advance was very unusual.[28] In another case where a customer bought artists' materials in a different shop, the use of cash was avoided by recording the payment as two debits, one to the customer's account at the Giglio and one to the Giglio's own account at the other shop.[29] In this way, the shop provided the credit facility, while the actual commodities came from elsewhere. Falling outside the sample period, by far the largest cash loan recorded was the fourteen florins paid by the apothecary to Guglielmo Altoviti on behalf of the painter Cosimo Rosselli in February 1492, probably for goods bought in bulk by Rosselli, a debt that was paid back a few months later.[30] By contrast, those who borrowed cash directly took only small amounts below one florin in value.[31] These include, for example, Mona Agnola di Sagramoro, who borrowed forty-five soldi, delivered to her by means of a local mercer,[32] or the barber Maestro Bartolomeo, who borrowed fifty soldi.[33] Overall, apart from a tiny proportion of clients who borrowed very small amounts, access to the cashbox was normally restricted to his immediate circle of shop staff. It is misleading to think of the apothecary as a sort of bank for petty loans.[34]

While on first sight the shop looks to be carrying a catastrophic amount of debt and making a loss, with the debts mounting each year, the credit offered by the shop was for goods that were mostly manufactured in the shop. Their retail prices were assigned nominal values by the apothecary, and they exceeded his costs in producing them. Without knowing more about production costs (rent, labour, fuel, taxes etc.), it is impossible to judge how profitable the shop was. However the available evidence suggests that labour costs in particular were insignificant compared to those of raw materials, and that profit margins could be very high, especially for medicines. This meant that the 'debt' carried by the shop was greatly inflated with respect to the actual amount of capital invested, something that may have been useful when protesting over taxation.

Most clients did not bother to discuss prices at the moment of transaction, and the apothecary therefore applied standard prices in the accounts that would be presented to the customer later. We know this because prices are generally uniform throughout the accounts; they do not usually vary in relation to the particular client or external factors such as the time of year (by contrast, the records of wholesale supplies show that the cost of raw materials could fluctuate considerably). The only variability was linked to the quantity of commodities sold, with discounts for substantial purchases in bulk. This contrasts strongly with the results of an analysis of a draper's shop retailing cloth in late fourteenth-century Pinerolo, where prices were personal and established through bargaining and by reference to the relationship between shopkeeper and client.[35] At the Giglio, prices were standard and very few clients sought to bargain with the apothecary at the moment of sale.[36] In contrast to costly sales of cloth, it was not normally worthwhile discussing the price for such a high number of low value transactions at the apothecary shop. Because the apothecary was carefully to record the 'agreed' price whenever this took place, it is possible to show that bargaining occurred in only one per cent of transactions during the sample year.[37] Many of these were poorer clients who had to pay on the spot, such as the carters mentioned above, [38] as when Falconiere the carter bought a single torch,[39] or when Mona Oretta bought a single purge.[40] People with credit rarely bothered to do this, with some exceptions for particularly valuable large transactions, as when other apothecaries bought commodities from the Giglio.[41] Interestingly, a number of married women haggled over prices, something which perhaps reflects their greater experience of marketplace practices and food shopping, in contrast to the more respectable premises of shops.[42] Lucrezia Mannini, a woman whose son was the account-holder, haggled with the apothecary over the price of theriac.[43] Bartolomea Gianfigliazzi, again the mother of a male account-holder, negotiated in the shop over the price of saffron and almonds.[44] The practices of the wholesale sector, where 'trade' prices were variable and always established through bargaining, and payment was made promptly and in full, stand in marked contrast to those of the retail sector, where prices were standardised and stable, and payment was delayed in time.

In the retail sector, prices were not normally discussed at the moment of sale – most clients did not haggle for each individual item. Perhaps to do so in the public environment of the shop would have damaged their reputation. Haggling over prices in the public environment of the shop was something considered unseemly by the patrician élite.[45] Apothecary goods were mostly low cost items, and only the very poorest clients were prepared to publicly display their concern about the cost of an individual julep, particularly if they were expected to pay for it up front. But this does not mean that bargaining did not take place – instead it was postponed to a later stage and regarded the settlement of the bill as a whole. The public space of the shop presented a façade where prices were equal for all, but clients received personal treatment when it came to determining how and when they would pay, something that took place behind the scenes as part of the private relationship between client and apothecary. Clients buying on credit generally did not bother to dispute the apothecary's prices at the moment of sale, for they could do so at a later stage.

These credit agreements were extremely loose and open. Key details such as the timing, extent and form of eventual payment were rarely specified up front. Instead, credit was granted, seemingly with no strings attached, and the details would only emerge as part of an evolving personal and credit relationship that allowed the debt to grow.[46] This can be seen even in an exceptional case where the apothecary took the trouble to establish terms at the moment of the sale. In September 1493, the carter Benedetto da San Donnino, after bargaining to establish the price of four lbs of costly azures at 360 soldi, agreed that he would pay back the debt within the next eight days. The subsequent record of payment shows that the apothecary might have been right to be wary of granting credit to such people, and also that such agreements had little force in practice as circumstances changed. Nearly a year later, Benedetto paid back two florins via a company of mercers, and he only settled the outstanding balance in February 1501, when he gave the apothecary six *staia* of millet worth a total of six lire.[47] The apothecary had been forced to wait nearly seven and a half years for final payment of a debt that was supposed to last only eight days.[48]

Interest was not charged on loans of cash or other commodities. When the apothecary lent twenty lbs of pepper to a customer for two and a half months, he was paid back in kind with no interest charged.[49] Nor was any interest applied to consumer debt. In the case of the carter Benedetto (see above), the apothecary obtained full repayment many years later, but normally he had to settle for less. This becomes clear if we compare payments and debts on a number of accounts that the apothecary struck through as 'settled'. The Spaniard Andrea di Parides obtained a discount of nineteen per cent on a debt of L1s11 that was over fifteen months old.[50] Similarly, Girolamo Niccoli obtained a discount of fourteen per cent on a debt of L2s6d8 that was over two years old.[51] In the case of a bigger debt, that of Simone Ginori for over eight lire, the discount was twenty-four per cent after a delay of more than nine years.[52] Giovanni di Messer Carlo Federighi, who had debts worth L18s12d6, settled these in a single payment of L14s10 around a year later, a discount of twenty-two per cent.[53] The miller Lionardo del Chiaro, whose debt was over six lire in May 1493, made payment of two lire in 1501, but only settled the debt in 1522 – in this case the discount was around fifteen per cent after nearly thirty years, long after Tommaso di Giovanni was dead.[54] It is possible that there are further payments not recorded in the accounts, as revealed in some cases by the 'reckoning' process (see below). This does not however detract from the strong evidence for the habitual discounting of debt: Luigi Calderini, who bought a single julep for eight soldi in August 1494, paid only six soldi five days later (a discount of twenty-five per cent), and this payment was specifically recorded as being for the julep.[55] Discounting was part of the process of negotiation over the payment of debts – on the one hand the apothecary offered discounts to encourage clients to settle, but on the other hand, clients obliged the apothecary to offer them discounts as a condition of payment. This appears to be the case with Benedetto degli Alessandri, where the apothecary specifically recorded that the client refused to pay the asking price for a delivery of sugar, obtaining a discount of fifteen per cent, 'because he did not want to give any more'.[56]

In a way, therefore, bargaining *did* take place at the shop, but it was mostly delayed in time and regarded the negotiation of payment, rather than the up-front price. The arithmetic principle of equal prices for all was applied at the moment of transaction, but geometrical principles were applied firstly at the level of access to credit and secondly in the negotiation of debt repayments.[57] Where credit was denied, as in the case of the clients lacking in wealth or connections, clients haggled over the up-front price at the moment of transaction; by contrast, where credit was available, bargaining took place at a later stage, at the moment of payment, and regarded the entire debt.[58] This was the contrary of the sort of market haggling that might have favoured the poor; rather, it was a form of occult negotiation that favoured the wealthy and the connected. The latter were able to obtain easy terms of credit, paying their debts years later, and with substantial discounts. For the shopkeeper, these were mostly steady clients who spent consistently, whose loyalty was worth buying by offering a discount, but there may have been other political and social advantages in offering credit to influential clients. As Weissman has argued, running a shop on debts was part of being an 'important man'. Business life was not autonomous, but was constrained by patronage and the need to maintain a network of contacts.[59]

The 'prices' stated in the books are nominal figures whose real value can only be understood in this context of delayed payment and negotiated reduction. It may be that the apothecary habitually exaggerated these prices so as to be able to make such discounts and remain profitable. As Molière put it in *The Imaginary Invalid*: 'twenty sous, in the language of apothecaries, means only ten sous'.[60] Studies of apothecary bills elsewhere have confirmed that bills were typically discounted at the moment of payment.[61] But the level of discount varied according to individual status and bargaining power – some clients paid in full, some obtained substantial discounts of around twenty per cent, and others failed to pay at all. Exaggerated nominal prices gave the apothecary a wide degree of flexibility in dealing with clients that was intimately bound up with personal relations. Behind the rigorous account-keeping of the ledgers lay a more human reality of flexible negotiation regarding the timing, extent and mode of payment.

A further aspect of this negotiation of debt repayment regarded the mode of payment. It was fairly common for payment to be made in kind, almost one third of the value of all payments.[62] Those who paid in kind obtained discounts of a different kind, by paying in a more convenient form, especially given the shortage of ready cash in the economy. It is inaccurate to regard this practice as 'barter', since such payments were characterised in most cases by their precise quantification of value in terms of money of account. Francesco Castellani for example records a number of payments to the apothecaries at the *Palla*, in several different forms: coins of various types (each precisely evaluated), barrels of oil and especially grain, all of it precisely quantified.[63] Only occasionally do we find transactions that explicitly go outside a commercial logic of precise quantification. When Bernardo di Piero del Palagio gave the apothecary two bushels of charcoal, the accounts specifically recorded that this was a gift, and no price was set in the accounts.[64]

Agricultural commodities such as grain, oil, firewood and wine were particularly important as a means of payment – this reflected the land ownership diffuse among Florentine society, and was particularly important for some of the big religious institutions. The Cistercians at Settimo and Cestello, with their large estates, paid the apothecary with grain and oil as well as with cash.[65] These sorts of products could be fairly easily redistributed among the apothecary's own immediate family circle and also circulated more generally in the economy, behaving to some extent as an alternative form of currency. When Giovanni Lapi made payment in the form of twelve *staia* of grain, this was delivered to the country villa of the apothecary's son-in-law Lapo Lapini, and debited to his account.[66]

Similarly, craftsmen were able to pay in the form of clothing and shoes that were then distributed among the apothecary and his immediate circle. We learn a great deal about how the apothecary, his family and employees were dressed, since many clients paid in the form of clothing, such as black woollen stockings,[67] or fur trimmings for a cloak.[68] Agnolo and Domenico di Paolo, shoemakers at the sign of the Fig, paid for their purchases of medicines, wax and pitch in the form of shoes, which the apothecary then used to pay his employees.[69] The stocking-maker Carlo di Bartolomeo paid his bill in the form of stockings that were distributed to both the apothecary himself and to his son Marco, and duly recorded in their separate accounts.[70] Similarly, the stocking-maker Cristofano di Paradiso paid his debts in the form of stockings that were in turn given to the apothecary's factor, Girolamo della Barba, and debited to his account.[71] In this same way Girolamo also received some wool cloth from a retailer,[72] and a doublet from a doublet-maker.[73] These sorts of goods were not normally circulated to the clientele in general, which would have transformed the shop into a general store, but only to the 'inner circle' of relatives, employees and business associates of the apothecary. Just as the contents of the cashbox were generally distributed among the shop staff, so the commodities received as payment in kind were distributed to the same close group of people. The circulation of such goods as forms of payment was not allowed to interfere with the identity of the shop as an apothecary business or intrude upon the circuit of retail.

The apothecary also accepted commodities that were directly related to the shop's production, as when a blacksmith settled his debt with fifty-three lbs of roses.[74] Particino Particini paid in the form of wood, which was probably burned in the shop's stove.[75] One client supplied a great deal of pine-nuts and almonds to the shop – he might have obtained these from his own lands or through trade.[76] The charcoal-burner Antonio di Lionardo made payment in the form of charcoal,[77] and the gold-beater Bernardo in the form of *oro di metà*, an inferior variety of gold.[78] Artisans might also pay in the form of work, as in the case of the engraver Cervagio Del Tasso, who carried out work on the shop's furnishings and fittings, including the desk, window frames and money box.[79] Similarly, the painter Giovanni di Chimenti Rosselli, nephew of the more famous Cosimo Rosselli, paid some of his old debts by painting panels for the apothecary (it is not clear whether these were in the shop or in the house).[80] A couple of builders also paid their debts in the form of labour.[81] The carpenter Matteo Bardelli made payments in the form of materials to repair a garden gate.[82]

Anyone could make payment in kind. So, for example, the *ossaio* Santi di Monte (probably a carver of ivory), paid his debts with a variety of different goods, including a 'courtesan's torch', some azure enamel of 'Jesus' quality, and three pairs of spectacles.[83] He had probably received these goods from his own clients as pledges or as payment. However, in practice, the facility of paying in kind worked to the advantage of a select group of habitual clients who regularly supplied goods that the apothecary needed. This was the case with Antonio and Francesco di Giano, a firm of stocking-makers who were among the Giglio's biggest clients. The high level of credit they enjoyed,[84] was probably related to the role they had established as suppliers of stockings to the apothecary and his family, paying their bills in kind.[85] This once more underlines the importance of long-term personal and business relationships in the retail trade: certain clients were able to benefit from privileged channels of exchange, paying with their own produce, manufactures or work, rather than having to obtain cash. Free of the need to pay with hard cash, they were able to consume more freely and enjoy a higher level of credit.

Rather than paying interest on the sum, long-term debtors were therefore able to obtain further discounts when negotiating the payment of their debts, with regard to the timing, level and mode of payment. The outcome of such negotiations was a function of the personal and business relations established between the parties over time. When the apothecary struck an account through as 'settled', this does not necessarily imply payment in full. Obtaining repayment of debt meant negotiation and compromise, but this was preferable to obtaining nothing at all. We have also suggested that some of the imbalance between receipts and 'sales' can be explained in terms of the inflated nominal prices that gave the apothecary room to manoeuvre in negotiating the terms of payment.

An alternative way of looking at the problem of debt is therefore to shift the focus from the imbalance of receipts and sales to look instead at how 'satisfied' the apothecary was in order to determine how many of those debts were actually 'bad'. This can be done by estimating the total value of the debt held in all customer accounts that are marked as 'settled'. This reveals a far more positive picture. Focusing first on the 'active clients' who consumed goods during the sample year, the vast majority (eighty-six per cent) of this debt was eventually struck through as 'settled' by circa 1504, even if it was not necessarily paid promptly or in full.[86] For example, the Badia of Florence, the shop's biggest debtor, eventually settled its account. However, if we extend this to include all the old debt registered in the accounts up to and including the sample period, then the figures are less promising: forty-two per cent of this debt was held in accounts that were never settled.[87] Particularly prominent bad debts include those of the monastery of San Donato a Scopeto and the Guild of Shoemakers, two of the biggest corporate debtors (see above), neither of which were active in the sample year aside from some small payments.[88] This suggests that while most of the shop's active clients did eventually settle their accounts, the shop had built up many bad debts over time, some of which would never be resolved.

Some of the debts that remained unpaid at the end of the 1490s were over thirty years old. The oldest recorded debts dated back as far as 1465, shortly after the shop began trading and were therefore probably its first customers, people like the baker Piero di Nardo, who owed over 1,200 soldi,[89] or the more modest debts of the painter Antonio di Tommaso, who owed just over sixty soldi.[90] While it was unlikely that these would ever be paid off, some clients did eventually do so, particularly when setting their affairs in order before death. Andrea da Monte Fiesole, for example, whose debts dated back at least as far as 1481, paid these off in full in 1503.[91] Some of these clients with old unpaid debts were even able to enjoy continued credit at the shop. Antonio d'Agnolo da San Casciano, whose debts dated back to at least 1483, was able to obtain a further extension of credit in 1497, when he bought two ounces of aniseed and coriander, despite not having been a regular client of the shop for years.[92] Nor is there any evidence that Agnolo subsequently paid these debts. Accounts remained open and debts were only written off altogether 'for the love of God' as a last resort, usually limited to poor monks, especially Franciscans.[93] Such cases of charitable debt relief included the monastery of San Francesco at San Miniato.[94] In most cases, the old debts stayed on the books, to be inherited by the apothecary's son-in-law and subsequently by the foundling hospital of the Innocenti, a bequest of book debt that was mostly so old as to be 'hopeless'.

In the face of persistent failure to pay, the apothecary had a number of options before embarking on legal action. Although sometimes the apothecary sent his apprentices to collect money from debtors, as from the papal mace-bearer Maestro Jacopo,[95] the extent of the debt and the number of clients involved also made it worthwhile for him to employ a *riscotitore* (debt-collector) called Ugenio di Tommaso Fiaschi. One of the short stories written by the Lucchese apothecary Giovanni Sercambi at the end of the fourteenth century describes an apothecary who employs a servant full-time to go around collecting debts.[96] Clients are often recorded as paying money or goods directly to Fiaschi, presumably as he made his rounds of shop debtors.[97] In March 1496, for example, the client Bernardo Ridolfi paid an ounce and a half of saffron to Fiaschi, an indication that he lacked ready cash.[98] These were recorded in Fiaschi's account as debts that he owed to the shop, in effect transferring the debts to Fiaschi for a further period, rather than immediately returning them to the apothecary.[99] Fiaschi was paid two soldi per day worked and a five per cent cut of all debts recovered,[100] and the accounts show that across a period of just over four years he was paid a salary of nearly twenty-one lire.[101] That was not much – only about a hundred soldi per year, which suggests that Fiaschi was probably not a 'professional' debt-collector, but rather someone who collected debts on a casual basis, rounding out his income through occasional work (though he may have worked for others as well). He was, in fact, a man of independent means and moderate wealth, rather than a servant – according to his tax entry of 1480, his net value was over 418 florins (more than twice that of Tommaso di Giovanni at 168 florins).[102] He was even elected Prior in 1496, although ineligible because due to being already a member of the Great Council.[103] The shop also employed a second debt-collector called Bardo di Taddeo,[104] whose services were paid for mostly in the form of red wine.[105] He was far less active than Fiaschi – in the sample period, he collected money only from the client Bernardo Vermigli, which was paid on his behalf by the silk manufacturer Ruberto Cavalcanti.[106] In both cases, the shop's debt collectors appear to have worked on an informal and personal basis, rather than as professionals.

The application of pressure from debt collectors did not necessarily imply that clients were denied credit. This can be seen with Bartolomeo di Tommaso and his brothers, described as wool manufacturers at San Martino,[107] whose debts dated back at least as far as January 1486.[108] In 1494 they continued to consume products at the shop, particularly for

Bartolomeo's sick daughter, and they did so intermittently all the way up to April 1497.[109] During the same period, the shop used Fiaschi to collect its debts, and the account records a number of payments made to him – one florin in September 1494, another florin in June 1495, five and a half *braccia* of purple woollen cloth in 1495, and nearly five ounces of cochineal in 1497.[110] Like other clients who had difficulties paying, they paid a little at a time, and often in kind. The fact that Fiaschi was calling on them while making his rounds did not preclude them from having continued access to shop credit. Rather, they may have reached a credit ceiling where further consumption was linked to making regular payments. The apothecary was not necessarily interested in closing accounts definitively and terminating relations with his clients, but rather in obtaining some concrete sign that he would be repaid in the future. (In this case, despite receiving some payments, the account was never struck through and the debts were left unpaid.)

A key procedure in the negotiation of debt was the *saldo*, a reckoning whereby the client and apothecary together examined their accounts and reached an agreement as to the extant value of the debt. Probably as a result of the fact that credits attributed to customers in accounts carried far more legal weight than debts, the apothecary was much less careful about recording payments than he was about recording debt. Pierfrancesco Guidi had to remind the apothecary about the rhubarb he had supplied him.[111] Similarly, the account of Cosimo Rosselli contains corrections suggesting that his payments were not always rigorously recorded.[112] A reckoning was an opportunity for both sides to compare their records and to calculate the remaining balance.

The reckoning process places shop debt in a wider context of personal and business transactions existing between the apothecary and his clients. The case of Cosimo Rosselli is particularly revealing and demonstrates how payments made by clients often went unrecorded. A reckoning of 27 September 1493 found that Cosimo Rosselli owed the sum of just over three lire.[113] Subsequently, Rosselli bought sweets, medications and wax, at times paying his bill with cash, at times borrowing money from the apothecary, mostly remaining in credit.[114] On top of this, Rosselli must have made payments to the apothecary in ways that are not recorded in the accounts, because a reckoning that took place two years later found that the shop now owed him a total of nine florins.[115] His account reveals a close business relationship, in which exchanges of raw materials, cash and favours were offset against his consumption of apothecary stuff. These complex transactions were disentangled and clarified through the periodic reckonings. When one of the shop's biggest debtors, Giuliano di Giovanni Marucelli, 'reckoned' his debt in 1495, this involved offsetting the debt against other credits that are not recorded in the apothecary's accounts, reducing it from over 344 lire to 215 lire.[116] This evidence suggests that the payments recorded in the account books were only part of the story, and that the imbalance that we have noted between the shop's book debt and payments received is significantly exaggerated by the apothecary's failure to rigorously record the income he did receive.

In a number of cases the agreements following a reckoning were actually signed by clients in the account book, giving them additional legal backing. So, for example, the accounts of Pierfrancesco Guidi, which list old debts of nearly sixty lire in 1492, and subsequently a number of payments in 1497 and 1499, in the form of rhubarb and red wine, also contain a written agreement that was reached with his brother Antonio in 1501.[117] Although the debts and credits recorded in the Giglio accounts suggest that the remainder of the debt was over thirty lire, the reckoning found the debt to be only fourteen lire, and his brother then signed the register to certify this agreement. These 'reckoned' debts were therefore more valuable in legal and financial terms, since their precise extent had been agreed by both parties, and usually signed by the debtor, and the apothecary was careful to identify them as such in his accounts.[118]

Nevertheless, a reckoning was no guarantee that payment would be prompt or that it would be made in full. Although Giuliano Marucelli (see above) promptly paid a hundred lire a couple of days after the reckoning of January 1495, his repayments subsequently slowed down and by the end of the year he had paid back only 184 lire 2 soldi.[119] Since his account was then struck through and the debt regarded as settled he was able to obtain a discount of nearly fifteen per cent by delaying repayment. In other cases, the account was reckoned but the debt remained unsettled with no further payments recorded. Antonio, innkeeper at Le Falle (in the Arno valley to the east of Florence), had old debts of around twenty-five lire, and his representative reached an agreement with the apothecary in 1493 by which the debt was reckoned at nineteen lire.[120] However, no payment was ever recorded and the debt remained unsettled. In the case of Ristoro di Piero and company, mercers, the accounts list an old debt of July 1481, valued at over eighteen lire.[121] A reckoning of 1487 reduced the debt to only twelve and a half lire, but there is no record of payment and the account was never settled.[122]

This problem could be countered in part by establishing terms of payment at the moment of the reckoning. A number of clients promised to settle the debt by a given date. In June 1496, Guido del Palagio, who had debts of around nine lire, met with the apothecary to go through the accounts and they reckoned the debt at seven and a half lire, which he promised to pay in full by the end of July.[123] Guido signed the book with his own hand to authenticate the contract, and the debt was subsequently struck through, suggesting that he kept to his word. Similarly Matteo Pollaiuolo, with debts of a little over three lire, agreed in August 1496 to pay the remainder of his debt, now rounded down to three lire, by the end of October.[124] The register shows that he subsequently paid back one lire on 19 November 1496, and this late and partial payment was only followed by a final unquantified payment around a year and a half later.[125] Although payment was late, his account was regarded as settled.

The apothecary usually reached settlements with clients who were unwilling or unable to pay, but this was a long process that might last many years. A further means of encouraging recalcitrant debtors to settle was to initiate legal action, for which the accounts contain evidence because the associated costs were added to a customer's debt. This involved only a tiny minority of clients (about one per cent), indicating that informal techniques were considered adequate in most cases.[126] Nevertheless, the sample suggests that this involved him in approximately five or six plaints per year. This evidence permits us to sketch in the legal options that were available to the apothecary – what size of debts were worth pursuing in court, which courts he used, how expensive it was, and what sort of results he could hope to obtain. For this he used three alternative courts: the Podestà, the tribunal of the apothecaries' guild and the Mercanzia.

The court of the Podestà was the cheapest option, incurring costs from around ten soldi for the very lowest claims and up to about thirty soldi, roughly in proportion to the size of the claim. The apothecary tended to use this court for particularly small debts in the range from fifty to a hundred soldi. Although this justice was cheap, this sort of litigation was not particularly economical since the costs were actually fairly high relative to the size of the debt. The opponent was usually liable to repay all associated legal costs if the sentence went in favour of the apothecary, but even following a sentence obtaining payment was not necessarily guaranteed. The Podestà, in particular, does not appear to have been particularly effective, since few of these actions resulted in a recorded payment – although this may be a problem of poor record-keeping. In the worst case the apothecary spent twenty-two soldi in an attempt to claim back only sixty-three soldi, and, although these costs were added to the claim, there is no evidence that the sentence led to payment.[127] What such cases demonstrate is that the apothecary was prepared to contemplate legal action even in the case of very small debts, and the threat of such action may itself have been an effective means of encouraging clients to settle. Litigation was not reserved solely for the biggest debtors but was based on the apothecary's valuation of his prospects of payment in each individual case.

Costs at the Guild and the Mercanzia were higher, typically around thirty to forty soldi, but were increasingly cost-effective in proportion to the size of claims. The apothecary used the Guild for claims from around a hundred soldi upwards, and the Mercanzia for claims from around 250 soldi upwards, limiting this sort of litigation to clients who had larger debts than average (see Chapter 3). In both cases, his biggest claims were around two thousand soldi. As far as this limited sample is able to suggest, actions at these courts tended to be more likely to result in repayment. The account of Bartolomeo D'Ambra gives a detailed breakdown of the kind of costs and times involved. He spent heavily during the sample year, mostly for his son's sickness and subsequent funeral,[128] along with debts from previous years, so that his total debt amounted to almost fifty-seven lire at the end of February 1494.[129] The account lists the stages of the legal process at the Mercanzia: L1s7 paid in October 1495 to the notary in order to register the lawsuit.[130] Further sums were paid when the shop accounts were presented in court in November 'to approve the book'.[131] A fee was then paid to hear sentence in December 1495.[132] This case progressed from plaint to sentence in just forty days, with costs of just over two lire, about four per cent of the value of the claim.[133] Other evidence confirms that obtaining a sentence at the Mercanzia was fairly swift, for example a plaint against Giovanni Sogliani, registered on 6 June 1494 resulted in a summons delivered on 14 June 1494 and was followed by a sentence on 17 June 1494. The costs in this case – a claim for 260 soldi – amounted to just over thirty soldi.[134]

Legal costs were scaled to the size of the claim, so one way of cutting costs for the biggest debts was to make claims for part payment. When the debt was around two thousand soldi or more, the apothecary tended to make claims for fifty lire – ie. a thousand soldi – as part payment. This was a cheap means of establishing the merit of the lawsuit, encouraging debtors to settle.[135] The main drawback was that this might potentially involve the apothecary in further litigation if the defendant subsequently contested the extent of the debt as well. This happened in the case of the most valuable debt for which the apothecary sued, the case of Alessandro di Paolo Federighi, from a high-status patrician family based in the Lion Rosso district of Santa Maria Novella.[136] His total debt at the shop in 1492 was around 2,500 soldi.[137] In October 1496, the apothecary recorded costs of fifty soldi at the Guild incurred obtaining a sentence against Alessandro's heirs for the sum of a thousand soldi, which was specifically as 'part payment' of a bigger debt, to which legal costs would also be added.[138] Since there were many other members of the Federighi family who were important clients of the shop, part of the motive here may have been to try to broker a solution. However, the Federighi family continued to contest the extent of the debt, and in January 1499, the apothecary recorded further costs incurred in having Guild experts evaluate the debt, which they established was almost four thousand soldi.[139] The debtor was liable for all these associated costs. On the same day, the accounts record a payment of just over two hundred soldi by the heirs to the apothecary for the cost of paying the *taratori* (the Guild evaluators).[140] Again, it must have helped Tommaso di Giovanni that, although not himself a member of the Guild of Apothecaries, many of his clients held influential positions in the Guild – for example, the evaluator in one of these cases was the Giglio client Benedetto Rigogli.[141] His personal and business contacts must have given him access to the sort of professional solidarity enjoyed by members of the guild.

Even a favourable sentence did not always lead to repayment. What typically happened was a pattern of further delays and partial payment that the apothecary was generally obliged to accept as better than nothing at all. In December 1493, the apothecary sued Goro Viviani at the Guild for debts of around 320 soldi, obtaining a sentence in his favour, but at a cost of thirty-three soldi.[142] Although, in theory, Viviani was now liable for these costs, the apothecary was obliged to pay them up front, and repayment was not guaranteed. Viviani paid fifty-six soldi in two payments to Ugenio Fiaschi in 1494 and 1495,[143] but these repayments amounted to little more than the costs and made little impact on the overall debt. This was never settled, remaining at nearly 300 soldi.[144] The painter Bernardo Rosselli,[145] who had debts of nearly five lire in February 1494,[146] for which proceedings were commenced at the Guild,[147] made some initial signs of paying,[148] but only settled his outstanding bill in 1520.[149] Another client, Giovanni de' Ricci, had debts of nearly twenty-five lire in 1490.[150] The apothecary commenced an action against him at the Mercanzia court in 1493.[151] This had little immediate effect, and Giovanni only began to pay back his debt several years later, with instalments in 1499 and 1511.[152] In this case, the total repayment amounted to about two thirds of the total debt and costs, and his account was struck through as 'settled'. Similarly, following legal action, Agostino di Pippo promised to pay his family's old debts, which dated back at least as far as 1484, by the end of September 1496.[153] But by March 1500, Agostino had paid only one and a half lire, and the debt remained on the books.[154] In cases like this, the debt was so small (four lire), that concerted legal action was difficult to contemplate, since even the cost of registering a plaint amounted to six per cent of the value. Even though justice was fairly cheap and efficient, it was not necessarily effective, and the practical difficulties of obtaining payment meant that the apothecary was often willing to accept further delays.

The evidence suggests that the apothecary preferred to work towards negotiated settlements of debt, rather than invoke the formal machinery of enforcement. Nevertheless, on occasion, the accounts record payment to a *toccatore*, a court official whose job it was to 'touch' the debtor, that is, to inform them of the final deadline for payment of debts that had been legally established. This was an essential stage prior to initiating enforcement procedures, such as the sequestration of property or goods, or imprisonment in the *stinche* (debtors' prison).[155] In the case of Francesco di Andrea Zati, who had debts of over two thousand soldi, part inherited from his father, towards which he had been making a number of the poorly documented payments of grain, the apothecary obtained a sentence for part payment at the Mercanzia in June 1497,[156] and subsequently paid sixteen soldi to 'touch' the debtor in February 1498.[157] (It is unclear if this was effective, since the debt remained unresolved.) Similarly, the apothecary successfully sued Andrea di Carlo, *galigaio* (a maker and repairer of shoes) for a debt of nearly ten lire at the Podestà,[158] and again he had to pay a *toccatore* to commence enforcement proceedings.[159] In the case of Girolamo d'Antonio, *gualcheraio* (fuller), with debts of over fifty-four lire, following a Mercanzia sentence of September 1498 against his heirs, a *tenuta* (occupation of property) was carried out, which finally encouraged them to settle the debt by making payment in the form of fourteen *braccia* of wool cloth, washed, sheared and dyed. The register notes how this payment was accepted on the express conditions that the debtors would not contest the extent of the apothecary's claim against them, an important condition since the original sentence was for part payment, and as we have seen, the values in the accounts were typically inflated.[160] Valued at sixty-three lire, this payment was sufficient to cover the entire value of the debt and the costs (L3s17 for the Mercanzia sentence and L5s10 for the *tenuta*).[161] This was paid on their behalf by a firm of wool-manufacturers, showing how clients who lacked ready cash could nevertheless arrange payments by transferring the debt elsewhere.[162] Whether this was possible would depend on their credit and personal relations with third parties prepared to take on the debt.

The difficulty of obtaining payment is well illustrated by a dispute with the heirs of Agnolo di Jacopo Tani. The bulk of the debt was inherited from their father, but also included a purchases of medicines in late 1493. The Giglio accounts record a total debt of almost 1,225 soldi, but following evaluation by the Guild *taratori* in May 1495, this was reduced to around 957 soldi, a discount of twenty-two per cent. This corresponds closely to the sort of discounts that clients were typically able to obtain when negotiating a settlement (as previously discussed), and further suggests that the prices recorded in the accounts were inflated.[163] The fee of nearly eighteen soldi paid by the apothecary to the Guild evaluators was also added to the debt.[164] Two years later, in May 1497, the apothecary obtained a sentence at the Mercanzia, which awarded him only two thirds of the outstanding amount (640 soldi), probably due to competing claims on the inheritance. Obtaining the sentence incurred further costs of almost seventy-four soldi, which were also added to the debt.[165] However, the continued refusal of the heirs to pay obliged the apothecary to pay much more to execute the sentence – he paid over 437 soldi to the Mercanzia for its 'military arm' to sequester the debtors' property by force.[166] This, at last, had the desired effect – the accounts subsequently record payment of eight florins in four instalments between February and July 1498.[167] In this case, although the total payment (1,072 soldi) exceeded the value of the debt as determined by the Guild evaluators (957 soldi), it failed to cover the legal costs (amounting to 529 soldi) that the apothecary had paid up front. The instalments ceased after July 1498, with the account still not regarded as 'settled', but no further legal action is recorded.

Despite the apparent differences produced by the shift into the public arena, litigation shared much in common with arbitration. The legal process must be considered parallel to the more informal process of private negotiation to reach a settlement. A legal sentence that confirmed the debt juridically was just one more instrument in this process of negotiation, bringing additional pressure to bear on debtors. Sentences were relatively cheap and could be quickly obtained, yet in themselves they were of limited effectiveness. They would have aided bargaining principally as a threat of further action. Executing a sentence was far more expensive, and could only really be effective if both the debt was substantial and the debtor had assets that could be constrained. For debtors with property, goods or financial assets, these could be seized and held until payment was forthcoming, or sold. Debtors could be constrained in the *stinche* until they or others settled the debt. But for poor debtors, who lacked either assets or anyone willing to pay on their behalf, there was little to be gained from having them thrown into the debtors' prison. Once imprisoned, they would be even less likely to pay the debt, since they would be unable to work and would face additional costs to cover their stay in prison. If clients were bankrupt, then competing claims on their assets might further reduce what the apothecary might expect to recover. As a result, although the costs of obtaining and executing sentences could theoretically be recovered, the apothecary had to pay them up front with no guarantee that this would happen. As we have seen, there is little evidence that, in practice, litigation led to recovery of the full value of the debt, let alone the legal costs. These factors therefore meant that although the apothecary made use of legal process, he usually did so as part of an attempt to find a negotiated solution, rather than to enforce the rigour of the law.

Conclusion

In this chapter the authors have examined whether, how and when customers paid for their purchases. In doing so it has been emphasised that the retail market was not a purely 'economic' sphere of impersonal transactions. It was deeply embedded in interpersonal relationships. The public face of the shop was that arithmetic principles governed the retail market, with fixed prices applied to all clients without regard to person. Bargaining was restricted to a small minority of clients who lacked credit and were therefore obliged to pay cash up front, people like Falconiere the carter. But in reality, this only postponed the negotiation process to a later moment – the time when debts were settled. Rather than negotiate each transaction at the moment of sale, in the apothecary sector, negotiation regarded the debt as a whole, and it was not restricted to simply the price of goods but might also involve the timing, extent and mode of payment. These practices contrast strongly with the wholesale sector, where prices were variable and had to be negotiated for every transaction, and transfer of goods was usually followed by prompt and full payment. In the retail sector, some clients paid years after the debt was incurred, sometimes long after the apothecary and the principal debtor had died; some clients made payment conditional on their obtaining substantial discounts; some paid the apothecary in the forms of goods, labour or other services; some never paid at all, or made only insignificant payments, and their accounts were never 'settled'. Behind the public façade of equal prices for all was an occult reality of personal terms regarding the payment of that debt, mediated via the sorts of personal factors examined in the previous chapter. Certain kinds of clients, in particular those producing goods or services regularly required by the apothecary, such as stockings or glassware, were able to establish privileged channels of exchange with the shop and obtain unusually high levels of credit. The practices of shopping in the Renaissance can only be properly understood in relation to the practices of consumer credit prevailing in each specific sector. It appears that retail credit was particularly important in the case of apothecary goods, where demand was characterised by irregular surges. Similar patterns can also be found in other trades in the medical sector, such as doctors, surgeons and barbers.[168]

From the point of view of the business, the situation at first sight appears disastrous, with outgoing sales of goods far exceeding incoming payments, and a huge volume of old debt that would never be wholly reclaimed. Examined more closely, it is apparent that the volume of debt recorded in the books was much higher than the capital invested – the apothecary did not normally lend cash, but sold manufactured goods whose recorded prices were nominal values that included a significant profit margin. These asking prices were inflated so as to establish a starting point for negotiation, so giving the apothecary sufficient manoeuvring space to offer discounts in return for payment. Furthermore, evidence from the reckoning process suggests that clients paid more than is apparent from these accounts. Particular care must be applied when examining the record – payments from clients were not rigorously recorded (because to do so was to give them legal confirmation), and accounting practices therefore exaggerate the imbalance. These contrasts in accounting practices correspond to the two different faces of the shop noted above. The rigorous recording of debt, like the public façade of standard prices, can be contrasted to the more *ad hoc* recording of payment, reflecting a more occult and human world of negotiation.

Despite the apparently huge volume of debt, most of the shop's clients only obtained petty credit. Just as consumption in the sample year was strongly polarised, with a small 'tail' of clients accounting for the vast bulk of sales, so too the shop's debt was strongly polarised, with most of it concentrated in the hands of a minority of clients. The shop's biggest debtors were corporate institutions like the Badia, or the Guild of Shoemakers. Only a minority of private clients were able to run up anything approaching this level of debt. Such relations may have been useful to the apothecary in other ways – his position in negotiating the terms of repayment might involve assessment of a number of personal factors outside a purely commercial logic. Debt created ties of obligation with powerful patrons that might prove advantageous; conversely, it might be particularly difficult to oblige the powerful to pay their debts. Most of the shop's active clients eventually settled their debts in some way that was satisfactory for the apothecary, but there were always some who failed to pay. Over time, a sizeable number of 'bad' debts accumulated on the books, to be inherited by subsequent owners of the shop and eventually by the Ospedale degli Innocenti.

In practice, the apothecary appears to have accepted this level of risk. There were a number of mechanisms available to help resolve disputes, certify debts and encourage payment, including, for example, the employment of debt collectors, the periodic reckoning of accounts, the signing of the accounts by debtors, oral and written agreements to pay in instalments, obtaining sentences at various tribunals, and, as a last resort, the execution of sentences – involving the constraints of debtors' property and person. In most of these cases, the apothecary appears to have used these methods not with the intention of terminating the relationship by constraining debtors to make full repayment but to reach a negotiated settlement that would allow the relationship to continue, only on a more solid basis of legally certified debt.[169] The apothecary recognised the difficulty that clients could have in paying the entire balance at once in a form acceptable to him, and preferred to set up schedules of repayment that managed the debt over time. In some cases it appears that such clients had reaching a ceiling on the amount of credit that the apothecary was prepared to offer without further certification. Rather than claiming the full amount of debts, and so calling their precise extent into question (something which might expose his own inflation of prices), he preferred to make claims for part payment, potentially allowing the debt to continue to grow but on a more solid legal basis. The cost of such a strategy was that some debts might become 'bad', but this was a risk associated with doing business on credit in this way. In any case, debts were never truly 'hopeless' (and were only written off altogether in special charitable circumstances), because even years later, it was still possible that people could pay.

Importantly, most of this discussion over credit has concerned the retail side of the Giglio's business where, as we have seen, prices were not normally negotiated at the moment of sale, but were standard values, applied to all customers alike. In the wholesale side of its operation, supply networks were partly commercialised and mediated by professional brokers, but remained dependent to a significant extent on *ad hoc* opportunities that arose primarily through personal connections. Apothecaries were able to purchase large quantities of stock as they became available, far in excess of their own needs, knowing that they could easily dispose of the surplus to other businesses (apothecary shops, hospitals and other trades), both within the city and in the wider regional state and importantly, rely on almost immediate payment. Similarly, they could make up any shortfall in supply by exploiting their contacts with other distributors.

These features of the wholesale trade show how important it was for the business to be integrated into a densely knit network of operators. This also permitted apothecaries to specialise to some extent, as the Giglio appears to have done in loaning funeral equipment. The possibility of specialisation raises questions about whether one shop can be representative of the whole market sector, but also shows how each shop did not stand alone, but was part of a broader network. In Florence, to participate in this network it was less important to be formally enrolled in the apothecaries' guild than it was to be well connected to other operators in the sector. Guild restrictions (such as the prohibition of trading on feast days, or limits on the recycling of wax products), were probably of very limited effectiveness against those who had the right connections.

Retailing was a different world, with its greater range of products and particular trading practices, most strikingly the provision of credit. The credit practices so dominant in this sector were a function of the highly variable nature of demand. Customers might buy nothing at all for long periods, and then spend intensely in short bursts of consumption in response to their specific needs. Although this applied to apothecary goods in general, it varied according to the nature of the commodities in question. By contrast, in the wholesale sector, prices were always negotiated at the moment of sale and therefore responsive to short-term market fluctuations. Here, the Giglio records show that payment was prompt (usually within one month) and almost always in full. The breaking open of bales and barrels transferred business to a different world. Moving on to examine the actual goods that were sold will require having to look at all these facets of the complex business of supplying the city with the goods its citizens needed.

Notes

1. E882, fo. 289v, 'Falchoniere di [BLANK] vetturale' 29 March 1493, s6d8 'dachordo' for a *falchola* of no specified weight (the apothecary did not bother to record this, because the taper was already paid for). Within the sample period there are *four* separate accounts in his name, see ff. 289v, 312r, 318r, 322r.

2. E882, fo. 31v, 'Jachopo di Vitale Vetturale', 26 July 1493, payment of 1 florin worth L6s10. He came to the shop every 3–4 days, making 14 visits across a period of 47 days from 27 July 1493 to 11 September 1493. Total spending across this period was s114.67, or s2.44 per day.

3. E882, fo. 291r, 'Domenicho dant.o detto montanello vetturale', 13 August 1494, s8d4 for a purge.

4. E882, fo. 291r, 18 August 1485.

5. E882, fo. 291r, 1 September 1494.

6. A minority of accounts (around 80) were closed simply with the formula 'Paid. Put in the cashbox' or occasionally just 'Paid', with no details of when, how much or in what form. For the purposes of estimating total payments to the shop, we have assumed that debts were paid in full in these cases. While the method is inaccurate, these were mostly petty debts and any error will therefore be insignificant. Assuming that all of these clients paid in full, the maximum amount they paid to the shop during the sample year was 1,193 soldi, not enough to make a significant impact on the total payment figures. The apothecary paid little attention to recording payments carefully in these cases because the debts were small and short-lived. For example, E882, fo. 352r, 'ser Franc.o di luigi di giovanni di messer stefano buonachorsi', with a debt of 67 soldi, the account was only open for a period of 22 days.

7. The total of all debt dated up to the end of the sample period, plus undated debt, was 627,735 soldi. From this we have subtracted the 137,924 soldi that was owed by the apothecary and his immediate circle of family and dependants, leaving a total of 489,811 soldi.

8. See also I. Naso, *Una bottega di panni alla fine del trecento: Giovanni Canale di Pinerolo e il suo libro di conti* (Genoa: Università di Genova, 1985), 58.

9. 123,901 soldi was owed by Tommaso alone. This accounted for 90% of the 137,924 soldi owed by shop staff.

10. E882, fo. 116r, 16 October 1493, purchase of spices 'per mandare in villa'.

11. E882, fo. 331v. 'Antonio diachopo nostro gharzone pestatore'. Like other shop employees, he was paid partly in goods supplied from the shop,

including 'spezie fine', perfumed soap, comfits, pennets, honey, pepper and
treggiea.

12. E882, fo. 34v, 'Fratti e monaci della badia di firenze', 14 May 1493, 1161
lire.

13. E882, ff. 34v, 79v, 220v, 257v, 309r, 329r, 342v, 350r, 'Frati e monaci della
badia di firenze', total spending of 5525 soldi in sample year.

14. E882, fo. 34v, 3 August 1493, for the only payment made by the Badia
during the sample year (10 florins). See also fo. 183r, 'Giovanni di [BLANK]
daruota sta al monte', 13 November 1495, L3s3, 'per lui dala badia di firenze
recho bastiano n.o sono per le partite della ciera'.

15. E882, fo. 350r, 27 January 1494 (m.f.), gives a total debt of L1372 s14 d10
at this date.

16. G. Bertoli, 'Librai, cartolai e ambulanti immatricolati nell'arte dei medici e
speziali di Firenze dal 1490-1600. Parte 1', *Bibliofilia*, 94, 2 (1992), 125–64:
132, for shops owned by the Badia. (The Badia does not appear to have
owned the site of the Giglio, since there is no mention of this in the
apothecary's tax declaration of 1480.)

17. E882, fo. 179r, 'Fratti e chonvento di san donato aschopeto', 8 May 1493,
11 June 1481.

18. E882, fo. 30r, 'Larte de chalzolai', 1 May 1491.

19. E882, fo. 44v, 'Antonio e franc.o di giano chalzaiuoli', 25 May 1493, debts
of L230s8d3.

20. E882, fo. 307r, 15 April 1494; fo. 326v, 7 June 1494.

21. E882, ff. 144v, 234v, 'Bartolomeo di niccholaio di ghino e chonpangni
bichierai'.

22. 18 out of 515 clients.

23. E882, fo. 131r, 'Lorenzo diachopo di mafio berti nostro gharzone', 17 April
1493, receipt of 1 florin 'disse per dare a m.a lesandra sua madre'.

24. Total cash advanced to clients was 3,512 soldi. Of this, 2,655 soldi (76%)
went to the apothecary's immediate circle of family, dependants and
employees.

25. Tommaso and his son Lorenzo together took cash advances of 1,486 soldi in
the sample year.

26. E882, fo. 249v, 'm.o Giovanni di raghugia', 26 May 1494, L8s13 paid to
client in cash 'chonte per risquotere il mantello'.

27. E882, fo. 249v, 23 April 1494, 1 florin 'in prestanza'; fo. 246r, 3 January
1493 (m.f.), L1s1 in cash 'disse voleva pagha e portatori chelgliaiutorono
sghonberare'.

28. E882, fo. 249r, 'Lando di [BLANK] tanalgli', 18 January 1493 (m.f.), 'e per
chonte s1d8 per chonperare semi chomuni chenoncienera'.

29. E882, fo. 203v, 'Dino di fran.co di bettino', 22 February 1486 (m.f.), a debt of L1s7d7 'sono per queste cose ebe dala bottegha di san giorgio ala nighittosa per nostro chonto'.

30. E882, fo. 111r, 'Chosimo di lorenzo rosselgli dipintore', 8 February 1491 (m.f.), payment of 14 florins to Guglielmo Altoviti on account of Rosselli 'ebe da tomaso di giovani n.o e quali disse aver paghati per lui a ghulglielmo di bardo altoviti'; 19 May 1492, repayment of 14 florins, 25 lire and 1 soldo. This money was probably to cover a wholesale transaction, since payment of the *tara* is recorded in undated credit of L3s3d4, 'fanno buoni per tara dela sopradetta ragione'.

31. Similar casual arrangements are illustrated in E. Welch, *Shopping in the Renaissance: Consumer Cultures in Italy 1400–1600* (New Haven: Yale University Press, 2005), 233.

32. E882, fo. 327r, 'm.a Angniola di saghramoro', undated debit, loan of L2s5 'porto lucha dalbizo'. Delivery of the money was made by another client, a mercer with a nearby shop, whose account is on fo. 175v, 'Lucha dalbizo merciaio nel chorso'.

33. E882, fo. 175v, 'm.o Bartolomeo di m.o vezano barbiere', 10 February 1493 (m.f.), L2s10 'in prestanza'.

34. There is little sign that customers could use the Giglio to provide a personal banking service for substantial cash advances, as the nearby Pinadori shop appears to have done – see D. Covi, 'A Documented Altarpiece by Cosimo Rosselli', *Art Bulletin*, 53, 2 (1971), 236–8: 238. For an apothecary lending small sums of money in Prato, see R.K. Marshall, *The Local Merchants of Prato. Small Entrepreneurs in the Late Medieval Economy* (Baltimore: Johns Hopkins University Press, 1999), 91–2; S. Rosati, 'Benedetto di Tacco da Prato speziale, 1345–1392: Vita, attività, ambiente sociale ed economico', graduate thesis, Facoltà di lettere e filosofia dell'Università di Firenze (1970–1), 213, 216–17, 223–4.

35. Naso, *op. cit.* (note 8), 64.

36. Accounts are predominantly recorded in terms of the weights of individual goods, with a total price given in the right column for the whole transaction.

37. Bargaining is recorded as taking place (with the formula 'd'accordo', followed by the agreed price) in only 88 out of 12,288 (1%) retail sales in the sample period. Where bargaining took place, the weight of goods was not usually specified.

38. E882, fo. 312r, 'Falchoniere di [BLANK] vetturale', 19 April 1494, purchase of 'piu chose' (no weight or items specified) for an agreed price of s9 'dachordo'. Again the bill was settled immediately 'pagho mese in chasa'. See also fo. 322r, 'Falchoniere vetturale', 9 May 1494, 21 May 1494; fo. 17r, 'Zanobi di Stefano Vetturale dasingnia', 2 April 1496, purchase of an unspecified quantity of 'olio di spigho e di chosto' and 2 doses of syrup for

an agreed price, 'dachordo s11d8'.

39. E882, fo. 289v, 29 March 1493, purchase of 1 'falchola' (no weight specified) for s6 d8 'dachordo'. The bill was settled immediately 'pagho messi in chasa' (see n.6).

40. E882, fo. 115v, 'm.a Oretta di giovanni solosmei', 28 September 1493.

41. E882, fo. 144v, 'Stefano di franc.o porcellini e chonpangni speziali'; fo. 97v, 'Franc.o di pagholo pinadori e chonpangni', 28 November 1493; fo. 99r, 'Ugholino di bartolomeo di chanbio e chonpangni speziali', 8 February 1493 (m.f.), 12 May 1494.

42. Welch, *op. cit.* (note 31), 212–20.

43. E882, fo. 82r, 'Adovardo di franc.o mannini', 28 September 1493, purchase of 3 oz of 'triacha fine' for s7, 'tolse e porto m.a luchrezia sua madre dachordo [soldi] 7'. See also entries for 7 December 1493, 'porto la luchrezia', and 1 December 1493, 'porto m.a luchrezia sua madre'.

44. E882, fo. 11r, 'Antonio e franc.o di niccholo gianfilgliazi', 23 December 1493, payment in the form of 3 oz of 'zaferano e mandorle' 'recho m.a bartolomea loro madre dachordo' for an agreed price of L4.

45. Welch, *op. cit.* (note 31), 216.

46. R.A. Goldthwaite, *The Building of Renaissance Florence: An Economic and Social History* (Baltimore: Johns Hopkins University Press, 1980), 314.

47. E882, fo. 103v, 'Benedetto di piero da san donnino vetturale', 20 September 1493 'e quadanari ci debe dare per di qui aotto di prosimi a venire'; 6 August 1494, payment of L13s2 'per lui da giovannmatteo e guseppe nelli e chonpangni merciai'; 12 February 1500 (m.f.) payment of 6 staia of 'panicho' valued at L1 per staio. Although arithmetic suggests the debt was settled at this point, the account was not struck through, confirming that the recording of clients' credits was not as rigorous as that of their debts.

48. Naso, *op. cit.* (note 8), 66–7, similarly notes that there was rarely any interest charged on payment by instalments, and pledges were only rarely required. These were usually simple verbal promises to pay by a certain date, often subsequently extended.

49. E882, fo. 240r, 'Luigi dant.o scharlatti', 20 December 1493, 'in prestanza'; 11 March 1494 (m.f.), for the payback.

50. E882, fo. 108r, 'Andrea di parides spangniuolo', 5 June 1492, records debt of L1s11; 26 September 1493, payment of L1s5 and the account is struck through.

51. E882, fo. 107v, 'Girolamo di [BLANK] niccholi', 30 May 1492, records debt of L2s6d8; 26 September 1494, payment of L2 'per resto di questo conto' and the account is struck through.

52. E882, fo. 110v, 'Simone di guliano ginori', 17 June 1492, records debt of L8s6d8; 15 November 1501, payment of L6s6 'chontanti per resto' and the account is struck through.

53. E882, fo. 45r, 'Giovanni di messer charlo federighi', 15 July 1493, 5 August 1493, 13 September 1494.

54. E882, fo. 150r, 'Lionardo delchiaro mungniao al ponte ala badia', 8 May 1493, records a debt of L6s3d11; 28 January 1500 (m.f.), payment of L2; 4 April 1522, payment of L3s6.

55. E882, fo. 194r, 'Luigi di christofano chalderini', 15 August 1494, 20 August 1494.

56. E882, fo. 55v, 'Benedetto di Bartolomeo delghalesandri', 13 February 1493 (m.f.), payment of L1s16, 'sono per la partita del zuc.o de [lire] 2 [soldi] 2 [denari] 4 perche non vole dare piu'.

57. S.C. Humphreys, 'History, Economics and Anthropology: The Work of Karl Polanyi', *History and Theory*, 8 (1969), 165–212: 189, 'Extension of credit is another way of introducing more flexibility into transactions at a 'fixed' price; both quantity variation and credit are important ways of favouring regular customers and fulfiling 'reciprocal' obligations while still nominally adhering to the market principle of the same terms for all comers.'

58. This qualifies the remarks given in Welch, *op. cit.* (note 31), 215, '…it was not simply the lower social classes who bargained. Purchasers of spices, silk or woollen cloth, antiquities, books or furnishings were just as if not more likely to negotiate as those buying basic foodstuffs whose prices were often fixed… bargaining took place at all levels…'. Whether bargaining took place at the moment of sale was strongly influenced by the credit practices that were specific to each market sector.

59. R.F.E. Weissman, 'Taking Patronage Seriously: Mediterranean Values and Renaissance Society', in F.W. Kent and P. Simons (eds), *Patronage, Art and Society in Renaissance Italy* (Oxford: Clarendon, 1987), 43.

60. Molière, *The Imaginary Invalid*, Project Gutenberg, 2005, Act I, Scene i.

61. O. Lafont, 'Comptes d'apothicaires normands', *Revue d'histoire de la pharmacie*, 35 (1988), 135–7: 135, found discounts from 6 to 17%.

62. During the sample period, payments totalling 16,758 soldi can be positively identified as payments in kind. This represents 29% of the total payments of just over 58,000 soldi. On this see also Rosati, *op. cit.* (note 34), 114.

63. F. Castellani, *Quaternuccio e giornale B (1459-1485)*, Biblioteca Italiana, Università degli Studi di Roma 'La Sapienza', 2005. [Florence: L.S. Olschki, 1995], entry for 1442, 'Speziale della Palla'.

64. E882, fo. 143r, 'Bernardo di piero del palagio', 28 September 1493, 2 bushels (*moggi*) of charcoal (*bracie*).

65. E882, fo. 95v, 'fratti e monaci di settimo eccestello', 1 September 1489 to 27 February 1492 (m.f.).

66. E882, fo. 190v, 'Giovanni di salvestro lapi', 28 October 1493, 'per valuta di staia [12] di ghrano dette per noi alapino n.o in villa sua a chasteletti a [s17] lo st.o dachordo posto lapino debi dare'.

67. E882, fo. 307r, 'Ant.o e franc.o di giano chalzaiuoli', 15 April 1494, 'chalze di panno nere'.

68. E882, fo. 333r, 'Tommaso di giovanni di piero nostro', 3 January 1494 (m.f.).

69. E882, fo. 123r, 'Angniolo e domenicho di pagholo chalzolai al ficho', 7 April 1495, 'sono per piu lavori auti da lui'. See also fo. 205v, 'Bastiano di giovanni da monte varchi nostro fattore', 2 May 1494, 'per lui a angniolo dalficho per un paio di scharpette', where the apothecary's factor took his pay in the form of shoes.

70. E882, fo. 147v, 'Marcho di tomaxo di giovanni nostro', 31 October 1494, 'chalze da chordellato paghonazo', 'ebbe per noi da charlo di bartolomeo chalzaiuolo'. See also fo. 146v, 'Charlo di bartolomeo chalzaiuolo fratello di franc.o da santo andrea', 3 January 1493 (m.f.), a pair of 'chalze di panno nere chiuse' which were 'dette per noi a tomaso di giovanni n.o posto debi dare i questo fol 30'.

71. E882, fo. 146r, 'Cristofano di paradiso chalzaiuolo', 23 November 1493, payment in the form of 'chalze di perpingniano paghonazo', which were 'dette per noi a girolamo di m.o piero della barba posto debi dare in questo fol 95'. See fo. 95r, 'Girolamo di maestro piero della barba nostro fattore', 23 November 1493, 'ebe per noi da christofano di paradiso'.

72. E882, fo. 95r, 21 November 1493, 'pano bigio fiandrescho bangniato e cimato' 'ebe per noi da rede di giovanni daghostino'. See also fo. 206r, 'Rede di giovanni daghostino', 21 November 1493.

73. E882, fo. 95r, 7 June 1494, 'farsetto dighuarnello tane' 'per lui a michele de chante farsettaio'. See also fo. 46v, 'Michele di chante farsettaio', 7 June 1494, 'per un farsetto dighuarnello tane dette per noi a girolamo di m.o piero delab[ar]ba n.o gharzone'.

74. E882, fo. 113v, 'Domenicho di [BLANK] fabro al poggio achaiano', 2 May 1495, 9 May 1495.

75. E882, fo. 18v, 'Particino di guliano particini', 4 July 1494, payment of ½ catasta of oak and bitter oak 'lengnie ghrosse mescholato quercia eccierro', valued at 6 lire.

76. E882, fo. 170v, 'Franc.o di christofano nacchianti', 2 December 1484 to 13 May 1486.

77. E882, fo. 185r, 'Antonio di lionardo charbonaio'.

78. E882, fo. 185v, 'Bernardo di [BLANK] battiloro', 12 August 1493. On *oro di metà*, see M. O'Malley, *The Business of Art: Contracts and the Commissioning Process in Renaissance Italy* (New Haven: Yale University Press, 2005), 288 n.30.

79. E882, fo. 257r, 'Ciervagio di franc.o del tasso lengniaiuolo', 8 January 1493 (m.f.), 'sono per piu lavori fatti a tomaso nostro in chasa e in bottegha cioe usci finestre scrittoi e lachasetta de danari', valued at L26s13. Fo. 333r, 6

149

December 1494, records L1s12d8 paid to a blacksmith for metal fittings and nails supplied to Del Tasso to fix Tommaso's desk in place, 'per lui a mariotto fabro per piu feramenti e aghuti dati per lui a ciervagio del tasso per aghonciare loschrittoio di tomaso'.

80. E882, fo. 184r, 'Giovanni di chimenti rosselgli dipintore', undated, 'per dipintura di palchi attomaso'.

81. E882, fo. 185r, 'Antonio di zanobi e mariotto muratori', undated, 'per lui atomaso di gio[vanni] per opera'.

82. E882, fo. 141v, 'Matteo di cristofano bardelgli lengniaiuolo', 15 May 1493, 'sono per toppe e aghuti chonpro per noi per luscio delorto della torre di villa'.

83. E882, fo. 108r, 'Santi di monte ossaio', 18 July 1490, 22 July 1488, 11 May 1489. He had old debts of around 50 lire, some dating back to the early 1480s and paid with a variety of goods in kind in the period 1488–90. The debt was subsequently 'reckoned' in October 193 and subsequently paid off in full in January and May 1494, when the account was finally struck through. See fo. 148r, 15 October 1493, 18 January 1493 (m.f.), 12 May 1494.

84. E882, fo. 44v, 'Antonio e franc.o di giano chalzaiuoli', 25 May 1493, debts of L230s8d3.

85. E882, fo. 307r, 15 April 1494; fo. 326v, 7 June 1494.

86. Of the 88,609 soldi recorded book debt from consumption in the sample year, 86% was on accounts that were eventually struck through as settled.

87. Of the 627,735 soldi recorded book debt up to and including the sample year, only 58% was in accounts that were eventually struck through as settled.

88. E882, fo. 179r, 'Fratti e chonvento di san donato aschopeto', 17 July 1493. Fo. 30r, 'Larte de chalzolai', 10 September 1493, 1 June 1493. Neither account was struck through.

89. E882, fo. 302v, 'Piero di nardo fornaio', 3 April 1465, records debt of L60s18d8.

90. E882, fo. 304r, 'm.o Ant.o di tomaso dipintore', 21 July 1465, records debt of L3s1d9.

91. E882, fo. 264v, 'Andrea di bartolo da monte fiesole', 18 August 1481, records debt of L3s16d4; 21 April 1503, payment of L3s16. For a similar case see fo. 267r, 'Lucha di ser bernardo dalancisa'.

92. E882, fo. 111r, 'Antonio dangniolo da sanchasciano', 19 January 1496 (m.f.).

93. E882, fo. 162r, 'Fratti di san franc.o da chastello san giovanni'; fo. 166r, 'fratte di san franc.o del palcho da prato', fo. 172r, 'fratte Lorenzo chorsi frate deloservanza di san franc.o'; fo. 175v, 'fra Nicholo dangniolo ghuardiano di bargha delordine di san franc.o'; fo. 190v, 'frate Bastiano frate

di san franc.o da fiesole'; fo. 193r, 'frate Bastiano in san franc.o a aserezana', all of which were 'cancelasi per lamore di dio'.

94. E882, fo. 17v, 'Frati e chonvento di San Franc.o da Saminiato'.
95. E882, fo. 233r, 'm.o Jachopo di [BLANK] maziere del papa', 22 January 1493 (m.f.), payment of L10 'per resto di questa ragione per noi a nicholo di marchionne del m.o ridolfo nostro gharzone'.
96. E. Coturri, 'Spunti di medicina e di farmacia nelle novelle di uno speziale toscano del trecento, Giovanni Sercambi (1348–1424)', in *Atti del IV convegno di studi AISF, Varese: 3–4 Ottobre 1959* (Pisa: Arti grafiche Pacini Mariotti, 1959), 6; R.A. Pratt, 'Giovanni Sercambi, Speziale', *Italica*, 25, 1 (1948), 12-14; A. West Vivarelli, 'Giovanni Sercambi's Novelle and the Legacy of Boccaccio', *MLN: Modern Language Notes*, 90, 1 (1975), 109–27.
97. E882, fo. 19r, 'Bernardo di [BLANK] [Ver]milgli', 16 March 1495 (m.f.); fo. 20v, 'Ghoro discholaio viviani', 10 June 1494; fo. 244r, 'Niccholo di charlo strozi', 6 February 1495; fo. 332r, 'm.a Andrevuola decierchi', 23 May 1495; fo. 338r, 'messer Bartolomeo di [BLANK] schala', 7 January 1494 (m.f.); fo. 349r, 'Bartolomeo di tomaso settecielgli e fratelgli', 25 September 1494, 2 June 1495.
98. E882, fo. 88v, 'Bernardo dinghilese ridolfi', 9 March 1495 (m.f.) 'disse non voleva dare piu'. Although the apothecary rated this as being worth only 21 of the 26 soldi owed, the client refused to pay any more, and the account was struck through as settled, representing a discount of nearly 20% on a debt that dated back at least four years. See entry for 7 February 1491 (m.f.) for the original debt of 16 soldi.
99. E882, fo. 349r, 'Bartolomeo di tomaso settecielgli e fratelgli', 25 September 1494, where the client paid a florin 'per noi a ugenio di tomaso fraschi n.o rischotitore posto ugenio debi dare i' questo c. 330'. See fo. 330v, 'Ugenio di tommaso fiaschi nostro rischotitore', 2 June 1495, for recording of this in Fiaschi's account. Further monies owed to Fiaschi were credited to his son – see fo. 190v, 'Tommaso dugenio fiaschi'.
100. E882, fo. 322v, 'Richordo choma ugienio di tomaso fiaschi veneastare chonessono per risquotter e per suo prezo gli dobiamo dare [soldi] dua aldi chelui serve la bottegha edeto essercizio [soldi] dua p[iccoli] e di ttutto quelo che i rischotese [soldi] unno per lira e degli achordi chelui fa[ce]si [soldi] una per lira quando si ritraesino el sopradett[o] uginio si sochrive di sua mano...', an agreement of 14 May 1494.
101. E882, fo. 138v, 'Ugenio di tomaso fiaschi', payment of L20s19d4 'e quali sono per suo salaro di danari ci afatto risquotere da di [1 May 1490] per insino adi [14 May 1494] dachordo'.
102. ASF, Catasto 1022, Microfilm 2474, fo. 397r, the net value placed on his property was fl.418 s17 d8.
103. Tratte 110041, 'Ugonio di Tommaso Fiaschi'.

104. E882, ff. 253v, 268r, 'Bardo di taddeo di stagio da ghiaccietto nostro rischotitore'. Note that this was probably Bardo di Taddeo di Stagio Barducci, born 1444 (tratte 402391). He may have been distantly related to the important client on ff. 31r, 118v, 'Stagio di lorenzo barducci'.

105. E882, fo. 253v, 6 October 1483.

106. E882, fo. 19r, 'Bernardo di [BLANK] [Ver]milgli', 8 March 1493 (m.f.), payment of 1 florin 'per lui da ruberto chavalchanti setaiuolo recho bardo'.

107. E882, ff. 90v, 349r, 'Bartolomeo di tomaso settecielgli e fratelgli lanaiuoli in samartino'.

108. E882, fo. 90v, 23 February 1491 (m.f.), transfer of existing debt of L295s14; 25 January 1485 (m.f.) for purchase of 51 lbs of aloe. In addition, a small amount of this debt was incurred as surety for another client – see fo. 159r, 'Lodovicho di franc.o di tomaso cini', the sum of L4s1 was transferred to the Settecieli and the account was struck through.

109. E882, fo. 349r, 6 April 1497.

110. E882, fo. 349r, 25 September 1494, 2 June 1495, 28 June 1497 and undated payment.

111. E882, fo. 127r, 'ser Pierfranc.o di ser luigi ghuidi', undated payment of L7 in the form of 2 drams of 'ribarbero fine', which, 'ci aveva renduto che non era fatto chreditore'.

112. E882, fo. 111r, 'Chosimo di lorenzo rosselgli dipintore', undated credit of L3s3d4, 'fanno buoni per tara dela sopradetta ragione', with the following crossed out 'sbattuto lacha ciaveva data e verderame aveva paghato insino a questo di' – a reference to red lake that he had supplied but that had not been recorded, and verdigris that he had already paid for.

113. E882, fo. 111r, 'edachordo faciemo restassi chreditore detto chosimo di [L3s2]'.

114. E882, fo. 161r, 'Chosimo di lorenzo rosselgli dipintore', 30 June 1494, payment of 3 florins; 16 October 1494, payment of 3 florins; 2 August 1494, Rosselli receives 2 florins.

115. E882, fo. 161r, saldo of 9 September 1495, 'e per suo resto gli demo [florins] nove… choma pare di suo mano ale portate [fol] 30 e chancielasi ongni ragione di nostre merchatantie a lui date in sino a questo di'.

116. E882, fo. 112r, 'Guliano di giovanni marucelgli', 25 June 1492, records debts of L344 s8 d3; the account further records 'saldammo la sopradetta ragione ogi [i.e. 5 January 1494 (m.f.)] et dachordo faciemo isbattuto il dato delavuto che detto guliano restassi nostro debitore di [L215]'.

117. E882, fo. 127r, 'ser Pierfranc.o di ser luigi ghuidi', 24 August 1492 records debt of L57s1d9; 1 June 1499, payment of L6s17; 16 September 1497, payment of L12 in the form of 6 barrels of 'vino vermiglio'; undated payment of L7 in the form of 2 drams of 'ribarbero fine'; 22 April 1501

'saldamo la sopradetta ragione chon ant.o di ser luigi suo fratello ogi e dachordo rimanemo ci restassi debitore di [L14]'

118. E882, fo. 221v, 'Zanobi di baldo e lorenzo di piero e chonpangni dipintori', the debt of L9s15 is recorded in the accounts as being already reckoned and signed, 'per saldo fatto dachordo e soschritto di suo mano'.

119. E882, fo. 112r, 'Guliano di giovanni marucelgli', 7 January 1494 (m.f.), and 27 May 1495, 2 November 1495, 12 December 1495 for further payments totalling 84 lire 2 soldi.

120. E882, fo. 150r, 'Antonio di ghuasparre oste alefalle', 8 May 1493, records debt of L23s19d2; undated entry records debt of L1s13d8; 26 October 1493 'saldammo', the debt was agreed at L19 and the client's legal representative 'Piero di ser Bartolomeo' signed the register.

121. E882, fo. 252r, 'Ristoro di piero e chonpangni merciai', 24 July 1481, records debt of L18s6d8.

122. E882, fo. 294r, 20 September 1487, records a saldo carried out on that date reckoning the debt at L12s10 (the old entry was struck through). The reduced debt was, however, never settled.

123. E882, fo. 136r, 'Ghuido di lodovicho del palagio', 25 December 1492, records debt of L9s3d4; 30 June 1496, 'saldamo la sopradetta ragione' the debt was reckoned at L7s10, which Guido 'ci promette dare e paghare per tutto il mese di luglio 1496'.

124. E882, fo. 173r, 'Matteo di domenicho pollaiuolo', 8 May 1493, records debt of L3s3d4; 2 August 1496 the debt was reckoned at L3 'sbattuto la tara e le spese fatte al palgio [sic] del podesta', and Marco signed his name in the register.

125. E882, fo. 173r, 19 November 1496, payment of L1; 10 July 1498, payment with no value given.

126. The accounts sample reveal recorded legal actions for 31 out of a total of 2247 clients (1%). If we consider only the sample year, the figure is 7 out of 515 active clients (1%).

127. E882, fo. 174r, 'Benedetto dandrea bifoli'.

128. E882, ff. 71v, 105v, 258r, 260r, 'Bartolomeo di ser franc.o da anbra', spent 1352 soldi during the sample year alone.

129. E882, fo. 258r, 23 September 1493, records debt of L15s18; fo. 105v, 6 September 1493, records debt of L8s9d4.

130. E882, fo. 260r, 31 October 1495, L1s7 'paghati per diritto ala merchatantia per ser giovanni di maso e per la richiesta'. This client can be found on fo. 83v, 'Giovanni di maso notaio ala merchatantia'.

131. E882, fo. 260r, 28 November 1495, s5d6 'paghati ala merchatantia per aprovare i libro'.

132. E882, fo. 260r, 10 December 1495, s8d8 'per la richiesta e udere sentenzia e per la tassa dela sente[n]zia che si dette detto di'.

133. E882, fo. 260r, total costs 31 October 1495 to 10 December 1495 recorded as L1s20d14.

134. ASF, Mercanzia 7320, n.p. 17 Jun 1494. See fo. 243r, 'Giovanni dandrea solgliani'. Claims could also presented to the Judge of the Mercanzia, rather than the 'Six', see, for example, ASF, Mercanzia 8133.

135. J.E. Shaw, *The Justice of Venice: Authorities and Liberties in the Urban Economy, 1550–1700* (Oxford: Oxford University Press, 2006), 191–3.

136. E882, fo. 127v, 'Alessandro di pagholo federighi'. A. Molho, *Marriage Alliance in Late Medieval Florence* (Cambridge: Harvard University Press, 1994), 389. Tratte 400704, 3092, 3093, 3091 – he was born in 1461, and elected Consul of the wool guild in two occasions, though too young to take office. He had died by 6 September 1492.

137. E882, fo. 127v, 30 August 1492, debts of L122s18d4 in his own name. He had also promised to cover the debts of a neighbour, see undated entry recording L3s17d4 'e quali ci promisse per lorenzo tesitore suo vicino'. On this see also fo. 77r, 'Lorenzo di [BLANK]', 4 October 1491.

138. E882, fo. 127v, 25 October 1496, L2s10d4 'sono per i spese fatte alarte degli speziali che detto di s[i] e[b]be la sentenzia chontro a redi e beni e posessori de beni dalesandro di pagholo federighi di [L] 50 per parte di maggior somma e delespese', an equivalent formulation is given on fo. 294r, 'Girolamo dant.o di simone ghualcheraio', 1 September 1498, 'sono per ispese fatte ala merchatantia che detto di avemo la sentenzia'.

139. E882, fo. 127v, 15 January 1498 (m.f.), L1s12d8, 'per la parte loro della taratura che monto tutto la ragione [L196s2d10]'. The Guild experts were named as Paolo Morelli and Bartolomeo di Biagio.

140. E882, fo. 127r, 15 January 1498 (m.f.), payment of L10s2s10, 'che tanti fu tarata la sopradetta ragione per taratori delarte che fu bartolomeo di biagio e pagholo moregli'.

141. For a similar evidence on the costs of paying *taratori*, see E882, fo. 58r, 'Rede dangniuolo diachopo tani' 25 June 1495, s17d8 'per loro anicholo da enpoli benedetto righogli taratori delarte perla parte loro dela tara dela sopra detta ragione' and n.166. One of these *taratori* was listed as a client, fo. 109r, 'Benedetto di [BLANK] righolgli e chonpangni speziali alangniolo rafaello'.

142. E882, fo. 20v, 'Ghoro discholaio viviani', whose debts amounted to s320.33 in December 1493. Entry for 11 December 1493, L1s13 'sono per i spese fattogli a larte delgli speziali che detto di sebe lasentenzia etasate le spese'.

143. E882, fo. 20v, 10 June 1494 'recho ugienio f[i]aschi'; 24 October 1495, 'presi per noi augienio di tomaso fraschi'.

144. After the final recorded payment in October 1495, the debt was s297.

145. E882, ff. 47v, 261v, 310r, 'Bernardo di stefano rosselgli dipintore'.

146. E882, fo. 310r, 27 February 1493 (m.f.), records debt of L4s10.

147. E882, fo. 310r, undated entry (but prior to 1499), records costs of L1s12d4, 'per piu spese fatogli alarte degli speziali'.

148. E882, fo. 310r, 7 December 1499, 20 December 1499, payments amounting to L2s3.

149. E882, fo. 310r, 31 May 1520, payment of L4.

150. E882, fo. 12r, 'Giovanni di rugieri de ricci', 20 September 1490 records debt of L24s9d6.

151. E882, fo. 12r, 7 November 1493, L1s16 to the notary 'per tanti fattolgli dispesa ala merchatantia per ser giovanni dimaso'.

152. E882, fo. 12r, 30 December 1499 [probable year], payment of L6s11; 25 January 1499 (m.f.), payment of L3s10; 8 September 1511, payment of L7.

153. E882, fo. 282v, 'Pippo dant.o e ant.o di pippo da san ghaggio suo figliuolo', 8 July 1484, records debts of L4; 1 August 1496, costs of s5 'per ispese fatte' (presumably legal expenses).

154. E882, fo. 282v, 10.March 1499 (m.f.), payment of L1s10.

155. ASF, Mercanzia 12, for a sixteenth-century description of the *tocco* and the role of *toccatori*.

156. He had significant debts of his own as well as inheriting further debts from his father Andrea, amounting to over 100 lire in total. E882, fo. 38r, 'Franc.o dandrea zati', 19 May 1491, an undated entry 'per una ragion i' andrea di franc.o suo padre', and 30 May 1483, for a total of 2191 soldi; 18 September 1494, payment of 10 staia of grain, valued at L13s16d6, followed by two further payments which have no price details; 15 June 1497, L3s13 'sono per ispese fatte ala merchatantia che detto di sebbe la sentenzia di [lire] 50 per parte di magiore somma per le mani di ser giovanni di maso notaio in detta chorte'.

157. E882, fo. 38r, 7 February 1497 (m.f.), s16 'per lui aghottior tochatore per farlo tochare'.

158. Old debt plus consumption August 1493 to September 1494 amounted to s191.2. E882, fo. 59v, 'Andrea dicharlo ghalighaio', entry for August 1496, L1s2 'sono per i spese fatte al palagio del podesta che detto di sebe la sentenzia per ser benedetto dalascharperia'. This notary listed as a client on fo. 149r, 'ser Benedetto di [BLANK] dalascharperia'.

159. E882, fo. 59v, 3 October 1496, s10, 'per lui a bruogio tochatore elchonpangnio chelotochorono detto di a nostra petizione'.

160. E882, fo. 294r, 'Girolamo dant.o di simone ghualcheraio', 13 May 1499, payment of L63 in the form of 14 *braccia* of 'panno rosetto bangniato e cimato', the agreement further specified 'chon patto che della nostra ragione dele chose date loro non si avessi a fare tara nessuna e chosi rimanemo dachordo chon domenicho e chon franc.o frategli e figliuoli di Girolamo sop[r]adetto'. The Mercanzia sentence of September 1498 was in fact for 40

lire, 'per parte di maggior so[m]ma', which left open the possibility of contesting the extent of the debt.

161. E882, fo. 294r, 1 September 1498, L3s17 'sono per ispese fatte ala merchatantia che detto di avemo la sentenzia chon figliuoli erede di girolamo dant.o di simone ghualcheraio e nominata ment[re] [qua] domenicho e franco sua figliuoli di L40 per parte di maggior so'ma per ser giovan[n]i di maso'; 13 May 1499, L5s10 'per le spese della tenuta che si sono fatte insino a ogi'.

162. E882, fo. 294r, 13 May 1499 'el quale avemo per lui da giovanni di ser filippo da sa'miniato e chonpangni lanaiuoli nela vignia'.

163. This may explain why the apothecary preferred to avoid litigation of this sort regarding the extent of the debt – see n. 160.

164. E882, fo. 58r, 'Rede dangniuolo diachopo tani', 'Fu tarata la sopradetta ragione adi [27 May 1495] per le mani di benedetto righogli e nicholo daenpoli alpresente taratori delarte delgli speziali e dachordo tarorone detta ragione [L13 s8] p[icco]li che sa[ran]no asbattere di [L61 s4 d10] diche restono debitori chome sivede quidisopra e piu ci [h]a[n]no a fare buoni [s17 d8] p[icco]li equali si paghorono per loro adetti taratori per la parte loro dela tara chenne sono fatti debitori quidisopra sotto di [25 June 1495] che detto di rischotemo laragione tarata', with recorded debt of L47s16d10.

165. E882, fo. 58r, 'E deono dare adi [29 May 1497] [L3 s13 d9] p[icco]li sono per ispese fatte alamerchatantia che detto di sebe la sentenzia di [L32] per dua terzi cioe per la parte deladonna di giovanbatista della tosa e per la parte del dona delchapitano desanti chefu: chechosi furono tassate lespese detto di'. These competing claims on the inheritance may refer to the wife of the client on ff. 338v, 345r, 355v, 'Giovanbatista di bernardo della tosa' and possibly to the widow of the client on fo. 180r, 'ser Piero di [BLANK] chapitano de fanti'.

166. E882, fo. 58r, 'E deono dare [L21 s17 d6] p[icco]li sono per piu spese fatte alamerchatantia per la sentenzia delbraccio milatare e per dare bando delasghonbro a lavoratori e piu altre spese chome si vede alibro di ser Giovanni di maso n.o prochuratore'.

167. E882, fo. 58r, 6 February 1497 (m.f.) to 3 July 1498, each a payment of 2 florins, each transaction evaluated at s13d8.

168. Shaw, *op. cit.* (note 135), 151.

169. *Ibid.*, 206.

PART THREE

PRODUCTS

6

Wax

Patterns of Consumption

With credit or cash at their disposal, what could the Giglio's customers buy? Answering this key question is more difficult than it might first appear. The shop's inventory, taken in 1504, is problematic, partly because it presents only a snapshot of stocks for which the supply was often extremely variable. Commodities with a long shelf life are sometimes overestimated, while those with a limited shelf life or that were made up on the spot are often absent. In addition, much of this stock was destined for the bulk distributive trade (see Chapter 3) and relatively few of the commodities listed were sold directly to clients. The retail trade was much more specialised than the inventory suggests, with a number of products manufactured in-house from raw materials. Honey, for example, was used to manufacture aromatic variants with roses or violets.[1] Many of the goods retailed at the shop, particularly in the medicinal sector, were unique items made for particular clients. The existence of so many specialist products makes analysis difficult, and in order to obtain some sense of the relative importance and weight placed on different items for sale, it is necessary to bundle these products into a number of broader categories[2] (see Table 6.1, overleaf).

Although a number of historians have suggested that medicines were a relatively unimportant aspect of the apothecary's trade,[3] the Giglio evidence clearly shows that this was the most important class of goods for retailing (forty-two per cent, mostly purges, syrups and electuaries), exceeding wax products (twenty-eight per cent, mostly candles and torches) and foodstuffs (twenty-five per cent, chiefly sweets). This matches the pattern at fifteenth-century Arles, although here medicines were even more important.[4] The sales figures show that the most important goods were manufactured goods – compare, for example, the sales of candles to those of unprocessed wax, or the sale of sweets to those of sugar or spices. Moreover, some of these goods, such as grain, were not normally 'on sale' but instead reflect diverse modes of payment.[5] As we have seen, many clients paid in kind, and these goods were often subsequently distributed to shop staff, as happened with stockings. Although these are indistinguishable from 'sales' in the accounts, this does not mean that the shop retailed grain or clothing to the general public. Such commodities did not represent the core business of the shop

Table 6.1

Retail Sales by Commodity Group

Category	Sub total (soldi)	As % of grand total	Commodity group	Sales (soldi)	As % of sub total	As % of grand total
Medicinal	37,005	42%	Purges	11,168	30%	13%
			Syrups	6,515	18%	7%
			Electuaries	4,662	13%	5%
			Juleps	2,091	6%	2%
			Clysters	1,823	5%	2%
			Epithems	1,443	4%	2%
			Pills	1,185	3%	1%
			Ointments	771	2%	1%
Wax	24,567	28%	Candles	15,433	63%	17%
products			Torches	8,215	33%	9%
			Wax	904	4%	1%
Food	21,970	25%	Sweets	11,676	53%	13%
and spices			Sugar	3,869	18%	4%
			Grain	2,103	10%	2%
			Spices	2,065	9%	2%
			Olive Oil	424	2%	–
			Honey	401	2%	–
			Rice	283	1%	–
Other	2,667	3%	Colours	603	23%	1%
			Miscellaneous	436	16%	–
			Funerals	346	13%	–
			Cloth	340	13%	–
			Receptacles	166	6%	–
			Cotton	145	5%	–
			Lead	91	3%	–
			Clothing	88	3%	–
			Incense	83	3%	–
Data unavailable[6]	2,400	3%				3%
Grand total	88,609	100%				100%

but rather the sort of side trading carried on by most of the economic operators of the period as a result of accepting payment in kind.

Strikingly, the sales figures show that the shop was open on every day of the year.[7] The base-line demand for apothecary products was consistent and clients were not to be denied – people even struggled out during the terrible snowstorm of 20 January 1494, when, according to Landucci, it was 'impossible to open the shops'.[8] The strict observance of religious feasts was similarly set aside in case of medical need, as on Good Friday 1494, when Girolamo Fortini bought a purge for his daughter.[9] Even churchmen participated: the Badia of Florence purchased pills, *manuschristi* and marzipan on Easter Sunday 1494,[10] and the Jeromites at Santa Caterina bought incense and drugs on Good Friday 1494.[11] Certain trades were exempted from the prohibitions on feast-day trading on grounds of public health,[12] and this applied to apothecaries for the sale of medicines.[13] The Guild statutes made specific allowance for this; for example, a lottery system was introduced in 1481 to determine which shops could open on holy days.[14] These restrictions were probably easy to evade, and the lack of resources – or will – to enforce them is particularly striking in the case of the Giglio, which was not even registered with the Guild. The apothecary perhaps kept up appearances by closing the shop door and windows on these days, opening up for trusted clients as a personal favour – a practice that was extremely difficult to police. This sort of private trading was usually tolerated so long as it took place out of sight, maintaining a façade of respect for the holy days. This sort of compromise can be found in older Guild regulations that forbade retailing on feast days but allowed the sale of medicines and funeral accessories in cases of 'vital' need. On such days, apothecaries had to close their shops but were permitted to trade through a *sportello* (a small opening in the door).[15]

That these were mostly petty transactions of an emergency nature, mostly for medicines, is confirmed by comparing sales figures to the festive calendar. This analysis shows that there were fewer customers on holy days,[16] and that their consumption was lower.[17] The pattern of sales over the week (Table 6.2) shows that business was slowest on Sundays, and steady during the rest of the week – averaging seventeen to nineteen transactions per day – with a slight rise on Saturdays to twenty-one transactions per day. More customers came to the shop on Saturdays, and they also consumed more, with average sales of 360 soldi per day. This suggests that although the flow of customers was fairly steady, they tended to stock up before the feast days. There is a corresponding, although smaller, peak of consumption on Mondays as clients came to shop again after the feast.

Table 6.2

Sales Figures by Day of Week, 1493–4

Day of week	Total sales (soldi)	Total retail transactions	Number of days in sample year	Average sales per day (soldi)	Average retail transations per day
Monday	14,948	900	48	311	19
Tuesday	11,335	795	47	241	17
Wednesday	12,789	918	49	261	19
Thursday	12,906	820	48	269	17
Friday	13,188	896	50	264	18
Saturday	18,350	1084	51	360	21
Sunday and other feast days[18]	8,606	618	72	120	9

Chart 6.1

Number of Clients per Month, 1493–4[19]

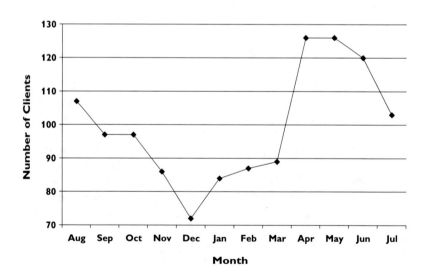

Chart 6.2

Retail Sales by Day, 1493–4

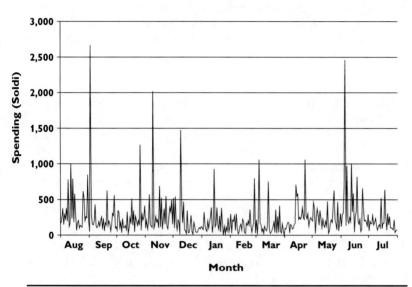

Examination of the number of different customers who came to the shop each month further shows that the shop was quieter during the winter (November to March), and especially December, but much busier in the spring and early summer (April to June).[20] These kinds of shifts in baseline demand were probably related to seasonal patterns of disease, in particular the prevalence of fevers in the spring (see Chapter 8).

Plotting sales figures over the year, rather than numbers of customers, reveals a very different pattern. As we saw in Chapter 4, most of the Giglio's clients were 'crisis' clients who bought goods in response to specific needs. Individual demand for apothecary products varied significantly – customers might not come to the shop at all for months, and then spend large amounts in only a few days. As a result of this erratic demand, the range of sales on any one day was enormous: from a minimum of twelve soldi to a maximum of 2,635 soldi (see Chart 6.2).[21] The religious calendar, weekly shopping rhythms and seasonal demand patterns can therefore explain only a limited proportion of the variation across the year. The most striking feature of the graph are the sharp peaks that stand out against a background of more steady consumption.

These peaks of consumption were almost entirely related to demand for a specific group of products – candles, torches and tapers, mostly purchased to celebrate funerals. One peak was produced by Taddeo di Giovanni Bisdomini, who bought nearly five hundred soldi-worth of torches, candles, tapers and funeral fittings for his mother's funeral,[22] and by Francesca Mormorai, who bought over eight hundred soldi-worth of wax products for her husband's funeral on the same day.[23] The only major peak not related to wax products resulted from an anomalous bulk sale of grain to a baker.[24] Most of the daily variation in sales figures was linked to fluctuations in demand for a specific group of products, and related to events in the family life of individuals (funerals) rather than season or religious calendar.

Consumer demand shows pronounced contrasts according to product group. Although the peaks of demand were very important for the business, they do not represent the ordinary day-to-day business of the shop or the consumption of the majority of clients. The extreme variability in demand for wax products, concentrated in the hands of only a few clients, can be contrasted to a more steady background demand for products like medicines, the consumption of which was more evenly distributed across the clientele. Less than twenty per cent of clients bought wax and wax products, making demand much more concentrated compared to the client base for foodstuffs (around sixty-seven per cent), or medicines (eighty-four per cent).[25] These differences in the nature of demand mean that analysis of the retail market must differentiate between the various product groups. The rest of this chapter looks more closely at production, retail and consumption of wax products, which was the most important commodity in the 1504 inventory[26] in terms of weight (eleven per cent) and value (nineteen per cent), a pattern common to most apothecaries of the period. It also accounted for a significant proportion of the cost of supplies (sixteen per cent). But the whole term 'wax' disguises what was a complex and important economic product in the period.

Wax and the dead

Although the Giglio sold a great number of medicinal products designed to keep its customers alive, it had an important sideline in goods associated with their deaths. The shop bought in all its raw wax and cotton wicks, and used these to produce a wide range of candles, tapers and torches for retail.[27] The inventory lists wax in both virgin and 'worked' forms, and also heavy cauldrons, copper pans and the stove needed for processing.[28] The process itself, although simple, was time-consuming and took place on the premises, in the kitchen to the rear. Tapers and candles were made by repeatedly dipping wicks into the liquid wax, or the wax could be poured into moulds.[29] An image from a late fourteenth-century *Tacuinum Santitatis* shows the sale

Image 6.1

'The Candle Shop' from Tacuinum Sanitatis,
Italian School, fourteenth century.
Osterreichische Nationalbibliothek, Vienna, Nova 2644 fo. 95v,
©Alinari// Réunion des Musées Nationaux

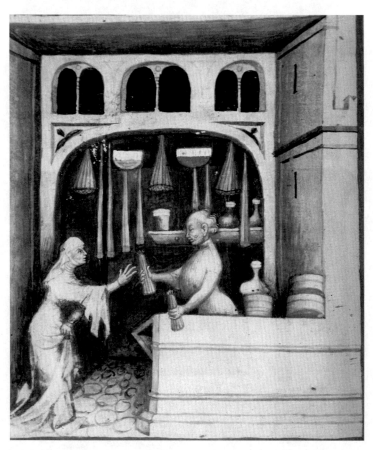

of candles, tapers and torches as well as oil lamps from a specialist shop (see Image 6.1).

The Giglio seems to have operated at what might be termed the high end of the wax market. Raw wax accounted for only a relatively small proportion (four per cent) of the total sales of wax products. Minor amounts of wax were also used to make medicinal products such as plasters and ointments (see Chapter 8), but most of the wax purchased by the shop was used in the

Image 6.2

'A Good Harvest': The shrine and market of Orsanmichele, Biblioteca Laurenziana, Florence. Photo: Biblioteca Laurenziana.

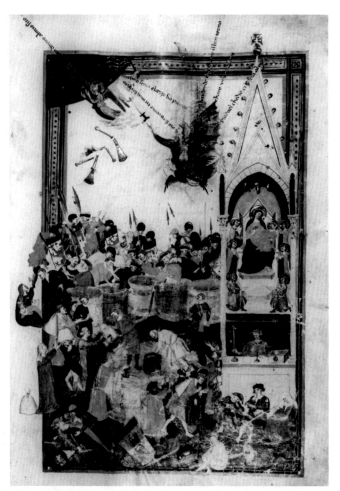

manufacture of candles, tapers and torches. These were made from beeswax, a product which, unlike tallow or oil, generated a clear consistent and sweet-smelling light.[30] This was in distinct contrast to the use of animal and kitchen fats that were used to create candles for cheaper domestic use. The two trades were normally quite separate – in early fifteenth-century London, for example, members of the newly established Chandlers' Guild dealt primarily in tallow candles as well as soap products which used similar fats, while a separate guild specialised in beeswax candles.[31] Similarly in Florence, tallow candles were probably retailed by butchers, while apothecaries specialised in beeswax candles. Beeswax candles were not normally used for household illumination, but rather to worship the saints, celebrate funerals and to commemorate the dead.[32] This is evident from the highly distinctive demand profile for wax products shown at the Giglio: a relatively small number of clients – compared to sweets or medicines – consumed very large quantities on an irregular basis, a pattern that was principally linked to funerals and commemorative services.[33]

The sale of candles to worshippers was a major source of income for many religious communities in fifteenth-century Florence. The shrine of Orsanmichele, for example, covered much of its day-to-day running costs by selling tapers to worshipers who wanted to honour the miracle-working Virgin.[34] The fourteenth-century illumination of the corn-chandler's account book shows these transactions already taking place when the image was in a simple enclosure in the marketplace and much of the construction cost of the elaborate marble shrine was covered by these sales (Image 6.2). Another important use of wax on this site was in the many votive images that were clustered around the tabernacle, symbols of either healing received or required. The churches, shrines and oratories that encouraged these devotions did not normally manufacture their own wax products. Instead they bought them from apothecaries or specialist chandlers for resale to pilgrims, or encouraged devotees to bring their own.[35] Relatively small wax objects, made in the shape of the arm, eyes, feet or other body parts can be seen for sale in the Issogne fresco of the apothecary's shop. Some wax specialists were capable of creating whole effigies which could be hung from the rafters of churches containing important miracle-working images, such as that of Santissima Annunziata.[36] The Giglio did not itself deal in these sorts of votive images but it did retail large quantities of candles, torches and tapers. In the sample year, it retailed a total of 1,762 lbs of wax and wax products. Its leading customer for these products was the Sacristy of Sant'Ambrogio, where there was an important cult based around a thirteenth-century miracle of the eucharist.[37] The relic was taken in an annual procession around the city – a scene represented in the fresco decorating the chapel by the Giglio's client, Cosimo Rosselli – and also displayed outside the church three times a year.[38] There were indulgences for visiting the relic and pilgrims would have lit candles at the chapel that housed the sacred blood as a sign of their devotion.[39] This sort of connection between apothecaries and religious sites was not unusual: the most important client of the fourteenth-century apothecary of Prato, Benedetto di Tacco, was the local monastery of San Domenico, which bought large quantities of candles and torches, far outweighing the importance of medicines for his business.[40]

This was a relatively expensive product. The wholesale price for yellow wax was generally from eleven to twelve soldi per lb, with the finer quality known as *zavorra* or 'ballast wax' at the top end of this range.[41] This wax, along with 'slav', or 'ragusan' qualities, was imported from the Balkans, and much of it was bought from Ragusan merchants who were probably based either in Venice or in the Marche.[42] White wax, sometimes specified as 'Venetian', was more expensive, costing over sixteen soldi per lb,[43] although the apothecary also bought a quantity of 'old' white wax for twelve soldi per lb.[44] The retail price of yellow wax was around fourteen soldi per lb, and, again, most of this was probably the better-quality Balkan wax that was taken directly from the bales.[45] By contrast, locally produced wax was an inferior grade that retailed for under twelve soldi per lb.[46] The retail price of white wax was around eighteen to twenty soldi per lb.[47] For both yellow and white wax, therefore, the margin was around fifteen to twenty per cent. In addition, specialist varieties of wax were available such as red wax and green wax – the latter specifically 'for making seals' – which retailed at twenty soldi per lb.[48] The green and red wax bought by an official of the Monte and sent to the Badia may have been for clerical purposes or for sealing jars in the dispensary.[49]

Candles and tapers retailed at a standard price for weight according to the grade: fourteen soldi per lb for yellow wax, and eighteen to twenty soldi per lb for white wax. They ranged from the tiny *candele da due denari* (these cost two *denari* each, and weighed only about four grams – they were so small that the Guild outlawed their production in 1501, probably because they constituted a fire hazard),[50] *candele da quattrino* (costing four *denari* each, these weighed about eight grams) and small candles sold in groups of twenty-four or sixteen per lire (each of which weighed twenty or thirty grams respectively), up through to white candles 'for the home' weighing two ounces (about fifty-seven grams). The smallest sizes in particular would have burned quickly and were intended to be placed before an altar.[51] *Falchole* (tapers) tended to be larger, were bought individually rather than by weight, and ranged from three ounces (eighty-five grams) to about twenty-four ounces (679 grams). Far bigger were the heavy devotional candles called *ceri*, which weighed anything from twenty ounces (about half a kilo) up to 192 ounces (over five kilos), and *doppieri* (formed from several candles twisted together) at seventy-one to ninety ounces (over two kilos).[52] The great range of sizes for these larger candles and tapers suggests that they may have been made to order.[53] In this respect, it is interesting that while the inventory of 1504 contained a great quantity of torches, there were no candles in stock.[54] Torches on the other hand tended to be slightly cheaper, retailing at eleven to twelve soldi per lb, and weighed from forty-seven to 115 ounces (around one to three kilos). These consisted of several cylindrical candles (usually four) that were fixed together and placed on a wooden support.[55] Smaller, more expensive, varieties called *torchietti* were also available, weighing from four to twelve ounces.[56] Some of these were specifically for holding in the hand during processions.[57] It is notable that the retail price of all these products was only slightly higher than that of wax itself.[58] There was no incentive for clients to buy wax in order to make their own candles at home; these kind of savings could only be made by buying wax in bulk. Indeed, raw wax was only bought by a tiny minority of clients (two per cent).[59] Total sales in the sample year amount to only 904 soldi (one per cent of total sales), and the vast bulk of this (sixty-five per cent) was accounted for by sales of burnt or 'broken' wax to the Sacristy of Sant'Ambrogio.[60]

Given the relative simplicity of the ingredients and processing techniques, it is possible to use these retail prices to make a rough estimate of the profit that the apothecary could make on wax products. Although there are evident risks in comparing wholesale and retail prices from different years, the margin on wax products can be estimated at around twenty per cent. Applying this to total retail sales (see Table 6.1), gives approximate profits of around thirty florins per annum for the retail of wax products alone,[61] around the income of a master builder.[62] Of course, there are other costs to consider in addition to the raw materials, such as shop rent, fuel and labour, and, most importantly, the typically long delays in payment. It is much more difficult to estimate margins for the other products on sale, but considering that the retail of wax products constituted only twenty-three per cent of the whole, the retail trade probably provided the apothecary with a good baseline income, perhaps around a hundred florins per year, which might further have been supplemented by earnings from the distributive trade.[63]

The function of these candles was primarily devotional. With Christ's description as 'the light of the world', the spiritual associations between illumination and devotion had roots that went back to Classical Antiquity. An important way of honouring God and the Saints was the donation of oil lamps and the oil that permitted the presence of an everlasting light before their images. Candles that could be lit as prayers were said were also very acceptable forms of worship. But there was an audience closer to home as well. As Sharon Strocchia has shown, the quantity of wax burned at funerals broadly corresponded to the social prestige of the deceased: ten to twenty lbs was the norm for artisans, fifty to sixty lbs for physicians and notaries, and five hundred lbs or more for the patrician élite.[64] Contemporaries took note of these quantities as a sign of the honour of the deceased.[65] Torches were needed for the procession as the body was carried to the church and place of

Image 6.3

Benedetto Bonfigli, The Gonfalone *or* Standard of St Bernadino of Siena,
fifteenth century, detail of men with candles,
Galleria Nazionale dell'Umbria, Perugia, Italy. The Bridgeman Art Library.

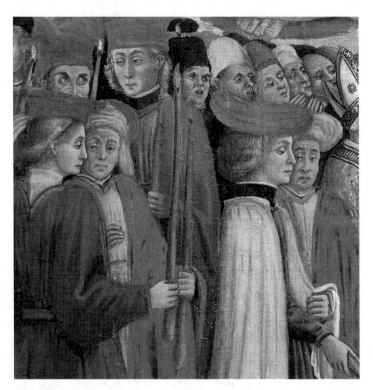

burial and for any vigil that might take place. Fifteenth-century images, such
as those commemorating the burial of St Francis, offer suggestions as to how
these long torches may have been used during the ceremony, while others
may have been left to burn in front of altars during the burial or
commemorative mass (Images 6.3 and 6.4). Jean Fouquet's illumination of
the service for the dead reveals just how elaborate such spectacles could be,
with the family coat-of-arms draped from large candles held proudly by the
accompanying mourners (see Image 6.5).

At the Giglio, the greatest volume was the 218 lbs (nearly seventy-five
kg) of candles, tapers and torches bought by Giovanni Niccolini for his
father's funeral, a visible sign of the family's prestige.[66] On a more modest
scale, Giovanni and Ser Girolamo di Bartolomeo, *bicchierai* (glassmakers)

Image 6.4

Domenico Ghirlandaio, The Death of St Francis,
scene from a cycle of the Life of St Francis of Assisi, 1486 (fresco), Sassetti Chapel,
Santa Trinita, Florence, Italy. The Bridgeman Art Library.

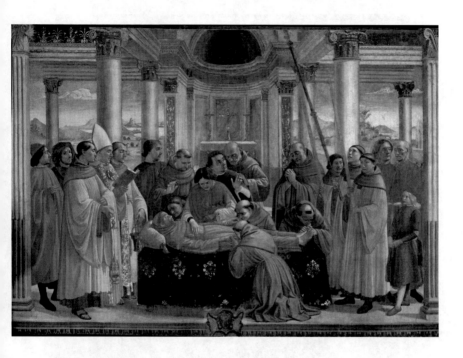

bought nearly forty lbs of 'big new torches' for the funeral of their father,[67] and the *galigaio* (leather-worker) Andrea di Carlo spent around 177 soldi for his brother's funeral on more than twelve lbs (just over four kilos) of candles, tapers and 'used torches', along with sixteen torch poles, a quantity appropriate for an artisan.[68] Although candles, tapers and torches were a costly luxury, these examples show that artisans were not entirely excluded from the market. The financial and social power involved in organising a great procession and burning large quantities of wax was an important marker of social prestige that remained beyond the reach of the bulk of populace, but the profile of consumption for these products was fairly similar to that for the shop clientele as a whole.[69]

Closely linked to expenditure on funerals, although less publicly visible than a procession through the streets with the bier, was the purchase of wax for masses for the dead.[70] Niccolò Guntini bought nearly fifteen lbs of

Image 6.5

Jean Fouquet, Service for the Dead,
c.*1480. Musee Conde, Chantilly, Ms 71 fol.27 Giraudon,
The Bridgeman Art Library* .

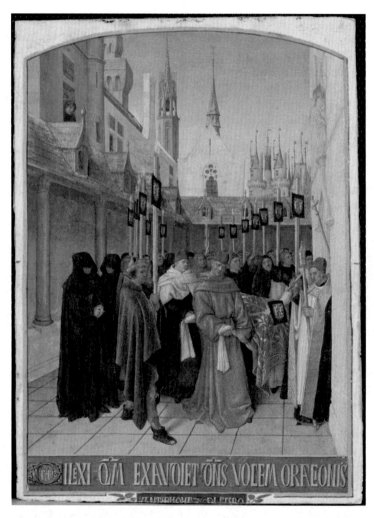

candles and tapers 'for masses',[71] and Mona Silvaggia, the widow of Filippo
Strozzi, bought twelve lbs of candles and yellow tapers to say a mass for her
dead husband.[72] Similarly, almost a week after his mother-in-law's funeral,
Antonio del Caccia returned to the shop to buy candles and tapers for a mass

for her soul.[73] Florentines took pride in spending appropriately for these functions and were careful to note their expenditure for posterity, as when Luca da Panzano recorded in his journal that he had held a mass for his wife's soul at Santa Croce in 1445 'with candles and as much pomp as possible'.[74] In this mercantile culture, the prospects for the deceased soul, the honour of the family and the devotion of the donor were in some way *quantified* through the amount of wax burned and money spent.[75]

The sort of 'conspicuous consumption' associated particularly with funeral processions, and masses for the dead to a lesser extent, was not always uncritically accepted. In a republican context there was some aversion to excessive spending of this sort, particularly when people were felt to have overstepped their social grade. Sumptuary limits were imposed on funerals, although in no very rigid fashion, since people were able to purchase exemptions from the restrictions, in effect reducing the legislation to a sort of tax on funerals. Strocchia suggests that the purchase of such exemptions, although initially marked by a fairly broad social participation, shifted towards a more polarised divide between the élite and populace by the mid-fifteenth century, with only a small minority of families willing or able to afford the expense of a really showy funeral.[76] There are also some indications of a growing doubt about the spiritual efficacy of such actions. The burning of candles came under increasing criticism in the later fifteenth century, being targeted, for example, by Savonarola and by Erasmus as empty signs of outward devotion that were no substitute for inner spiritual reform.[77] Savonarola's attack was particularly pointed:

> By the ass we are to understand the simple people. They are led in the way of sin by the ceremonies of the lazy, since they are not thought fit for the worship of the heart, and must be led by masses, penance, and indulgences, and they throw away what might be of profit for money and for candles. The lazy give them council in their sermons: Give some vestment, build a chapel, and thou wilt be freed from any danger of going to hell.[78]

For Protestants, the use of candles remained a key symbol of an unthinking or superstitious religion during and after the Reformation,[79] but Catholic thinkers also reconsidered these practices in the era of reform.[80] Nonetheless, the Giglio's customers, some of whom were clearly sympathetic to Savonarola's religious programme, continued to invest in the spiritual benefits of buying and burning candles for their deceased relatives.

Strocchia shows that surplus candles and torches were often donated to the church after the funeral, allowing them to benefit either from the free illumination or to resell the wax.[81] But Giglio clients were often more concerned to recuperate their costs. This is important because it provides a very different context for the 'conspicuous consumption' described above. The primary value was the light that a candle generated and the fact that once used, it was gone forever. This was genuine consumption where the item was completely consumed in its use, leaving little or nothing left over.

However, Giglio clients could make a substantial investment in expensive, heavy candles; they could light them for a specific period of time, perhaps during the procession and funerary services or the mass, and then quickly extinguish them. The wax was then re-usable either by selling the half-burnt taper to a new customer or simply by melting it down and remaking it into a new candle. Given that the majority of the cost of the candle lay in the raw material rather than the labour, this was a very effective form of recycling.

Clients were able to return not just the unused candles, tapers and torches, but even 'burnt' ones, which the apothecary was able to resell at a slightly lower price. Comparing the value of new and burnt torches suggests that clients lost relatively little on these exchanges. Ottaviano Doni, who bought a 'piece of torch' for eleven soldi per lb, was able to sell it back to the shop for 9.2 soldi per lb after burning.[82] These items were resold again at a cheaper price, with the price ranging from eight to twelve soldi per lb according to their condition.[83] For example, Taddeo Bisdomini bought a 'piece' of burnt torch priced at ten and a half soldi per lb.[84] Buying 'used torches' offered some clients a further way of cutting costs, but most of the shop's old and burnt wax, candles and *moccoli* (candle stubs) were sold to the Sacristy of Sant'Ambrogio, its key customer for the disposal of these materials and its biggest customer outright. So, for example, in June 1494, the Sacristy bought nearly thirty-two lbs of 'burnt candles and tapers', and in October 1494, it bought forty-one lbs of 'burnt candle stubs'.[85]

There was a lively trade in such recyclable materials, establishing strong business ties between the shop and religious institutions.[86] Churches themselves could raise money by selling off these materials, as in the case of Ser Guido, priest and chaplain, who was paid two florins for supplying used candles, torches and stubs to the shop, which may in turn have recycled them or sold them to the Sacristy.[87] Candles were generally extinguished at a determined height to help reduce the risk of fire, and the wax could then be recycled (this may explain why the smallest varieties of candles were outlawed in Florence in 1501).[88] For example, the accounts dealing with candles at Rouen Cathedral even commence with a recipe for the recycling of 'used candles'.[89] The records of Florence Cathedral's board of works show how, in common with many other religious institutions of the period, it too made money from selling off used candles and torches.[90] For example, in 1417, the Cathedral sold wax offered for the feast of the Virgin Annunciate to the apothecary Matteo Palmieri.[91] To some extent this sort of recycling conflicted with the devotional functions of wax products – Guild regulations attempted to impose tight quality controls on their manufacture of candles and torches, partly to protect consumers from fraud, but also as a 'guarantee' of their ritual efficacy.[92] However, the Giglio evidence suggests that some customers were prepared to accept lower quality products in order to cut their costs.

In practice, this meant that funeral 'pomp' was available at a discount, since the value of unused or partially burnt wax goods would be deducted from the bill. The rates of return were often significant. Giovanni Niccolini returned seventy-nine lbs of burnt candles and torches to the shop after the funeral, shaving nearly a thousand soldi from his bill (thirty-two per cent of the total).[93] Similarly, Andrea di Carlo returned three and a half lbs of 'used torches' and thirteen torch poles to the shop, discounting nearly forty soldi from his bill (twenty-two per cent of the total).[94] Properly celebrating a funeral in proportion to a family's prestige could be prohibitively expensive, but returns allowed clients to cut costs while keeping up appearances. During the sample period, over five thousand soldi-worth of wax products were returned to the shop, amounting to twenty-one per cent of total retail sales of these goods.[95] Our estimate of the total value of retail sales and relative importance of wax products to the business must be corrected accordingly.[96]

One of the major expenses of funerals was the cost of buying funeral fittings, which were commonly donated to the church afterwards.[97] Again the shop offered a cut-price option for clients seeking to economise, allowing clients to hire funeral fittings rather than purchase them outright.[98] These included a canopy, drapes, mattress and cushions for the corpse, usually hired for a flat rate of around twenty-five soldi and delivered by a *becchino*.[99] Retailing these type of products may have been a natural progression from selling medicines, since the accounts show that expenses for treating the sick might be immediately followed by those for their funeral.[100] Along with the sale of candles and torches, apothecaries were therefore sometimes involved in the funeral trade more generally. This was the case with Benedetto di Tacco in fourteenth-century Prato,[101] and such items were also stocked by Leonardo Falorni in Florence in 1425.[102] However, in 1490s Florence, the hire of funeral fittings appears to have been a speciality of the Giglio, since the shop regularly let them out to other apothecaries (usually at a lower rate of fifteen soldi, but also sometimes at thirty soldi or more for the 'good drape'), which they hired in turn to their own clients. At least seven other shops were involved in these exchanges: the shop *al canto alle rondine*,[103] *colonna*,[104] *luna*,[105] *diamante*,[106] *croce*,[107] *sole*,[108] and the shop of Giovanni Baroncini.[109]

With the possibility of hiring funeral fittings, candles, tapers and torches, the Giglio therefore offered ways of celebrating funerals at a lower cost. This is important because the expense of celebrating a funeral in relation to social expectations could be ruinously expensive: Antonio and Ser Francesco Masi had to sell all their household goods to pay for their father's funeral in 1405, which cost 140 florins.[110] One of the functions of Florence's religious confraternities was to provide a sort of 'funeral insurance' to help cover these costs for their members.[111] Deaths in the family were often unexpected, and credit was a further mechanism that helped people to confront these expenses. This can be seen at a personal level: for example, the journal of Francesco Castellani records 176 soldi spent on goods from an apothecary for the funeral of his tenant, the tailor Piero di Giovanni, 'for which I must be satisfied by whoever is the heir', as he took care to note.[112] Similarly, the journal of Bernardo Machiavelli records how Francesco Bizini had paid for 'doctors, medicines, apothecary and funeral' for Zanobi, the son of Tommaso Deti, credit amounting to eleven large gold florins.[113] Just as masters often helped their dependents to buy medicines, so they might also help them to pay for funerals. The Giglio also offered generous credit facilities to its trusted customers, allowing them to hold a proper funeral without ruinous expense. Shop credit was a response to the irregular nature of demand for apothecary goods, which was particularly marked in the case of wax products for funerals.

Wax products were involved in a variety of other ritual functions, although these were far less important than funerals in terms of sales. Candles and torches were sometimes bought singly to celebrate baptisms, and traditionally placed in the hands of the infant or the godmother as a sign of the faith.[114] Lando di Giovanni Tanagli bought a candle and a small torch 'for a baptism', along with comfits for the party afterwards.[115] Similarly, Ser Zanobi di Jacopo di Borgianni bought a small yellow torch 'to baptise a baby girl'.[116] This can also be seen in the journal of Francesco Castellani, who records buying a single taper and a single candle for a baptism.[117] Wax products also acted as ritual gifts. The shoemaker Antonio di Benedetto took seven lbs of candles 'for the presentation of the consuls', presumably marking the election of new guild leaders.[118] They might also be donated to religious institutions and leaders. Giovanni de' Libri bought a large church candle of yellow wax which he sent to the Abbot of Santa Trinità.[119] Giovanni Bettini bought three lbs of candles and torches for donation to a confraternity, 'the company of purity'.[120]

It is, however, difficult to relate the consumption of wax products to the ritual calendar. The most notable exception was 24 June, the key Florentine festival of the nativity of San Giovanni. On the day of the feast, the apprentice Girolamo da Volterra took a yellow candle to offer to San

Giovanni at Montescudaio, where there was a Benedictine monastery.[121] The communes of Tremuleto and Favuglia bought candles for the feast of San Giovanni, presumably obtaining these at the shop prior to their traditional presentation in the procession as tokens of their submission to Florentine power.[122] In the early fifteenth century, Goro Dati described how in this procession 'a marvellous and countless quantity of large candles are offered, some of 100 lb, some of 50 lb, some more, some less, down to 10 lb. They are carried, lit, by the peasants of the villages who offer them.'[123] Candles were also sold in somewhat higher numbers around the feast of All Souls, the traditional festival for the dead.[124] A few other religious feasts are also mentioned – Mona Silvaggia bought four tapers 'for the Feast of the Assumption',[125] while the nuns of San Niccolò 'della via del cocomero' bought tapers and incense to 'raise the Lord' on Pentecost.[126] Beside these few examples, there was little relationship between consumption and the liturgical calendar. Surprisingly, there is no indication that clients bought large quantities of candles for Candlemas, a feast traditionally celebrated with great displays of blessed candles.[127] The only purchase linked to this feast was when the Spaniard Giovanni Salamanca bought four lbs of white candles,[128] which he had decorated by a painter.[129] The consumption of wax products was primarily linked to private funerals and only to a minor extent to public rituals.

Conclusion

This chapter has analysed the retail market for wax and wax products as a case study in the irregular nature of demand, showing how it varied principally in response to irregular events in private family life rather than season or public rituals. As we shall see, in contrast to this, products such as medicines constituted a more steady background demand, constant throughout the year, with some seasonal variation. Wax and wax products were distinct because they were so expensive, and because they were required in such large quantities relative to goods such as foodstuffs and medicines. In the absence of alternative forms of support (such as a confraternity), shop credit was a key mechanism that permitted trusted clients to confront the costs of a funeral appropriate to their social station. The apothecary could expect to make a decent profit from the retail of wax, but it was a trade that required considerable capital investment: keeping the shop well stocked with wax in sufficient quantity to meet sudden surges in demand, and offering generous terms of repayment, often delayed for years. A number of features of the retail trade further stimulated demand by helping customers make a good show on the cheap: selling back used and unused candles and torches to the shop, buying inferior quality goods produced from recycling, and hiring the funeral fittings. The evidence suggests that these efforts had some effect, since although wax products were an expensive luxury, they were accessible by a clientele broadly similar to that for the shop as a whole. Artisans and shopkeepers were able to participate in this market, even if to a lesser extent than the richest families. Nevertheless, concerns about the expense and the social exclusiveness of such practices may have helped to drive the shift to new forms of spirituality in the 1490s, rejecting an emphasis on outward forms that were publicly quantifiable, in favour of an inner spirituality.

Notes

1. E878, fo. 19r, lists two 'Pentole verde grande da mele rosato'.

2. There are a number of tricky methodological problems related to drawing these boundaries; for example, it is particularly difficult to distinguish between 'dietary' and 'medical' products (see Chapter 7).

3. A. Astorri, 'Appunti sull'esercizio dello speziale a Firenze nel quattrocento', *Archivio storico italiano*, 147 (1989), 31–62: 61–2; E. Diana, 'Medici, speziali e barbieri nella Firenze della prima metà del '500', *Rivista di storia della medicina*, 4, 2 (1994), 13–27: 18.

4. J.-P. Bénézet, *Pharmacie et médicament en Méditerranée occidentale: (XIIIe–XVIe siècles)* (Paris: H. Champion, 1999), 242, the retail market breaks down as follows: medicines 72.9%, wax 9.2%, foodstuffs 13.8%, other 4.1%. Bénézet suggests such extreme specialisation in medicines was unusual.

5. The surprisingly high figure for sales of grain is the result of a single large transaction to one client, reflecting the mixture of wholesale trading with the retail records that may have been an accounting slip.

6. 3% of consumption remains impossible to assign, because the accounts are recorded in terms of weights of individual commodities with a total price for the transaction as a whole. Where particular commodities were always bundled together with other items, it can be impossible to establish, or even estimate, a price for them. This is particularly important for goods in the 'medicinal' category due to the complexity of these products.

7. The only days on which no sales took place were 24 January 1494 and 31 March 1494, neither of which were holy days.

8. L. Landucci, *A Florentine Diary from 1450 to 1516*, A. De Rosen Jervis (trans.), (London: J.M. Dent & Sons, 1927), 55–6, 20 January 1494. The terrible weather did not stop Taddeo Bisdomini from buying stomach ointment and syrup – see E882, fo. 238r, 'Taddeo di Giovanni Bisdomini', 20 January 1493 (m.f.). Nor did it stop another client from buying candles to celebrate a mass for his mother-in-law – see fo. 248v, 'Antonio di giovanni del chaccia', 20 January 1493 (m.f.), two entries describing purchase of candles 'per le mese della suocera'.

9. E882, fo. 164v, 'Girolamo di bartolomeo fortini', 28 March 1494. For the date of Easter in 1494, see G. Ciappelli, *Carnevale e quaresima: Comportamenti sociali e cultura a Firenze nel rinascimento* (Rome: Edizioni di storia e letteratura, 1997), 303.

10. E882, fo. 257v, 'Frati e monaci della badia di Firenze', 30 March 1494.

11. E882, fo. 4v, 'Fratti di San Girolamo in Santa Chaterina', 28 March 1494, 'incienso e diemoronne'.

12. Ciappelli, *op. cit.* (note 9), 20, n.5, lists trades that were exempted from feast day observations.

13. R. Ciasca (ed.), *Statuti dell'arte dei medici e speziali* (Florence: L.S. Olschki, 1922), 175, quotes 1349 statutes, 'ogni uno della detta arte possa la sua bottega aprire e delle cose della detta arte vendere, si tali cose vendere fosse tale necessità, che, se non se ne vendesse o desse, ne potesse venire alcuno pericolo'.

14. *Ibid.*, 407; Diana, *op. cit.* (note 3), 18; Landucci, *op. cit.* (note 8), 32, 22 August 1481, 'We apothecaries arranged that we should not keep our shops open on holidays till 22 in the evening (6pm), as had hitherto been the custom, but that four shops in the whole city (to be chosen by lot) should remain open all day.'

15. Ciasca, *op. cit.* (note 13), 174–8.

16. Across the sample period of one year there were a total of 6,031 retail transactions (recording all entries except payments and debt transfers), a mean of 16.5 per day. Mean transactions were 8.6 on holy days compared to 18.5 on ordinary days.

17. Mean sales were only 120 soldi on feast days compared to 285 soldi on ordinary days.

18. These figures have been adjusted by grouping all feast days together with Sundays, which allows the pattern to emerge more clearly.

19. This graph counts the number of different customers buying something from the shop in each month.

20. Bénézet, *op. cit.* (note 4), 347, found the shop in Arles was most busy during the summer months June to August.

21. Sales for 2 March 1493 (m.f.) were 12 soldi. Sales for 2 September 1493 were 2,634.7 soldi.

22. E882, fo. 238r, 'Taddeo di Giovanni Bisdomini', 9 December 1493 entries, spending 486.7 soldi 'pel mortoro della madre'.

23. E882, fo. 238v, 'm.a Franc.a donna fu di luigi mormorai e giovanbatista suo figliuolo', 9 December 1493 entries, spending 834.7 soldi 'pel mortoro di luigi di nicholo mormorai'.

24. E882, fo. 218r, 'Jachopo di ristoro fornaio a san brachazio', 9 November 1493.

25. 94 out of 515 active clients (18%) bought wax or wax products in the sample year. 344 out of 515 active clients (67%) bought goods in the 'foodstuffs' category (mostly sugar, spices and sweets) in the sample year. 435 out of 515 active clients (84%) bought 'medicines' in the sample year.

26. P. Suardo, *Thesaurus aromatariorum* (1536) [Milan: 1496], similarly dedicates separate chapters to sweets ('De artificio zuccari') and to wax products ('De artificio cere').

27. For purchases of wicks, see E541, fo. 15v, 'Zanobi di biagio daprato', 9 January 1500 (m.f.), s193.5 for 43 lbs of 'lucingnioli leghati'; fo. 15v, 'Iachopo di benedetto daprato', 9 January 1500 (m.f.), s152 for 38 lbs of 'lucingnioli datorchi leghati'. The total cost of wicks across the three-year sample period was 345.5 soldi.

28. E878, ff. 19v–20r, under 'Masserizie' the inventory lists: 'chaldara grande daciera' weighing 120 lbs, 'chaldara mezana daciera' weighing 57 lbs, 'schaldaruola di rame da ciera biancha' weighing 22 lbs, 'pentola di rame da lavorare cera biancha' and also mentions a 'stufa della ciera'.

29. C. Vincent, *Fiat Lux: Lumière et luminaires dans la vie religieuse du XIIIe au XVIe siècle* (Paris: Editions du Cerf, 2004), 116–18.

30. J. Frith, 'Sweetness and Light: Evidence of Beeswax and Tallow Candles at Fountains Abbey, North Yorkshire', *Medieval Archaeology*, 48 (2004), 220–27.

31. G. Phillips, *Seven Centuries of Light: The Tallow Chandlers Company* (London: Book Production Company, 1999), 69–70.

32. Vincent, *op. cit.* (note 29), 72.

33. 94 out of 515 active clients (18%) bought wax products during the sample year.

34. B. Cassidy, 'The Financing of the Tabernacle of Orsanmichele', *Notes in the History of Art*, 8 (1988), 1–6.

35. Vincent, *op. cit.* (note 29), 113, 173,

36. See also Bénézet, *op. cit.* (note 4), 257.

37. H.P. Horne, 'A Newly-Discovered Altarpiece by Alesso Baldovinetti', *Burlington Magazine* 8, 31 (1905), 51–9: 51; E. Borsook, 'Cult and Imagery at Sant'Ambrogio in Florence', *Mitteilungen des Kunsthistorischen Institutes in Florenz*, 25 (1981), 147–202: 148–9.

38. S.T. Strocchia, 'Sisters in Spirit: The Nuns of S. Ambrogio and their Consorority in Early Sixteenth-Century Florence', *Sixteenth Century Journal*, 33, 3 (2002), 735–67: 744, 753.

39. *Ibid.*, 744–5.

40. R.K. Marshall, *The Local Merchants of Prato. Small Entrepreneurs in the Late Medieval Economy* (Baltimore: Johns Hopkins University Press, 1999), 42–3.

41. R. Ciasca, *L'arte dei medici e speziali nella storia e nel commercio fiorentino dal secolo XII al XV* (Florence: Leo S. Olschki, 1927), 432. Ciappelli, *op. cit.*

(note 9), 162, n.176 shows that in 1405, 100 lbs of imported Romanian wax cost 10.5 gold florins. By comparison, E541, fo. 28v, 'Girolamo di nicholo darghugia [sic]', 11 March 1501 (m.f.), shows that the price agreed for 'ciera zavorra' was slightly cheaper almost one hundred years later, at 8 florins per 100 lbs (equivalent to about s11.2 per lb).

42. E541, average prices: 'ciera' s10.0 per lb; 'ciera zavorra' s12.0 per lb; 'ciera schiava' s11.5 per lb; 'Ciera rachugia' s11.9 per lb; 'ciera gialla' s11.6 per lb. On Ragusan merchants, see J.-C. Hocquet, 'Commercio e navigazione in Adriatico: Porto di Ancona, sale di Pago e marina di Ragusa (xiv–xvii secolo)', *Atti e memorie della deputazione di storia patria per le Marche*, 83 (1977), 221–54; V. Ignacii, 'Relazione commerciale tra Ragusa (Dubrovnik) e le Marche nel trecento e nel quattrocento', *Atti e memorie della deputazione di storia patria per le Marche*, 82 (1977), 197–219.

43. E541, fo. 11v, 'Giovanni di guliano di govencho demedici', 7 September 1500, 209 lbs of 'ciera biancha viniziana'; fo. 22r, 'Franc.o di guliano di giovencho de medici e chonp.a lanaiuoli', 18 August 1501, 183.5 lbs of 'ciera biancha', in both cases with a price of s16.5 per lb.

44. E541, fo. 35v, 'Giovanfranc.o di girolamo da milano', 12 November 1502, 371 lbs of 'ciera biancha vechia' at s12 per lb.

45. E882, fo. 123r, 'Angniolo e domenicho di pagholo chalzolai al ficho', 12 August 1494, L1s1 for 1.5 lbs of 'ciera zavorra di balla', price s14 per lb.

46. E882, fo. 353v, 'Bernardo di bartolomeo doffi', 30 October 1494, 'ciera nostrale', at s11.75 per lb.

47. E882, fo. 260v, 'Chimenti di franc.o del tasso lengniaiuolo', 25 February 1493 (m.f.).

48. E882, fo. 183r, 'Giovanni di [BLANK] daruota sta al monte', 2 October 1493, 13 November 1493, 'ciera rossa'; fo. 256v, 'Andrea di simone chapponi', 6 February 1493 (m.f.), 'ciera verde da sugiellare'. Ciappelli, *op. cit.* (note 9), 162, n.176, states that the retail price of 'red' wax was s13 per lb in 1361.

49. E882, fo. 183r, 'Giovanni di [BLANK] daruota sta al monte', 2 October 1493, 23 October 1493, 13 November 1493, 13 November 1495 'sono per le partite della ciera'

50. L. Landucci, *Diario fiorentino*, Biblioteca Italiana, Università degli Studi di Roma 'La Sapienza', 2004. [Florence: Sansoni, 1985], 'E a dì 9 d'ottobre 1501, noi Speziali facemo all'Arte degli speziali che noi non potessimo fare più candele di due danari.'

51. A. Firenzuola, *Ragionamenti*, Biblioteca Italiana, Università degli Studi di Roma 'La Sapienza', 2003. [Rome: Salerno editrice, 1971], 'mi fanno abbruciar più ratto che non fa una candela d'un quattrino ad un altare!'. Vincent, *op. cit.* (note 29), 93, refers to tiny candles 'de denier' which similarly took their name from the price.

52. Vincent, *ibid.*, 88–90, on various types of wax products. *Doppieri* were formed from several candles joined together; in France these were known as 'bougies torquées', which were 'constituées de plusieurs unités torsadées ou enlacées.'

53. *Ibid.*, 93.

54. E878, there were 453 lbs of torches in stock in 1504, but no candles or tapers.

55. Torches were large items weighing 8 to 9 lbs each. On torches see Bénézet, *op. cit.* (note 4), 367–8; Vincent, *op. cit.* (note 29), 92; P. Thornton, *The Italian Renaissance Interior, 1400–1600* (London: Weidenfeld & Nicolson, 1991), 276.

56. The weight of *torchietti* ranged from 4 to 12 oz and the price was s14 per lb. Transaction 5049 for 'torchetti da tavola' weighing 4 oz each and retailing at s14 per lb.

57. E882, fo. 106v, 'Angiolino di lorenzo chapponi', 17 October 1493, L9s16 for 14 lbs of 'chandele gialle e falchole e ii torchietti gialli per imano', 'porto lorenzo suo nipote pel mortoro del figliuolo'.

58. Yellow candles typically retailed at s14 per lb, whereas the crude wax, often described as 'di balle' ie. coming from the bale of wax, retailed at an average of s13.4 per lb.

59. 12 out of 515 active clients (2%) in the sample year bought wax.

60. E882, fo. 102r, 'La saghrestia di santo anbruogio', 5 June 1494, L14s16 for 37 lbs of 'ciera rotta e nera' at an agreed price of s8 per lb; 5 June 1494, L14s11d8 for 20lbs 10oz of 'ciera biancha arsicciata' at an agreed price of s14 per lb. These two transactions, totalling 588 soldi, account for 65% of all retail sales of wax in the sample year. On Sant'Ambrogio, see Borsook, *op. cit.* (note 37).

61. Total retail sales of wax and wax products in the sample year was 19,396 soldi (after allowing for returns of 5,171 soldi on total sales of 24,567 soldi). Assuming a margin of 20%, this leaves an operating profit of 3,879 soldi per annum for wax products alone, about 30 florins.

62. S. Tognetti, 'Prezzi e salari nella Firenze tardomedievale: un profilo', *Archivio storico italiano*, 153, 2 (1995), 263–333: 331, gives an average wage of 14 to 16.2 soldi per day for a master builder in 1493–4. Assuming a maximum working year of c.250 days (*idem*, 265), this gives an annual salary of around 3,775 soldi, almost 29 florins per annum.

63. On this estimate see also Chapter 3, note 107.

64. S.T. Strocchia, *Death and Ritual in Renaissance Florence* (Baltimore: Johns Hopkins University Press, 1992), 128–9. For further comparison, I. Ait, *Tra scienza e mercato: gli speziali a Roma nel tardo medioevo* (Rome: Istituto Nazionale di Studi Romani, 1996), 88, gives the example of 326 florins of candles bought for the funeral of Callisto III in 1458; D. Balestracci, *The*

Renaissance in the Fields. Family Memoirs of a Fifteenth-century Tuscan Peasant, P. Squatriti and B. Merideth (trans.), (Pennsylvania: Pennsylvania State University Press, 1999), 66, for funeral expenses paid by a Tuscan farmer in the mid-fifteenth century for his wife's funeral; P. Jackson, 'Pomp or Piety? The Funeral of Pandolfo Petrucci', *Renaissance Studies*, 20, 2 (2006), 240–52: 245–6, for funerals in early sixteenth-century Siena.

65. Landucci, *op. cit.* (note 50), 'E a dì 15 d'ottobre 1495, si fece l'onoranza di Monsignore di Lilla, e fugli fatto un grande onore. Sotterrossi a' Servi. Ebbe 280 torchi, e predicossi sopra el corpo in sulla Piazza di Sa' Lorenzo.' See also Vincent, *op. cit.* (note 29), 497–8.

66. E882, fo. 65r, 'Giovanni di lapo di lorenzo niccholini'. 30 August 1493 entries 'pel mortoro di lapo suo padre': 31.5 lbs of 'torchi nuovi ghrandi', 'chandele perimano e perapichare', L1s5 for hire of 'baldacchino ghuanciali e materassino', 2 September 1493 entries: 29.5 lbs of 'chandele e falchole perapichare', 'chandele perimano', four 'torchi nuovi ghrandi' weighing a total of 31 lbs for L18s12, thirty-six 'torchietti ghrandi' weighing a total of 36 lbs; forty-seven 'torchietti mezani' weighing a total of 22 lbs; twelve 'torchietti' weighing a total of 6lbs; 8lbs of 'chandele perimano'; L3 for hire of 'drappo bello el ghuanciale'. Total cost: 3,012 soldi. Giovanni Niccolini was Prior in 1504 and 1514 – Tratte 300414, 118655.

67. E882, fo. 248r, 'Giovanni e ser girolamo di bartolomeo di nicholaio di ghino e chonpangni bichierai', 18 July 1494, L20s19d10 for four 'torchi nuovi ghrandi' weighing 38 lbs 2 oz, 'pel mortoro di bartolomeo loro padre'.

68. E882, fo. 59v, 'Andrea dicharlo ghalighaio', 1 September 1494 entries, amounting to s177.33.

69. Excluding corporate clients, clients with surnames accounted for 58% of individual consumption of wax and wax products (10,230 out of 17,641 soldi); this was equal to their proportion for all products (58%). Excluding corporate clients, clients with occupational titles accounted for 25% of individual consumption of wax and wax products (4,399 out of 17,641 soldi); this was lower than their proportion for all products (31%).

70. S.T. Strocchia, 'Remembering the Family: Women, Kin, and Commemorative Masses in Renaissance Florence', *Renaissance Quarterly*, 42 (1989), 635–54; S.T. Strocchia, 'Death Rites and the Ritual Family in Renaissance Florence', in M. Tetel, R.G. Witt, and R. Goffen (eds), *Life and Death in Fifteenth-Century Florence* (Durham: Duke University Press, 1989), 120–45.

71. E882, fo. 320r, 'Niccholo di [BLANK] guntini', 7 February 1494 (m.f.), purchase of 14 lbs 8 oz of 'chandele e falchole per le messe'.

72. E882, fo. 104v, 'm.a Silvaggia donna fu di filippo strozzi', 3 December 1493, purchase of 12 lbs of 'chandele e falchole gialle tra per apichare e per tenere imano', 'disse per fare uno uficio perlanima di filippo strozzi'. On women

paying for funerals see S.T. Strocchia, 'Funerals and the Politics of Gender in Early Renaissance Florence', in M. Migiel and J. Schiesari (eds), *Refiguring Women: Perspectives on Gender and the Italian Renaissance* (Ithaca: Cornell University Press, 1991), 155–68.

73. E882, fo. 248v, 'Antonio di giovanni del chaccia', 14 January 1493 (m.f.) entries for the funeral of his mother-in-law 'pel mortoro di m.a pipa sua suocera'; 20 January 1493 (m.f.) entries for candles and tapers 'per le mese della suocera'.

74. G.A. Brucker, *The Society of Renaissance Florence: A Documentary Study* [1971], repr. (New York: Harper & Row, 1998), 45.

75. J. Bossy, *Christianity in the West, 1400–1700* (Oxford: Oxford University Press, 1985), 28; E. Cameron, *The European Reformation* (Oxford: Clarendon, 1991), 389.

76. Strocchia, 'Death Rites' (note 70), 121, 130; Strocchia, *op. cit.* (note 64), 128. For sumptuary laws on funerals in Cortona, see Vincent, *op. cit.* (note 29), 519.

77. D. Erasmus, *Praise of Folly*, B. Radice (trans.), (Harmondsworth: Penguin, 1971), 139, 'Think of the many who set up a candle to the Virgin, Mother of God, and at midday too when it isn't needed, and of the few who care about emulating her chastity of life, her modesty and love of heavenly things. Yet that is surely the true way to worship and by far most acceptable to heaven.'

78. G. Savonarola, 'The Ascension of Christ', in G. Kleiser (ed.), *The World's Great Sermons* (Project Gutenberg, 2004), http://www.gutenberg.org/files/11981/11981.txt

79. Vincent, *op. cit.* (note 29), 526; E. Duffy, *The Stripping of the Altars: Traditional Religion in England, c.1400–c.1580* (New Haven: Yale University Press, 1992); Hobbes, *Leviathan*, Part 4, ch. XLV, analyses the use of images and burning of candles as survivals of pagan tradition.

80. Vincent, *ibid.*, 536. See *The Canons and Decrees of the Sacred and Oecumenical Council of Trent*, Hanover Historical Texts Project, 1995. [London: Dolman, 1848] 'They shall wholly banish from the Church the observance of a fixed number of certain masses and of candles, as being the invention of superstitious worship'; L. Dolce, *Dialogo della istitutione delle donne*, Biblioteca Italiana, Università degli Studi di Roma 'La Sapienza', 2006. [1545], Book 3, 'la cura d'i Mortorij (che noi Vinitiani diciamo Baldachini) la condition delle sepolture, e la pompa delle esequie, sono più tosto conforto de vivi, che beneficio de morti... Ma vorrei bene, che conoscendosi i marmi, i bronzi, gli ori, gli intagli, i grandi epitaphij, e le statue; onde si fabricano e adornano le sepolture; a morti inutili; la spesa, che in queste vane pompe, e pegni della nostra superbia si consuma, s'impiegasse nelle opere di charità: le quali sono le limosine, che si fanno a bisognosi...'

81. Strocchia, *op. cit.* (note 64), 34–5, 128–9; Vincent, *op. cit.* (note 29), 176–7.

82. E882, fo. 16r, 'Ottaviano di Jachopo Doni', 30 March 1493, L2s5 for 'un pezo di torchio' weighing 4 lbs 1 oz; 30 June 1494, payment in form of 'un pezo di torchio arsiccio' weighing 3 lbs 11 oz, valued at L1s16. However, the price was much reduced if the goods were damaged – see fo. 23v, 'Girolamo di pagholo federichi', 26 July 1493, with a price of only 0.6 soldi per lb for 7 lbs of 'broken burnt torch'. The shop also retailed *calo di torchio*, which sometimes appeared in medicines, and retailed at the same price as candles, 14 soldi per lb. (This price is based on extrapolation from fo. 53r, 'Indacho raghugieo', 16 August 1493).

83. A similar practice is found in fourteenth-century Prato, see S. Rosati, 'Benedetto di Tacco da Prato speziale, 1345–1392: Vita, attività, ambiente sociale ed economico', graduate thesis, Facoltà di lettere e filosofia dell'Università di Firenze (1970–1), 105, 119–21.

84. E882, fo. 64v, 'Taddeo di Giovanni bisdomini', 7 December 1493, L1s3d8 for a piece of burnt torch weighing 2lbs 3oz, price 10.5 soldi per lb.

85. E882, fo. 102r, 'La saghrestia di santo anbruogio', 5 June 1494, L49s2 for 31 lbs 10 oz 'chandele e falchole arsicciati' at an agreed price of s12 per lb; 29 October 1494, L24s12 for 41 lbs of 'mocholi arsicci'. Total spending of the Sacristy on wax and wax products in sample year was 5,891 soldi, including both new and old materials.

86. Strocchia, *op. cit.* (note 64), 35; Bénézet, *op. cit.* (note 4), 358.

87. E882, fo. 205r, 'ser Ghuido di stefano prete e chappelano in sa'michele bisdomini', 29 November 1493, 2 florins paid to client; 27 November 1493, he supplied 23.5 lbs of 'torchi arsicci' valued at L9s8; 29 November 1493, he supplied 9lbs 3oz of 'dopieri chorti' valued at L3s14; 29 November 1493, he supplied 15lbs 8oz of 'mocholi arsicci', valued at L7s16d8; 21 October 1494, he supplied 38lbs of 'mocholi arsicci', valued at L19.

88. Vincent, *op. cit.* (note 29), 169 and see also Landucci, *op. cit.* (note 50).

89. Vincent, *ibid.*, 171.

90. For sales of wax by the Duomo see the online source, M. Haines (ed.), 'Opera di Santa Maria del Fiore, Firenze. Gli anni della Cupola, 1417–36', http://duomo.mpiwg-berlin.mpg.de/, index entries for 'speziale'.

91. *Ibid.*, AOSMF, II 1 70, c.14v.

92. Ciasca, *op. cit.* (note 13), 40; E. Cingolani, 'Il Ricettario fiorentino e le disposizioni relative alla professione farmaceutica', *Atti e memorie della accademia italiana di storia della farmacia*, 16, 3 (1999), 122–32: 124; Vincent, *op. cit.* (note 29), 119.

93. E882, fo. 65r, 'Giovanni di lapo di lorenzo niccholini', 2 September 1493 entries: L6s12 for 8lbs of candles, L10s10 for 15 lbs of 'torchietti', L17s10 for five 'torchi arsicci' weighing 35 lbs in total, L9s16 for 14 lbs of candles; 3 September 1493 entries: L3s17d6 for a piece of burnt torch weighing 7 lbs 9

oz, L96 'per resto di qu.o chonto del mortoro di lapo'. Total value: 965.5 soldi. This was 32% of the total cost of 3,012 soldi.

94. E882, fo. 59v, 'Andrea dicharlo ghalighaio', 6 September 1494, goods returned to value of 39.5 soldi. This was 22% of the total cost of 177.33 soldi.

95. Wax products to a maximum value of 5,171 soldi were returned to the shop during the sample period.

96. Before correction, wax products represented 28% of retail sales (see Table 6.1). Correcting the consumption figures for wax (and those for total consumption), reduces wax products to 19,396 out of 83,438 soldi (23%). To a far lesser degree, returns also took place for sweets, approximately 158 soldi in value and receptacles, approximately 61 soldi in value (see Chapter 7). The relative importance of medicines and foodstuffs increases to 44% and 26% respectively. The difficulty of distinguishing 'returns' from 'payment in kind' makes it extremely difficult to incorporate the data with the sales figures, and so we have left these as estimates.

97. Strocchia, *op. cit.* (note 64), 35.

98. E882, fo. 221r, 'Giovanni di bartolomeo baroncini e chonpangni speziali', 18 May 1497.

99. These comprised items described as 'baldacchino', 'ghuanciali', 'materassino', and 'mantello'.

100. E882, fo. 247r, 'Bernardo di piero del palagio', 17 January 1493 (m.f.), L5s14d4 for 8 lbs 2 oz of 'chandele e falchole gialle per imano e per apichare', 'tolse ghuido del palagio pel morto di piero di bernardo'. The expenses associated with his son's medical treatment can be followed on the same folio.

101. Funeral fittings were also hired out by an apothecary in fourteenth-century Prato. Marshall, *op. cit.* (note 40), 41–2; Rosati, *op. cit.* (note 83), 197–203.

102. ASF, *Pupilli avanti il Principato*, n.159, cc.143v–144v, 'Rede di Leonardo di Niccolò Falorni, 1425' also lists this sort of equipment, 'federa di ghua'ciale di drappo fighurato', 'federa di drappo righato'

103. E882, fo. 107v, 'Giovanbatista e chonpangni speziali al chanto alerondine', 18 March 1493 (m.f.), s15 for hire of 'baldachino' 'porto domenicho bechamorto pel mortoro di Giovanni di lotto'; 22 December 1494, s15 'pel baldachino le choltre el ghuanciale', 'pel mortoro di piero misero'; 14 April 1493, s35 'pel drapo bello', 'disse pel mortoro diachopo bentini'.

104. This shop was owned by the Del Troscia and had close links to the Giglio. E882, fo. 109v, 'Niccholo e baldino trosci e chonpangni speziali ala cholonna', 9 January 1493 (m.f.), s15 for hire of 'le choltre el ghuanciale e baldachino' 'porto michele di piero bechamorto, pel mortoro di m.a nana di riciardo chavalchanti'; 25 August 1494, s15 'pel baldachino le choltre el

guanciale' 'pel mortoro di lionardo giachomini'; 4 August 1492, s15 'per le medesime choltre'.

105. E882, fo. 169r, 'Morello di giovanni e chonpangni speziali ala luna', 10 January 1497 (m.f.), s25 'pel baldachino le choltre e ghuanciale pel mortoro di messer alesandro davanzati'.

106. E882, fo. 187r, 'Piero di [BLANK] lorenzi speziale al diamante', 6 March 1494 (m.f.), s25 for hire of 'baldacchino ghuanciale choltre elmantello' 'porto michele bechamorto disse pel mortoro di luigi portinari'; 27 May 1497, s25 for hire of 'baldachino choltre elghuanciale', 'porto giovanni di bart.o bechamorto pel mortoro dela sorella di ser stefano di banbello'.

107. E882, fo. 208v, 'Bernardo di giovanni mini e chonpangni speziali alla chrocie', 17 May 1494, s30 for hire of 'baldachino choltre e ghuanciale' 'porto michele becchino pel mortoro del figliuolo di marcho del m.o ugholino'.

108. E882, fo. 249v, 'Domenicho di franc.o e chonpangni speziali al sole', 16 January 1493 (m.f.), s30 'pel drapo bello le choltre el ghuanciale'; 1 April 1494, s18 for hire of 'baldachino el ghuanciale elecholtre'; 16 May 1494, s18 for hire of 'baldachino el ghuanciale elecholtre'.

109. E882, fo. 221r, 'Giovanni di bartolomeo baroncini e chonpangni speziali', 18 May 1497, s25 'per prestatura' of 'baldachino ele choltre'.

110. Strocchia, 'Death Rites', *op. cit.* (note 70), 130.

111. R.F.E. Weissman, *Ritual Brotherhood in Renaissance Florence* (New York: Academic Press, 1982), 202; Strocchia, *op. cit.* (note 64), 34.

112. F. Castellani, *Quaternuccio e giornale B (1459–1485)*, Biblioteca Italiana, Università degli Studi di Roma 'La Sapienza', 2005. [Florence: L.S. Olschki, 1995], 'Paolo d'Antonio speziale agl'Alberti e compagni ebbono a dì 27 di genaio lb. otto e s. 16 per più cose si tolsono da la bothega loro per l'exequio di Piero di Giovanni da Montechio, e di tanti mi debbe satisfare chi sarà suo herede.' The journal also records 'Al Pulcino becchamorto a dì 10 di detto g° sei per sepellire Piero di Giovanni da Montechio sarto mio pigionale morì insin a dì 4 e sepellissi detto dì, e detti g° sei mi debbe restituire la redità sua. lb. 1 s. 13 d.'

113. B. Machiavelli, *Libro di ricordi*, Biblioteca Italiana, Università degli Studi di Roma 'La Sapienza', 2004. [Florence: Le Monnier, 1954], 1484, 'mi diede in casa sua di Firenze fiorini xj larghi d'oro in oro perchè io gli dessi domane, o come prima io potessi, al detto Francesco Bizini per intero pagamento di tutto quello che lui avessi speso in medici e medicine e speziale e mortoro e altro di Zanobi suo figliuolo; e così mi commise che io gliel dessi.'

114. S. Antoniano, *Educatione Christiana dei figliuoli*, Biblioteca Italiana, Università degli Studi di Roma 'La Sapienza', 2005. [1583], Book 2, ch.18, '...la candela bianca accesa, che si dà in mano al battezzato, ò per lui à la commare, significa la sincera fede infiammata di carità, la quale ci è data nel

bettesimo, et debbiamo nutrirla, et accrescerla con lo studio delle buone operationi, sino alla fine della vita.'

115. E882, fo. 254r, 'Lando di giovanni tanalgli', 24 April 1494 entries: s8d4 for a candle and a 'torchietto' weighing 7 oz, 'per battezare'; L1s1 for 6 oz of 'anici inbrattati' and 1 lb of 'mandorle e pinochi chonfetti'.

116. E882, fo. 239r, 'ser Zanobi diachopo di borgianni', 20 December 1493, 'torchietto giallo' weighing 6.25 oz, 'per battezare una banbina'.

117. Castellani, *op. cit.* (note 112), 'À batteziere a dì detto g° j°, e per una falcola g° j°, e a' poveri per Dio g° 1, e al chericho e jᵃ candela g° j. Nota per un altra volta. lb. 1 s. 2 d.', 'A candele e fiasco j° di trebiano a dì detto. lb. s. 18 d.'

118. E882, fo. 153r, 'Antonio di benedetto chalzolaio', undated entry, candles 'per presentare chonsoli'.

119. E882, fo. 319r, 'Giovanni di maffeo de libri', 6 May 1494, L5s12 for a 'ciero giallo dacielebrare' weighing 8 lbs 'porto lorenzo di lolo sta cho le monache di faenza e tolse labate di santa trinita chome disse detto giovanni'.

120. E882, fo. 308r, 'Giovanni di ser ant.o bettini', 9 May 1494, 'per lui ala chonpangnia della purita'.

121. E882, fo. 319r, 'Girolamo di tomme da volterra nostro gharzone', 24 June 1494, 'tolse e detto per monte schudaio chontado di pisa per oferire a san giovanni'.

122. E882, fo. 339v, 'Chomune e vuomini di tremuleto', 24 June 1494, a yellow candle 'oferto a san giovanni'; fo. 339v, 'Chomune e vuomini di favuglia', 14 June 1494, purchase of 16 lbs of 1 'ciero giallo', 'oferto a san giovanni'. On the procession see Ciasca, *op. cit.* (note 13), 390; R.C. Trexler, *Public Life in Renaissance Florence* (New York: Academic Press, 1980), 257–8.

123. Quoted in T. Dean (ed.), *The Towns of Italy in the Later Middle Ages* (Manchester: Manchester University Press, 2000), 74.

124. E882, fo. 102r, 'La saghrestia di santo anbruogio', 31 October 1493; fo. 116r, 'Lapino dangniolo lapini nostro', 31 October 1493; fo. 144v, 'Bartolomeo di niccholaio di ghino bichieraio', 31 October 1493. For Ognissanti, see fo. 5r, 'Lorenzo di Tommasso di Giovanni nostro', 1 November 1493; fo. 182v, 'm.a Andrevuola de cerchi', 1 November 1493; fo. 95r, 'Girolamo di maestro piero della barba nostro fattore', 1 November 1493. On the festival see Bossy, *op. cit.* (note 75), 32–3.

125. E882, fo. 254v, 'm.a Silvaggia donna fu di filippo strozi', 22 August 1494, 1 lb 8 oz of four 'falchole gialle', 'disse per la festa delasunzione'.

126. E882, fo. 311v, 'Munistero e donne di san nicholo dela via del chochomero', 17 May 1494, two 'falcholoni gialli' 'per levare il singniore' and s8 for 6 oz of 'incienso bian, cho'. Pentecost, or 'Pasqua dello Spirito Santo', was on Sunday 18 May 1494.

127. Ciappelli, *op. cit.* (note 9), 161, 164; L. Artusi and S. Gabbrielli, *Le feste di Firenze* (Rome: Newton Compton editori, 1991), 34.

128. E882, fo. 120r, 'Giovanni Salamancha spangniuolo in chasa andrea lapi', 1 February 1494 (m.f.) (the eve of the feast), L3s12 for 4lbs of white candles. On the same day the records also note the purchase of 2lbs of cheap candles by a priest, which may have been for the Candlemas feast – see fo. 205r, 'ser Ghuido di stefano prete e chappelano in sa'michele bisdomini', 1 February 1494 (m.f.).

129. E882, fo. 120r, 1 February 1493 (m.f.), L1s1 'per dipintura di dette chandele al dipintore'.

7

Sugar and Spice

After wax, sugar was the Giglio's second largest commodity for sale (see Image 7.1, overleaf). The inventory of 1504 shows that the shop had 927 lbs of sugar in stock – about 315kg – with a value equal to about seven per cent of the total stock, second behind wax – nineteen per cent. Sugar was by far the most important commodity purchased by the shop, accounting for over one third of all supplies. Unlike wax, which could be obtained from local sources, sugar was an imported luxury that raised moral as well as financial concerns. When, for example, the Florentine traveller Leonardo Frescobaldi travelled to Egypt and the Holy Land in 1384–5, he was impressed by his first encounter with a banana, which he described as something like a cucumber, but 'sweeter than sugar'. There was a guilt associated with such sweetness: 'they say it is the fruit in which Adam sinned'.[1] He went on to describe the production of sweets at Damascus:

> [H]ere there are many master confectioners, who make nothing else and who labour to make fine conserves of sugar, honey, ginger and other things; they have there many shops that do nothing else all year than sell flowers, violets and roses and they are much more odorous than ours, and there they make the best rose-water in the world.[2]

Frescobaldi's awe at the wares of these specialist confectioners and apothecaries indicates something of the oriental appeal of sweetness in the late fourteenth century. Less specialised than the shops at Damascus a hundred years earlier, Florentine apothecaries in the late fifteenth century combined the arts of chandler, grocer and pharmacist with those of the confectioner. The production, retail, social use and symbolic functions of sugar was to make this one of the most interesting products for sale at the Giglio.

The shop bought mostly 'Portuguese' sugar, produced on Madeira and the Azores, and imported wholesale by Florentine merchants. This was relatively new: sugar had previously been imported to Florence from Spain and Sicily, but in 1471, the Florentine apothecary Luca Landucci recorded how, 'I bought some of the first sugar that came here from Madeira; which island had been subdued a few years before by the King of Portugal, and sugar had begun to be grown there....'[3]

Image 7.1

'Sugar' from Tacuinum Santitatis,
*Italian School, fifteenth century, from private collection.
Courtesy the Conway Library, the Courtauld Institute.*

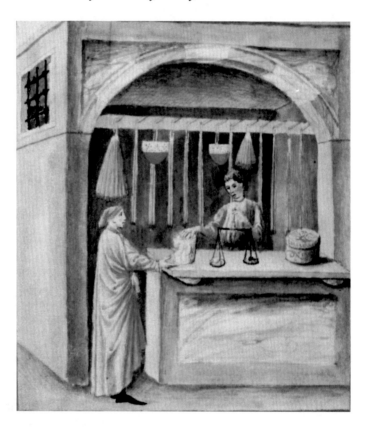

The first Portuguese settlers had, in fact, arrived in Madeira in the 1420s, and the first water-powered sugar mill was set up in 1452.[4] By 1472, when Landucci was writing, annual production on Madeira exceeded 165 tonnes per annum, and by the first decades of the sixteenth century it was around ten times higher.[5] To put these figures into perspective, the Giglio alone probably absorbed nearly 0.1 per cent of total production on Madeira, purchasing, on average, 3,716 lbs of sugar per year (1,262 kg). The rapid expansion of this industry went hand-in-hand with slave labour – the

Portuguese Atlantic colonies of the late fifteenth century have been described as the 'laboratories' of European imperialism.[6]

As a result, sugar was far more readily available in the 1490s than in Frescobaldi's day, leading to a dramatic fall in price: English data show that sugar was almost six times cheaper in the 1490s than it had been at the start of the century.[7] The Giglio data show that the wholesale price of sugar in Florence *c.*1500–2 averaged nine to ten soldi per lb.[8] At retail level most purchases were of 'refined' white sugar, with the price varying according to the grade of refinement: sugar that had been cooked once cost twelve soldi per lb;[9] 'twice cooked' sugar cost eighteen soldi per lb,[10] but most clients bought 'thrice cooked' or 'refined' 'white sugar', recommended by doctors,[11] for which the retail price was typically around twenty soldi per lb, twice the wholesale price. The finest 'Valencian' sugar cost even more – twenty-four soldi per lb. As with wax, this processing appears to have been carried out in-house, and the profit could therefore be significant, with margins of one hundred per cent or more.[12] Despite the fall in price across the century, sugar was therefore still expensive in the 1490s: a pound of white sugar (ie. 340 grams) cost more than a skilled craftsman could earn in a day.[13] In fact, sugar made an excellent gift, supplied in presentation boxes sold at the shop, such as the 'Venetian' sugar box with lock and key that was bought by a stocking-maker.[14] Yet as this example suggests, although sugar was a luxury, not something people consumed every day, it was nevertheless within the reach of middling groups of the urban population.

A much more expensive and exclusive form of sugar was 'sugar candy', large crystals imported wholesale for an average cost of twenty-five soldi per lb,[15] and probably originating in Damascus, since it was often referred to as 'damascene' candy. It typically retailed at sixty soldi per lb, illustrating the very high margins possible on luxury products, even when no processing was involved.[16] Since it had no application in cooking, it is best considered simply as a sweet. It was sometimes specifically described as being for sucking – 'to hold in the mouth' – and was therefore perhaps thought of as able to sooth a sore throat.[17] Only tiny amounts were sold – between three and four lbs in the sample year – to a limited number of customers.[18] Other medicinal varieties of sugar were those aromatised with flower essences such as rose or violet (see Chapter 8), which again retailed at around twenty-four soldi per lb.[19] An inferior quality of 'red sugar', bought wholesale at around six soldi per lb, and used exclusively in medicines, especially clysters (also see Chapter 8), retailed at twelve soldi per lb.[20] The Badia of Florence bought large stocks of red sugar during the sample year, probably for its own dispensary.[21]

Most of what was bought retail was refined white sugar. Most clients typically bought this in tiny amounts of two to six ounces (50 to 150 grams),[22] and more rarely up to about two to three lbs for a whole 'loaf' (almost one kilo).[23] Stefano di Francesco Porcellini & Co., apothecaries, bought nearly seven lbs of refined sugar from the Giglio in a single transaction, perhaps because their stocks were running short.[24] But these sorts of purchases were unusual – most client bought white sugar in small amounts, probably for use in cooking,[25] adding it to foods like a spice.[26] The contemporary dietary manual by Platina (1474) quotes a common proverb to this effect: 'no kind of food is made more tasteless by adding sugar' – what seems rather indiscriminate to us today was simply regarded as beneficial, and many contemporary recipes contain sugar along with other spices.[27] Sweet and savoury were not yet seen as contradictory flavours: the idea that sweetness should be a distinct realm of taste, entirely separate from the main meal, or wholly confined to a special 'sweet' course, was a subsequent development.[28]

Recipe books give the impression that sugar was much used in contemporary cooking, but the levels of consumption are so low as to suggest that it was actually quite unusual. Selecting only non-medicinal types of sugar, sales in the sample year amounted to about 120 lbs, about three per cent of the annual supply (3,716 lbs).[29] This was also a relatively small proportion of the retail market (three per cent of sales overall).[30] Sugar was bought by only a moderate proportion of clients, although the social profile reflects that of the shop's overall sales.[31] This suggests that recipe books may be misleading as a guide to daily practice: sugar was used in preparing dishes for special occasions, but was not for everyday consumption. The function of such books was set out clearly by Cristoforo di Messisbugo, who introduced his recipe collection by declaring that he would not describe things like vegetable soup, which 'any vile woman knows how to make perfectly well', but only the 'most notable and important dishes', the sorts of things used to make a feast.[32]

The most obvious alternative to sugar was honey, which was also sold at the Giglio. Despite being much cheaper than sugar, with a retail price of around three soldi per lb, sales were even lower, amounting to just over sixty lbs in the sample year, making honey insignificant for the retail trade as a whole.[33] There is therefore no indication that honey was a popular alternative to expensive sugar, or that the poor bought honey while the rich bought sugar. However, it should be remembered that Florentine consumers were probably able to obtain honey from their own estates, or directly from local producers, just as the shop itself obtained supplies from nearby areas such as San Donnino, San Casciano, Calcinaia, and San Gallo.[34] This is a clear indication that, at least from the point of view of retail, the apothecary shop was associated with exotica rather than everyday products, which could be obtained elsewhere at lower prices or made at home. It was primarily a place for special, unusual products, whose symbolic power was related to their rarity. Similarly, contemporary recipe books listed foods for special occasions rather than for everyday consumption, and they too placed the emphasis on sugar, although honey was sometimes mentioned as a cheap alternative.[35] Dishes involving sugar, which would need to be obtained from a specialist supplier, were potent symbols used to mark special events and a family's social status.

A similar pattern to sugar is found with spices, which were also prominent in the inventory, constituting 4.5 per cent of the value of stock (see Tables 7.1 and 7.2, overleaf). The most important were ginger and pepper, with cinnamon, cloves and saffron of lesser importance.[36] Spices accounted for twelve per cent of wholesale supplies, consisting mostly of pepper, though saffron and ginger were also important, and there were minor amounts of cloves, cinnamon and nutmeg.[37] Turnover was probably particularly high for pepper, saffron and nutmeg, where annual supplies greatly exceeded stocks; by contrast, cinnamon and ginger were probably fairly slow-moving. As with sugar, these spices were mostly obtained from Florentine trading companies, with the notable exception of saffron, which was produced locally.

Although there was no expansion of production, as in the case of sugar, the fifteenth century was generally a positive period for the spice trade, largely as a result of the efforts of Venetian merchants. Florence saw some expansion of its maritime trade after acquiring the port of Livorno in 1411,[38] but it remained dependent on Venice for the majority of its spice supplies, transported overland via Ferrara or Faenza.[39] Tuscan apothecaries sometimes even travelled to Venice in person to acquire supplies, as did the apothecary Antonio Domenichi of Pistoia in 1428.[40] Although Tommaso di Giovanni normally obtained his supplies in Florence from merchants there, in 1491 his son Lorenzo went to Venice to buy supplies in the company of Ferrando di Castro, a Spanish carpenter.[41] As Venetian merchants consolidated their trade routes – mainly through Alexandria, and, to a much lesser extent, Beirut – the supply of pepper and other spices expanded, leading to a steady fall in prices across the fifteenth century.[42] Pepper prices fell by about fifty per cent over the period 1420–50, only increasing after 1498, when the opening of the Cape Route disrupted the existing channels of supply and caused prices to increase.[43] Comparison of the retail price (1493–4) with the wholesale (1500–2) and inventory prices (1504) shows some of the impact of the increase in prices after 1498, a factor which should be borne in mind when comparing prices across the columns for pepper and other exotic spices that tended to travel in the same cargoes.

Table 7.1

Spices: Comparison of Data from the Inventory and Wholesale Records

	Weight (lbs)	Value (soldi)	% of total value of spices	Average Price (soldi per lb)
Inventory				
Pepper	39.0	1,326	30%	34.0
Saffron	1.1	153.5	4%	139.5
Ginger	114.2	1,998	46%	17.5
Cloves	12.4	209.5	5%	16.9[44]
Cinnamon	13.5	584	13%	43.3
Nutmeg	0.3	12	0%	40.0
Cardamom	-	-	0%	-
Galingale	-	-	0%	-
Coriander	3.0	3	0%	1.0
Cumin	0.7	2.7	0%	3.8
'Fine Spices'	2.0	80	2%	40.0
'Camelline Spices'	0.3	10	0%	33.3
'Mixed' Spices	-	-	0%	-
Total	186.5	4,378.7	100%	
Wholesale supplies				
Pepper	210.0	6,642.3	58%	31.6
Saffron	13.7	1,808.0	16%	132.3
Ginger	70.0	1,466.5	13%	21.0
Cloves	14.7	698.5	6%	47.6[45]
Cinnamon	8.3	466.7	4%	56.0
Nutmeg	10.6	297.1	3%	28.1
Cardamom	0.2	13.3	0%	60.0
Galingale	0.2	7.3	0%	44.0
Coriander	1.0	2.0	0%	2.0
Cumin	0.3	1.7	0%	5.0
'Fine Spices'	-	-	0%	-
'Camelline Spices'	-	-	0%	-
'Mixed' Spices	-	-	0%	-
Total	329.0	11,403.4	100%	

Table 7.2

Spices: Data from Retail Records

	Retail Sales (soldi)	% of total sales of spices	Retail Price (soldi per lb)
Pepper	792	38%	24 to 28
Saffron	172	8%	c.288
Ginger	47	2%	24 to 64[46]
Cloves	76	4%	72 to 80[47]
Cinnamon	158	8%	96
Nutmeg	28	1%	s1 each
Cardamom	-	0%	
Galingale	-	0%	
Coriander	-	0%	3
Cumin	2	0%	8
'Fine Spices'	607	29%	48
'Camelline Spices'	96	5%	
'Mixed' Spices	86	4%	
Total	2,064	100%	

As with sugar, retail sales of spices at the Giglio amounted to a small proportion of the whole, only 2,065 soldi (two per cent of sales). Throughout this book we have preferred to translate *speziale* as 'apothecary' rather than 'spicer', because the retail of spices was so insignificant compared to other products such as medicines or sweets. Of these spices, the most important was pepper. The shop purchased, on average, 210 lbs of peppercorns per annum, by far the bulk of its supply of spices (fifty-eight per cent of the total). Pepper was also the best-selling spice in terms of retail (thirty-eight per cent of sales),[48] but the volume of sales was much lower, only thirty-three lbs in the sample year. Most of the pepper bought by the shop must have been distributed in bulk, or used in manufacturing. It was the cheapest exotic spice on sale at the Giglio, retailing at around twenty-four soldi per lb for ground pepper, and twenty-eight soldi per lb for whole pepper, making it a little more expensive than the best sugar.[49] It has been suggested that because the price of pepper fell across the fifteenth century, it came to be used much more widely, and began to lose something of its exotic appeal, with élite consumers shifting to more exclusive spices such as clove, nutmeg and cinnamon.[50] The Giglio evidence supports this to some extent, because although pepper was bought by only a limited number of clients (seven per cent, much lower than sugar),[51] these tended to be from lower social groups.[52] Although pepper was by no means an item of mass consumption, it was no longer an exclusive status symbol.

Other spices were far less important in terms of sales. Saffron, which comes from the stamens of the crocus and was collected in the nearby Val d'Elsa,[53] was by far the most expensive spice, retailing at 288 soldi per lb,[54] amounting to about nine per cent of sales.[55] It was bought by only a tiny minority of clients, and despite its very high price, there was a pronounced tendency toward lower social groups, as found with pepper.[56] However, consumption is likely to have been higher than Giglio figures suggest, because clients could have obtained saffron from alternative local sources – some clients even used saffron to help pay their bill.[57] Cinnamon, also fairly costly at ninety-six soldi per lb, was of similar importance, at eight per cent of sales.[58] Of much lesser importance were cloves (four per cent),[59] ginger (two per cent),[60] and nutmeg (one per cent, always sold whole by number). The shop also bought in very small quantities of galingale and cardamom, but since neither of these were kept in stock or retailed to clients their use was probably confined to the manufacture of drugs. Finally, locally produced 'spices' such as coriander and cumin, despite being very cheap, were almost totally insignificant in terms of the retail market, although the former was an extremely important ingredient in confectionery, as we shall see.[61]

Rather than buying individual spices, clients often preferred to buy ready-made mixtures of spices composed by the apothecary himself. The most popular was 'fine' spices (thirty per cent of the retail market), which cost about twice as much as pepper.[62] Another, less popular, mixture was 'camelline spices'.[63] In addition to these standard types, many clients had special mixtures made to order, such as 'nutmeg, cloves and pepper', or 'saffron, pepper and spice'.[64] The consumption of blended spices helps to explain some of the discrepancy between stocks and retail sales, particularly striking in the case of ginger (forty-six per cent of stock but only three per cent of retail sales), which was a key ingredient of both 'fine' and 'camelline' spices. These mixtures were always made in the shop rather than being bought in, and therefore do not appear among the wholesale supplies. Only small quantities appear in the inventory because such mixtures would have had a very limited shelf life.

Spices were primarily bought by clients for use in cooking, as when the Badia of Florence bought one and a half lbs of currants and a half lb of fine spices 'for the kitchen'.[65] However, for most clients, the consumption of spices was confined to special celebrations rather than constituting a regular part of the diet, as when Fruosino da Verrazzano bought pepper, cinnamon and cloves for his sister's wedding, along with sweets.[66] Most clients bought spices in small quantities in powdered form, suggesting that consumption was linked to specific events, since the aroma would quickly fade.[67] Cloves and cinnamon were almost always bought as powders, for example. The main exception was pepper, which retailed mostly as peppercorns, suggesting that some households kept a stock that could be ground for use as required.[68] Again, this suggests that the richly spiced recipes found in contemporary cookbooks were probably for special occasions rather than the everyday diet.[69] There is also some indication that people adjusted their consumption of festive foods according to season. Sales of 'fine spices', for example, although spread across the year, were highest in the autumn and winter.[70] The few sales of ginger were almost entirely concentrated in the period October to January,[71] while sales of pepper were highest in October and November.[72] This corresponds to the idea of balancing the cold and wet season by eating hot and dry foods.[73]

Overall, this evidence suggests that spices were a niche product for the Giglio. Only a modest proportion of clients (sixteen per cent) bought spices during the sample year,[74] fewer than those who bought wax products, and fewer than those who bought sugar. People tended to buy spices occasionally, linked to special occasions, rather than on a regular basis, with the exception of a tiny minority of clients such as the Badia of Florence, by far the biggest customer for spices.[75] This suggests that spices, even pepper, remained a luxury, rather than something for everyday use.[76] However, there is no indication that this was a luxury restricted to the élite: spices were available to a minority of middling clients from across a fairly broad social range, excluding only those clients who used the shop solely to buy medicines.[77]

The quantities of sugar, honey and spices bought by the shop far exceeded the small amounts that were retailed directly to clients. As suggested in the previous chapter, much of this was related to the shop's bulk distributive trade, supplying other businesses in Florence as well as the wider region. The retail records contain only a few examples of this side of the business, probably entered there by error, as in the case of 103 lbs of Madeira sugar sold to Agnolo Acciaiuoli. This was a bulk transaction, far exceeding the ordinary volumes sold at retail, and the price was therefore much lower, only eight soldi per lb.[78] A considerable proportion of these commodities must also have been used in manufacturing, although it is impossible to estimate this since we lack precise details of the composition of most of these products. These included medicinal products such as syrups, purges, clysters electuaries and juleps. In addition, sugar, honey and spices was also used to make sweets. It is clear from the wholesale records that sweets were hardly ever bought in and so must have been manufactured on the premises.[79]

The data suggest that much more sugar, spice and honey was consumed in the form of sweets than in their raw form. Sweets were certainly far more important than sugar and spices in terms of the retail market (thirteen per cent of all sales compared to four per cent for sugar and two per cent for spices), about three times as much, and they were bought by a wider range of customers.[80] Sales of sweets far exceeded the stocks in the inventory, suggesting a high turnover and regular production.[81] Although medicines dominated the retail trade and the Giglio should not, therefore, be considered *primarily* as a sweet shop,[82] nonetheless manufactured sweets were an important sector of business.[83] Table 7.3 gives details of the relative importance and price of the wide range of sweets on sale, with the category 'Comfit' including *confetti, inbrattati, pizzichata* and *treggiea*.[84]

At the top of the list, accounting for over half of sales of sweets, were *confetti* – comfits made from spices, seeds or nuts coated in sugar.[85] The best-selling varieties were made from aniseed, coriander, almonds and pine-nuts, and retailed at fourteen to sixteen soldi per lb – they were cheaper than refined sugar because of their relatively lower sugar content, despite the additional processing involved in making the comfits. Specialist varieties of comfits were made with 'common seeds'[86] (ie. pine-nuts, almonds, pistachios and hazelnuts, retailing at sixteen to twenty-four soldi per lb), cinnamon (twenty-four to twenty-eight soldi per lb) and tamarinds (forty soldi per lb, these probably had medical applications), combining sugar with a wide variety of both local and exotic ingredients. They were bought by a wide range of clients (twenty-eight per cent of the total).[87]

Comfits were manufactured by placing the spices or nuts in a pan and repeatedly coating them with sugar syrup. Each layer had to be allowed to dry before the next was applied, and sometimes the comfits were heated in a stove to harden them between coatings. The forms varied according to the number of coatings and the consistency of the syrup; for example, one basic distinction was between 'smooth' and 'crisp' forms,[88] and other varieties were 'pearled' and 'ragged' comfits – the latter were to become particularly popular in the seventeenth century. These precise terms were not used at the Giglio, but *inbrattati* (seven per cent of sales), were 'smeared' or 'dirtied' comfits, made from aniseed or coriander seed and probably just a few rough coatings of syrup, costing the same as standard types.[89] Other special comfits, though not particularly significant in terms of sales, were called *pizzicata*, made with coriander seeds at the Giglio. The name suggests that these were small enough for people to take a 'pinch' of sweets[90] – they may have been similar to the sugar-coated spices served in Indian restaurants today. These were more expensive, retailing at twenty soldi per lb, probably because their small size gave them a higher proportion of sugar relative to seed.

In second place behind comfits (seventeen per cent) was marzipan, little cakes made of sugar, almond paste and – according to Quirico de Augusti – a small quantity of rose-water.[91] The shop produced marzipan in the form of large cakes, each weighing two thirds to one kilo, which were sometimes sold

Table 7.3

Sweets: Consumption 1493–4, in Order of Importance

Total (soldi)	No. of Sales	Sweets	Share	Price (soldi per lb)	
5,641	362	Comfits	53%	14–16	(anici confetti, coriandoli confetti, mandorle confette, pinocchi confetti)
				14–16	(treggiea, tregiea chon cienamo, tregiea ghrossa)
				12–16	(anici inbrattati, coriandoli inbrattati)
				16–24	(semi comuni confetti)
				18–20	(churiandoli chonfetti inpizichata)
				24–28	(cannella confetta)
				40	(tamerindi confetti)
1,936	252	Marzipan	17%	13–16	(marzapane)
1,279	239	Manuschristi	11%	24	(standard)
				32	(coral)
				48–56	(perlato, orato)
658	28	Pine-nut cakes	6%	14–16	(pinochiato, pinochiato biancho, pinochiato orato)
570	32	Pepper bread	5%	2.67	(pane inpepato)
525	67	Savonia	5%	24	(savonia, savonia frescha, savonia chon semi chomuni e mandorle etc)
350	94	Pennets	3%	16	(penniti, penniti bianchi)
74	8	Berrichucholi	1%	4	
72	16	Quince jelly	1%	22–26	(chotongniato in zucchero)
34	5	Candied fruit	0%	4	(ciederno chonfetto, ciederno e ranciata e zuchata, zuchata e ciederno)
otal 11,658	1,103		100%		

whole but more often cut into pieces for retail.[92] Around the same price were *pinochiati* (six per cent of sales), small individual cakes made from pine-nuts and sugar,[93] weighing from one a half to three oz, ie. about forty to eighty grams.

These three types of sweets in particular – comfits (including *inbrattati*), marzipan and pine-nut cakes – were often purchased together in assortments for use in festivities. In 1493, Fruosino da Verrazano bought ten lbs of assorted comfits, two oz of confected cinnamon, and four lbs of aniseed *inbrattati* to celebrate his sister's wedding.[94] A couple of days later he was back for a further four lbs of almond and pine-nut comfits and fifty white pine-cakes in a presentation box.[95] In November 1494, the Chancellor of Florence, Bartolomeo Scala, bought comfits, marzipan and pine-cakes, 'to give a dinner for the French' – French soldiers were the 'guests' of Florentine households following their invasion of the city.[96] The second-hand dealer Francesco di Francesco di Lotto bought tapers, spices, sugar and sweets to celebrate his sisters-in-law taking their vows as nuns.[97] Sweets might also be coated in gold for special occasions, as when Scala bought nine lbs of gilded *pinochiati* for the wedding of his daughter Alessandra to the 'soldier-poet' Michele Marullo.[98] Similarly Lorenzo Lanino bought five lbs seven oz of assorted comfits with gilded *pinochiati* for his own wedding.[99]

To understand the role of sweets in this context we can look at a wedding party recorded by Giovanni Rucellai in his *Zibaldone*, a hotchpotch of memoir, chronicle and paternal advice. It was a proud moment in his life – in June 1466 his son Bernardo married Nannina, the daughter of Piero di Cosimo de' Medici. The formation of this key alliance to the leading family of the city required a suitable, very public celebration, and Rucellai describes the event at length. The wedding party was held outside the house, on a platform that filled the square between his palace and loggia Rucellai, which was beautifully decorated with cloth hangings, garlands, a canopy, emblems of the Medici and Rucellai families, and most notably 'a great dresser full of silver items, very rich'.[100] As Rucellai puts it: 'this was considered the most beautiful and genteel display ever made for a wedding party.'[101] It was a feast for at least five hundred people, dancing, celebrating and dining on the platform, accompanied by pipes and trumpets. Among the details recorded by Rucellai to demonstrate and in some way quantify the size of the feast was the serving of sweets: he specifically noted how during the 'collations' (light repasts served between the main meals), 'twenty boxes of pine-nut cakes and candied fruits went out onto the platform.'[102]

The party may have looked something like a wedding feast represented by Botticelli in a series of paintings (Images 7.2 and 7.3), which have been linked to the marriage of Giannozzo Pucci and Lucrezia Bini in 1483.[103] The picture shows many elements similar to those identified by Rucellai – a

Image 7.2

Sandro Botticelli, The Story of Nastagio degli Onesti
[Third Episode: Nastagio Arranges a Feast at Which the Ghosts Reappear],
1483, Prado, Madrid, Spain. Giraudon/The Bridgeman Art Library.

Inset: detail of sweetmeats

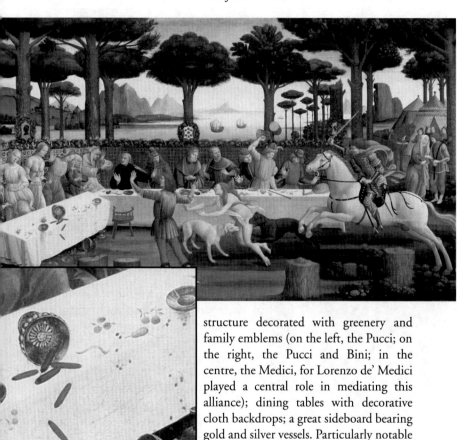

structure decorated with greenery and family emblems (on the left, the Pucci; on the right, the Pucci and Bini; in the centre, the Medici, for Lorenzo de' Medici played a central role in mediating this alliance); dining tables with decorative cloth backdrops; a great sideboard bearing gold and silver vessels. Particularly notable here is something also found in Rucellai's text: the serving of sweets to the guests. Confectionery was one of the markers used to distinguish the feast, like the silver and bronze vessels, the greenery and emblems, the cloth backdrops, the jewellery and clothing of the guests, and the forks – particularly rare and precious in this period.[104] In this painting, the sweets serve a key function in bringing the viewer to participate in the scene. As Patricia Rubin notes, the servants stand at the

Image 7.3
Sandro Botticelli, The Story of Nastagio Degli Onesti
[Fourth Episode: The Wedding Feast of Nastagio degli Onesti], 1483,
private collection. The Bridgeman Art Library.

Inset: with detail of servants carrying trays of sweets.

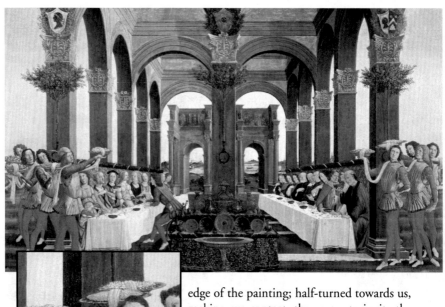

edge of the painting; half-turned towards us, making eye contact, they seem to invite the viewer to join the feast and take a sweet from their bowls. As we have seen, comfits were particularly popular for wedding feasts, and in Botticelli's illustration, the group of servants on the right of the picture appear to be carrying bronze *confettiere* filled with comfits of various types (the servant at bottom left of this group appears to be serving pine-nut cakes). On the other side of the painting, two of the servers appear to be carrying bowls of candied fruits, and these are also scattered across the table, where the guests are using forks to eat them.

Feasting was a form of public social display, the number and type of dishes were recorded by diarists alongside other details such as the number of guests, their dress, or jewellery.[105] A related social function at the level of relations between individuals or families was the role of sweets as gifts.[106]

Girolamo della Barba, one of the apothecary's factors, bought two lbs of spice-bread as a gift for Mona Ginevra.[107] The apothecary himself sent sweets to the convent of the Murate, including raisins, marzipan and aniseed comfits with added musk.[108] Presentation was particularly important for gifts, and these sweets were often gilded, for 'magnificence' and 'pleasure'.[109] Selvaggia Gianfigliazzi, the widow of Filippo Strozzi, bought a huge gilded *pinochiato* weighing nearly seven lbs (over two kilos) as a gift for Piero Soderini, the future life *gonfaloniere*.[110] The shop also sold presentation boxes for those wishing to make gifts which were probably similar to the containers shown in the Issogne Fresco[111] (see Image 3.2). Bartolomeo Lapi bought nearly six lbs of assorted comfits with cinnamon in a new box as a gift for Giuliano Orlandini.[112] The stocking-makers Antonio and Francesco di Giano bought an assortment of comfits with gilded cinnamon in a presentation box to send to their *compare* at Sesto.[113] What is interesting here is the social mix of consumers, from members of the social and political élite, such as Selvaggia Gianfigliazzi and Bartolomeo Scala, to stocking-makers, people without surnames and of middling wealth.

All the sweets on sale at the shop conformed to standard types. Although there was some variation in form, composition and presentation, such as the consistency and number of sugar coatings, the use of different nuts and seeds, gilding, and the addition of musk or cinnamon, these were the sort of things listed in apothecary's manuals. There is no evidence that the shop produced elaborate sugar sculptures, something that Mintz emphasises for élite feasting at the very highest level.[114] The diary of the Florentine apothecary Luca Landucci records with amazement the gifts presented by the King of Portugal to Pope Leo X in 1513 – the latter was himself a Florentine, Giovanni de' Medici. These consisted of:

[A] sugar Pope, with 12 Cardinals all in sugar, as big as real men, 300 sugar torches each 3 *braccia* long (about 1.75 metres),[115] 100 cases of sugar and many cases of fine spices, of cinnamon, cloves and other things, a white horse that exceeded all others for its beauty; and he also sent a moor, one of those of Calicut, 4 *braccia* tall (about 2.3 metres), with many jewels attached to his ears and all over....[116]

It was symbolic acknowledgement of the association of sugar and slavery being developed by the Portuguese at that time.

Italian confectioners were to become masters of elaborate sugar sculpture in the sixteenth and seventeenth centuries, with many leading artists involved in designing banqueting pieces, but the Giglio of the 1490s was a more basic sweetshop and drugstore. From this evidence, and from Botticelli's image, it seems that fifteenth-century Florentines served fairly simple sorts of sweets, even at élite celebrations. Gifts and banquet pieces suitable for popes and kings were hardly appropriate for a republic.[117]

If we plot the consumption of sweets over the year, there is, again, no link to the pattern of liturgical feasts or changes in season. It might be expected that more sweets would be consumed during Carnival, but average spending was actually lower during the Carnival period (nineteen soldi per day) than it was during Lent (twenty-five soldi per day).[118] The opposition between Lent and Carnival was based around the consumption of meat, wine, cheese, and fat, rather than sugar or spices;[119] the higher consumption of fish during Lent may even have encouraged people to eat more sweets, nuts and spices – all of which were considered to be hot and dry – as a corrective against the phlegmatic – cold and wet – humours associated with fish.[120]

The only identifiable seasonal pattern that can be identified is for pepper bread, a cheap product (at two to three soldi per lb, it cost less than honey) which accounted for about five per cent of sales of sweets, and which was consumed only in the winter.[121] This was perhaps because the heat of the pepper was thought to counteract the cold weather, but it was also strongly associated with the feast of All Souls, with a heavy concentration of sales on 31 October. The consumption of pepper also tended to increase at the same period of the year, suggesting that some clients may have made their own pepper bread at home.[122] Although the product was cheap, the client base was limited, much lower than that of comfits.[123] It also tended to be bought by lower social groups.[124] Another kind of spice bread were *berrichucholi*, little spice cakes made with flour, honey, and a mixture of spices, retailing at four soldi per lb.[125] These were a Sienese speciality and only of limited popularity in Florence.[126] Sales amounted to only seventy-four soldi in the sample year and, like pepper bread, were wholly confined to the winter months, October to December.

Despite these examples, the most striking peaks in demand for sweets were not linked to the ritual calendar but to private family celebrations – weddings, baptisms and the like.[127] By far the greatest peak of consumption was due to a family party held by Niccolaio Lapi, for which he spent over six hundred soldi on sweets.[128] Consumption was also linked to corporate feasts, as with one hundred pieces of pine-nut cake bought by the Guild of Doctors and Apothecaries, eight of which were gilded (presumably for the consuls).[129] Demand for sweets therefore surged in relation to private family and corporate celebrations – weddings, baptisms and the like – events marked through hospitality and shared consumption. As with wax products, demand for sweets was irregular, characterised by peaks of consumption related to special events.

Lapi's party is particularly interesting because he subsequently brought back some of the comfits to the shop.[130] As with candles and torches, clients were encouraged to over estimate their consumption needs, enabling them to put on a good show for family celebrations and then return any unused goods to the shop for a full refund.[131] Since the presentation boxes could also be returned, this meant that clients were effectively able to hire them for free for their parties.[132] Similarly, the journal of Francesco Castellani describes how he took five lbs of almond and pine-nut comfits to celebrate a wedding and later returned over half that amount in leftovers to the apothecary.[133] At the Giglio, the rate of return on sweets was much lower than that of wax products, with only a limited impact on the sales figures.[134] Nevertheless, the example provides further demonstration of how, as we have seen for funerals, it was possible to be 'flashy' on the cheap. This was particularly so when we recall that clients only had to pay for their consumption at a later stage and usually obtained further discounts when they did so.

Sweets also played a prominent role in medicine. Marzipan and comfits were not only used for wedding parties, but were also bought for sick people along with their medicines,[135] as when Antonio Del Caccia bought comfits and medicines for his sister.[136] Another client sent dragées, marzipan, *manuschristi* and nutmeg, all in a 'new box' to a pregnant woman in the country as her time approached.[137] Similarly, Francesco Castellani recorded how he commissioned an apothecary to make a large comfit 'loaf' to send to his relative Ginevra after she had given birth to a boy. This was a gift to a family and a celebration of their fortune, but it also had roots in a medical function of providing sustaining foods for the mother.[138] The records of the hospital of Santa Maria Maggiore in Pistoia show how sick patients were typically administered sweets such as comfits and *manuschristi* along with their medicines.[139] This makes the imposition of 'medicinal', 'alimentary' or 'festive' categories of consumption problematic. Dragées were, for example, a type of small comfits,[140] sold at the shop, and sometimes flavoured with cinnamon. Although they were normally bought as simple sweets, special medicinal varieties also existed: for example, the recipe book of Santa Maria Nuova includes a variety for treating diarrhoea.[141]

Sweets were not only pleasurable but had dietary functions linked to contemporary ideas about the digestive process and its role in health. As has been seen, the use of spices in cooking was limited to a small group of clients and usually linked to special occasions. Nevertheless, their consumption in confectionery was much more widespread. This reflected medical advice – most spices were considered so powerful that they were harmful if used alone; instead, their strength had to be 'tempered' by combination with sugar or honey. So, for example, Bartolomeo Sacchi warned that coriander seed 'should not be eaten alone on account of its innate harmfulness' because of its 'great force'. Instead, he recommended that it be either combined with honey or raisins, or 'prepared in vinegar and rolled in sugar'.[142] This was reflected at the Giglio, where coriander seed was hardly ever retailed direct, but commonly appeared in the form of 'smeared' and *pizzicata* comfits, as recommended by physicians.[143] The other main form in which people consumed spices was, of course, as ingredients in drugs, where their potentially 'dangerous' effects were again tempered by combination with other ingredients. Similar principles governed the consumption of spices in combination with sugar and honey in the form of sweets.

As Sacchi recommended, particular kinds of sweets were typically eaten during the 'third course', after the end of the main meal.[144] The stomach was popularly conceived as a sort of oven in which foods were 'cooked', and it was important to add different foods in the right order.[145] The function of the first 'aperitive' course was to light the 'fire', and open the digestive channels. 'Slow-cooking', or raw foods, particularly those of a cold and wet nature, like melons or salad, needed to be consumed at this point.[146] The 'second course', or main part of the meal, consisted of cooked foods, which were easier to digest. Finally, the function of the 'third course' was to close the mouth of the stomach, placing a sort of lid on the 'oven' and so preventing the 'fumes' from the digested food and 'vapours' from the wine from reaching the brain. Astringent and sour foods such as quince and coriander were particularly appropriate at this point.[147] In addition to coriander comfits, one of the other sweets retailed at the Giglio and linked to this dietary function was *cotognato*, a 'quiddany' or quince jelly retailing at twenty-four soldi per lb, which was traditionally eaten after the meal.[148] Another astringent food typically eaten in the third course was raisins.[149] These were typically retailed at the Giglio in small amounts from six to twenty-four ounces, for around three soldi per lb.[150] More expensive products that appear less frequently were currants and a variety called *zibibo*, especially the 'damascene' variety, which retailed for around six soldi per lb.[151] Customers usually bought them along with other items associated with the third course, such as almonds, comfits, pomegranate wine, marzipan and white sugar. There were also medical justifications for eating comfits in the third course, particularly following a meal of fish, when it was important to conclude with dried fruits (almonds, walnuts, hazelnuts, pistachios) in order to correct the excess of humidity.

In addition to the special functions played by 'astringent' and 'dry' spices, fruits and nuts, tempered by combination with sugar and sweets, generally were considered appropriate for the end of the meal since the sugar content made them 'warm' foods, easily 'cooked' and digested by the body.[152] They were typically eaten separate from the main meal, as part of a distinct third course, known in English as a 'void', justified by dietary theory, but also serving an important social function as the key moment of display to guests, where the display of expensive confections confirmed the status of the host (Cristoforo di Messisbugo rather disparagingly suggested that 'middling' gentlemen might have to make do with smaller amounts of spices and sweets in the third course than he suggested).[153] In the sixteenth century, this medieval tradition was to develop into the more elaborate form of the 'banquet', for which the company would retire to a separate, more private room.[154] Alternatively, as at the Rucellai wedding party, sweets might be served entirely separately from other foods in elaborate 'collations', which usually consisted of comfits and candied fruits accompanied by sweet aromatic wines.[155] Although some doctors frowned on 'collations' between meals, on the grounds that they might 'open up' the stomach and so interfere with the digestion of food that was still 'cooking',[156] others regarded them as harmless, since sugar and sweets were not really 'food' at all, but medically beneficial substances that could be easily digested.[157] Sweets were a sort of perfect food that could be exempted from the normally strict rules of order.

Sweets could therefore combine festive, dietary and medicinal functions. Nevertheless, it possible to distinguish between sweets that were bought exclusively for the sick from those that were also used for festive purposes. Certain kinds of sweets were never bought for wedding parties: their functions were primarily dietary or medicinal (a distinction that refers to their preventive or therapeutic functions respectively). The most important example of these 'medicinal' sweets were *manuschristi* (eleven per cent of sales). These were of a more strongly medicinal nature, being classified as 'cordial' sweets that were good for the heart, and unlike most sweets, listed in the *Ricettario fiorentino*.[158] The standard variety was made from sugar boiled with rose-water,[159] which gave them a red colour (linked to their 'cordial' function), and retailing at around twenty-four soldi per lb.[160] All sorts of more expensive varieties were available:[161] with cinnamon,[162] powdered coral (thirty-two soldi per lb),[163] gold,[164] pearls (around forty-eight soldi per lb)[165] or precious stones (fifty-six soldi per lb).[166]

A similar sort of 'medicinal' sweet, again made from sugar boiled with rose-water but with a softer 'soapy' consistency due the inclusion of starch, was *savonia* (five per cent of sales). It was particularly popular in Venice and might be further flavoured with ginger or sweet almonds.[167] Like *manuschristi*, this retailed at twenty-four soldi per lb, around the price of the best sugar. In addition to the standard product, the Giglio made special varieties to order – usually involving the addition of oils, nuts and spices, in contrast to the sort of 'cordial' ingredients that were added to *manuschristi*.[168] *Savonia* was more strongly associated with banqueting than with medicine, and not listed in the *Ricettario*, but the Giglio records list variants clearly intended to address medical conditions: one product made with sugar, liquorice extract, pistachios, quince seeds 'and other things', was described as an 'electuary of *savonia*'.[169] Some magisterial varieties of *savonia* even incorporated compound drugs, an effective way of 'sweetening the pill'.[170]

A further type of sweet with medicinal applications was the 'pennet', twisted sticks of pulled sugar, mixed with starch and oil of sweet almonds, probably used to comfort the stomach.[171] These cost sixteen soldi per lb and were a fairly cheap and popular form of medication.[172] Pennets could also be ground down and combined with spices and nuts to make a medicinal confect called *diapenidion*, also retailed at the shop.[173] These examples show how the boundary between sweets and drugs is a hazy one, because most medicines also contained sugar, spices and honey. In distinguishing them for analysis, the best solution is to adopt the categories used in contemporary manuals and recipe books. So, for example, *manuschristi* and *savonia* are clearly classified as sweets, despite their medical applications, whereas *morselletti*, little balls of drugs and sugar (see Chapter 8), are described as 'electuaries' in the *Ricettario fiorentino*. The Giglio recipes confirm that the latter almost always contained drugs and probably therefore required a doctor's prescription.

Conclusion

In his magisterial work on sugar, Mintz argued that the product's status was part of its attraction for the lower social orders in the early modern period. One of the reasons sugar tasted so good, in his view, was that it tasted of power. However, he regards this process of emulation as commencing in a later period. In the fifteenth century, despite the fall in price, he argues that sugar remained 'beyond the reach of nearly everyone'.[174] Rather than the increased supply widening the consumer base, Mintz suggests that the rich were simply eating more sugar. The Giglio evidence suggests, on the other hand, that the falling price of sugar in the fifteenth century had permitted the development of broader group of consumers in Florence than Mintz suggests. For sweets in particular, by far the most common mode of consuming sugar and spice, there was a fairly broad clientele. The customer base broadly corresponds to that of the shop as a whole, although with some tendency towards the middling sort of skilled artisans and shopkeepers – shoemakers, stocking-makers, barbers, second-hand dealers, butchers, bakers, painters, goldsmiths, tailors, smiths, etc. – and even a small number of maidservants, manual labourers and fishermen.[175] Among the biggest consumers of sweets were the stocking-makers Antonio and Francesco di Giano (579 soldi in the sample year), and Niccholaio Lapi (624 soldi in the sample year). Only the poorest clients were unable to afford sweets at all, limiting their consumption to medicines proper.[176] The consumption of sweets, spices and sugar was not confined to the feasts of the rich and powerful; by the end of the fifteenth century they had become more widely available to middling groups of the population. Although they remained far too expensive to be items of everyday mass consumption, as luxuries to mark special occasions, their usage was fairly widespread.

Flandrin has suggested that the taste for sweetness was something that people 'discovered' in the fifteenth century as the price of sugar fell.[177] This process of discovery may have taken place principally through the sweet therapy of contemporary medical practice. Many drugs resembled sweets, and many 'sweets' were taken by patients along with drugs as part of a programme of cure. As a result, middling groups – artisans and the like – may have been *introduced* to sweets through their medical treatment. Although sweets remained a luxury, where the highest peaks in consumption were linked to family celebrations, there was also a steadier background consumption linked to medical treatment. (By contrast, there are a very few cases of middling clients who bought sweets *without* buying any medicines, unless it was for a special occasion. The unnamed heir of the engraver Giovanni d'Agostino was a man of middling rank who habitually bought sweets for pleasure alone, but he is an exceptional case.[178])

Reflecting on this connection to medicine, this snapshot of the market practices in the 1490s can be placed in the broader context of medical thinking about sugar. The 1490s were the highpoint of the consumption of sweets, the height of the Arab medical tradition. Sugar and sweets were regarded as naturally good for the body – they were considered to be warm and moist, increasing the blood, and easily assimilated by the body, a sort of miracle food that was always useful, whatever the medical condition.[179] As Aristotle put it: 'nothing can nourish the human body unless it participates in some sweetness.'[180] Platina recommended it in terms of taste as a sort of universally 'good' flavouring for food, and Michele Savonarola, doctor at the court of Ferrara, recommended it as being good for the stomach, nutritious and clearing out blockages, reflecting standard medical opinion from Galen onwards.[181] Sweetness was simply good, a pleasure to be enjoyed happily, knowing that it was also good for the body. At the same time, with the price of sugar dropping, this kind of sweet therapy was more readily available than ever before. Not only were sugar and sweets recommended by all the best doctors, and dominant in culinary and medical recipe books, they were also increasingly accessible to consumers of middling rank.

This was to be followed in the early decades of the sixteenth century by a period of guilt about food in general. In the fifteenth century, Albala argues, dietary science had generally accommodated itself to taste and established practices, arguing that if something *tasted* good, it probably *was* good for the body. This was replaced in the rationalising drive of the early sixteenth century with a more cautious approach to food. The body's natural

211

instincts were no longer to be trusted – instead the rational mind must take control. People must *learn* to eat what was good for them, not what tasted good. Albala suggests this may be linked to the puritanical and moralising drive of the Reformation era.[182] Sweets came to be regarded as a luxury that was a corrupting moral influence.

This shift was also related to the impact of Hellenising medical theory, seeking to return to the purity of the original Galenic texts. The rejection of Arab medical learning had grave consequences for sugar and sweets in particular, which came to be regarded as difficult to digest and obstructive, easily converted into bile.[183] Sugar was generally bad for the body, especially because it 'burned' the blood and corrupted the teeth.[184] Sweets became a symbol of Arab decadence and luxury, to be rejected in a puritanical drive to get back to the pristine and healthy diet before the Fall, before artificial delicacies like marzipan were invented.[185] In 1537, Michele Servetus (1511–53), theologian, humanist and physician, wrote a tract on the use of medicinal syrups, which he argued that Arab physic had used in excess and indiscriminately:

[L]ike one returning home he has delivered the citadel which had been held by the forces of the Arabs, and he has cleansed those things which had been bespattered by the sordid corruptions of the barbarians.[186]

Servetus saw the struggle between Galen and the Arabs in terms of a battle, in which the use of sugar represented a corruption to be eliminated. These changes in medical thinking did not imply that Europeans gave up eating sweets and sugar – on the contrary, they ate more of them than ever before as the price continued to fall. But they could no longer do so with a clean conscience. Sweets were now associated with guilt, with the breaking of the rules of good diet. As sweets became more readily available, therefore, they were also subject to criticism by doctors. This may, of course, have made the sweets attractive in a rather different way, as a sort of wicked pleasure.

In the Florentine context, there may have been other reasons for sweets to fall from favour after 1494, following the expulsion of the Medici. The sort of vastly expensive wedding feasts described by Rucellai and painted by Botticelli, both linked to the Medici, were not appropriate symbols of Republican values. When Francesco Guicciardini's daughter Simona was born in 1509, he records that he specifically asked people *not* to send sweets, to avoid the expense and 'ostentation'.[187] In part, this went back to an traditional concern of Florence's merchant class to invest patrimonies carefully, rather than fritter them away on ephemera. Bernardo Machiavelli had held a deliberately low-key celebration for his daughter's marriage in the fifteenth century: '…so that I wouldn't have to spend anything'.[188] But it was also about cultivating an image of sober restraint and prudence in the era of reform. Piero de' Medici had scattered comfits from the windows in November 1494 to generate popular support,[189] but in the more sober era that followed the collapse of the Medici, the Guicciardini family no longer felt it appropriate to show off their status with ostentatious feasts. Sweets provided a clear message, but it wasn't always a positive one.

Shifts in the consumption and symbolic role of spices are less easily tracked. In the sixteenth century, spice prices were to fall further, and they increasing became an everyday necessity rather than an exotic luxury. Spices were less strongly associated with the Arab medical practice and so European medical thinking remained broadly attached to the use of exotic spices in diet and medicine until the seventeenth century, when doctors increasingly placed less emphasis on their positive role in aiding digestion and more on the need for moderating their use.[190] Such medical revisionism was, in part, a response to shifts in taste, away from exotic spices to the use of local herbs in cooking.[191] Their role as symbols of the exotic in the European imagination was to be replaced by new commodities in the seventeenth and eighteenth centuries, such as coffee and tobacco, and subsequently tea and chocolate.

The Giglio records, therefore, preserve a moment in which sugar and spices were more readily available than ever before, but in which their symbolic power had not yet been diluted by this greater availability, and they continued to be regarded as beneficial from a medical point of view. The role of medical theory in the dynamics by which commodities came into and fell from fashion is striking here. Medicine played a role in building acceptance for new commodities, constructing taste through therapy and encouraging consumption of costly and exotic ingredients. Sugar subsequently came to be rejected by medical theory, just as its consumption became more widespread. Commodities such as alcoholic spirits, tobacco and coffee were similarly first promoted by doctors and subsequently rejected as their consumption threatened to become a popular vice.

Notes

1. L. Frescobaldi, *Viaggio in Terrasanta*, Biblioteca Italiana, Università degli Studi di Roma 'La Sapienza', 2004. [Florence: Ponte alle Grazie, 1990], para 54, 'Quivi è una generazione di frutte che le chiamano muse, che sono come cedriuoli e sono più dolci che 'l zucchero. Dicono che è il frutto in che peccò Adamo, e, partendolo dentro per qualunque modo, vi trovi una croce; e di questo ne facemo prova in assai luoghi.'
2. *Ibid.*, para 245, 'Ha pella terra molti maestri di fare confezioni, che non fanno niuna altra cosa e sforzansi di fare buone conserve di zucchero, di

mêle, di gengiovo e di più cose; hanvi molte botteghe che non fanno tutto l'anno altro che vendere fiori, viole e rose e sono molto più odorifere che le nostre, e là si fa la migliore acqua rosa del mondo.'

3. L. Landucci, *A Florentine Diary from 1450 to 1516*, A. De Rosen Jervis (trans.), (London: J.M. Dent & Sons, 1927), 9, 26 May 1471.

4. H.C. Silberman, 'Les formulaires des pharmaciens Manlius di Bosco Quiricus de Augustis et Paulus Suardus et la place importante qu'y prennent les sucreries', *Atti e memorie della accademia italiana di storia della farmacia*, 18, 1 (2001), 17–22: 22; A.W. Crosby, *Ecological Imperialism: The Biological Expansion of Europe, 900–1900* (Cambridge: Cambridge University Press, 1986), 74.

5. Crosby, *op. cit.* (note 4), 77.

6. *Ibid.*, 100.

7. H.C. Silberman, 'Sugar in the Middle Ages', *Pharmaceutical Historian*, 28, 4 (1998), 59–65: 64.

8. E541, average price of sugar was s9.4 per lb.

9. R. Ciasca, *L'arte dei medici e speziali nella storia e nel commercio fiorentino dal secolo XII al XV* (Florence: Leo S. Olschki, 1927), 393; E882, fo. 255r, 'Tommaxo di giovanni di piero nostro', 9 May 1494, L1s4 for 2 lbs of 'zuc.o duna chotta'; fo. 11r, 'Ant.o e franc.o di niccholo gianfilgliazi', 31 August 1493, s6 for 6 oz of 'zucchero duna chotta'.

10. E882, fo. 308r, 'Giovanni di ser ant.o bettini', 24 May 1494, it is possible to calculate a price of s3 for 2 oz of 'zuc.o di dua chotte'.

11. M. Savonarola, *Libreto de tutte le cosse che se magnano*, Biblioteca Italiana, Università degli Studi di Roma 'La Sapienza', 2004. [Stockholm: Almqvist & Wiksell International, 1988], ch.18, 'E per somegiante dir debiamo delo invechito che quanto è più vechio, è più secco e cussì anco se varia in sua complexione, dove concludendo: il megliore è il biancho de tre cocte.'

12. The shop records some purchases of 'refined' sugar, which cost just over 16 soldi per lb wholesale, eg. E541, fo. 26v, 'Rinieri di giovanni quaratesi', 7 January 1501 (m.f.), 'zuc.o fine rifatto di valenza', costing 16.8 soldi per lb. However, the shop only bought small quantities of this (about 5% of the total), perhaps in response to stock shortages. An annual average of 185 out of 3,716 soldi-worth (5%) of sugar was bought in a refined form, for an average price of s16.3 per lb. The same product typically retailed for s24 per lb, so even here the margin was significant.

13. S. Tognetti, 'Prezzi e salari nella Firenze tardomedievale: un profilo', *Archivio storico italiano*, 153, 2 (1995), 263–333: 331, around 8 soldi per day for a manual labourer in the building trade, and 16 soldi per day for a master builder.

14. E882, fo. 309v, 'Vespino di [BLANK] chalzaiuolo', 7 July 1495, L1s10 for a 'chassa da zuchero viniziana cholatopa echolachiave'.

15. For wholesale purchases of sugar candy, see E541, fo. 9r, 'Franc.o di lionardo
    cienti da pistoia', 26 June 1500; fo. 9v, 'Taddeo dangniolo ghaddi e
    chonpangni', 9 July 1500; fo. 30r, 'Girolamo daghostino maringhi', 26 April
    1502; fo. 24r, 'Franc.o e ser piero di pagholo pinadori e chonpangni speziali
    ala pina', 31 December 1501. The total cost over the three-year sample
    period was 992 soldi for 39 lbs, giving an average price of 25 soldi per lb.
16. E882, fo. 179v, 'Ghuido di maestro ant.o di ghuido', 18 April 1494, s2 for 1
    quarro (ie. 1/4 oz) of sugar candy (s96 per lb); fo. 350v, 'Duccio di zanobi
    tolosini nostro schrivano', 18 July 1494, s2d4 for 0.5 oz of sugar candy (s56
    per lb); fo. 288v, 'Vespino di [BLANK] chalzaiuolo', 14 April 1494, s5 for 1 oz
    of sugar candy (s60 per lb); fo. 349r, 'Bartolomeo di tomaso settecielgli e
    fratelgli', 8 August 1494, s1d4 for 1 quarro (ie. 1/4 oz) of sugar candy (s64
    per lb); fo. 331v, 'Antonio diachopo nostro gharzone pestatore', 1 February
    1494 (m.f.) s2d8 for 0.5 oz of sugar candy (s64 per lb). In most other cases
    the price was s60 per lb.
17. E882, fo. 288v, 'Vespino di [BLANK] chalzaiuolo', 14 April 1494, 1 oz of
    'zuc[cher]o chandi', 'per tenere in boccha'.
18. Total sales of sugar candy in the sample year amounted to 3.6 lbs, valued at
    230.6 soldi. 37 out of 515 active clients (7%) bought sugar candy during the
    sample year.
19. P. Suardo, *Thesaurus aromatariorum* (1536) [Milan, 1496], fo. xxxiii, on the
    properties of these sugars.
20. E882, fo. 52v, 'Ghaleotto di Niccholo masi', 14 August 1493; fo. 60v,
    'Guliano diberto dasingnia', 25 August 1493; fo. 45v, 'Andrea di domenicho
    buti', 13 August 1493, specifically refer to 'zuc.o rosso per archomenti'. Red
    sugar cost around 6 soldi per lb wholesale (see E541, fo. 6v, 'Benvenuto di
    domenicho benvenuti', 8 May 1500) and retailed at around 12 soldi per lb,
    about half the price of refined white sugar. It was also used in medicinal
    drinks – see fo. 247v, 'Ghaleotto di nicholo masi', 13 January 1493 (m.f.),
    s16 for a 'bevanda' made with 4 oz of 'fiori chordiali folglie di sena e pittamo
    pulipodio uve passule e ciennamo' and 3.5 oz of 'zuc.o rosso per bere'.
21. E882, fo. 309r, 28 May 1494, L7s12 for 12 lbs 8 oz of red sugar; fo. 350r,
    10 September 1494, L7s4 for 12 lbs of red sugar; fo. 257v, 1 March 1493
    (m.f.), L5 for 8 lbs 4 oz of red sugar. During the sample year the Badia
    bought a total of 366 soldi worth of red sugar. This was an exception to the
    standard pattern that red sugar was always retailed in small doses.
22. The median weight of sugar retailed directly was 3 oz (ie. 85 g).
23. E882, fo. 319v, 'Fruosino di ciecie da Verrazano', 6 September 1494, L2 to
    buy 2lbs of white sugar; fo. 46r, 'Bartolomeo di nicholaio dalaquila', 8
    August 1493, L3s7 for a whole 'pane' of 'zuc.o rifatto' weighing 2 lbs 8 oz
    (905 g).

24. E882, fo. 144v, 'Stefano di franc.o porcellini e chonpangni speziali', 3 March 1493 (m.f.), L5s6d8 for 6lbs 8oz of 'zuchero rifatto'.

25. This was made explicit in as in the case of 2 lbs of sugar that one client sent to his sister – E882, fo. 96v, 'Giovanbatista di benedetto dighoro', 20 June 1494, L1s8 for 2lbs of 'zuc.o da zucherini', 'disse per la piatanza dela sirochia'.

26. S.W. Mintz, *Sweetness and Power: The Place of Sugar in Modern History* (New York: Sifton, 1985), 86.

27. B. Sacchi, *Platina, On Right Pleasure and Good Health: A Critical Edition and Translation of De honesta voluptate et valetudine*, M.E. Milham (ed.), (Tempe: Medieval & Renaissance Texts & Studies, 1998), 157; K. Albala, *Eating Right in the Renaissance* (Berkeley: University of California Press, 2002), 173.

28. J.-L. Flandrin, 'Le goût et la nécessité: sur l'usage des graisses dans les cuisines d'Europe occidentale (XIVe–XVIIIe siècle)', *Annales: E.S.C.*, 38, 2 (1983), 369–401: 378.

29. Total volume of 'white sugar', 'Valencia sugar' and 'sugar' retailed directly in the sample year (ie. not including sugar added to purges, electuaries etc.) was 119.4 lbs. By comparison, the average annual supply of sugar in the sample period 1500–2 was 3,716 lbs.

30. These sales were valued at 2,263 soldi (only 3% of total retail sales of 88,609 soldi in the sample year).

31. 101 out of 515 active clients (20%) bought some of this sugar in the sample year. Most of these (56 out of 101) bought this sugar on only one occasion. Excluding corporate clients, clients with surnames accounted for 62% of individual consumption of sugar (1,214 out of 1,973 soldi); this was slightly more than their proportion for all products (58%). Excluding corporate clients, clients with occupational titles accounted for 36% of individual consumption of sugar (707 out of 1,973 soldi); this was slightly more than their proportion for all products (31%).

32. C.d. Messisbugo, *Libro nouo nel quale s'insegna a'far d'ogni sorte di viuanda secondo la diuersità de i tempi, cosi di carne come di pesce* (Venice, 1564), 39v. '[I]o non spenderò Tempo, o fatica in descrivere diverse minestre d'hortami, o legumi, e insegnare di frigere una Tencha, o cuocere un Luzzo su la gratella, o simili altre cose, che da qualunque vile feminuccia ottimamente si sapriano fare. Ma solo parlerò delle piu notabili vivande, & piu importanti....'

33. Total volume of 'honey', and 'white honey' retailed directly in the sample year (ie. not including sugar added to purges, electuaries etc.) was 60.8 lbs, valued at 210 soldi. Only 19 out of 515 active clients (4%) bought some of this honey in the sample year.

34. E541, ff. 11r, 11v, 13v, 'Franc.o delciba vetturale dasandonnino' (for honey); fo. 25r, 'Bartolino di giovanni da san donnino' (for honey); fo. 21v, 'Andrea

di pagholo da san donnino' (for boxes); fo. 6r, 'Tommaso di pippo di vaggino da sanchasciano' (for honey); ff. 4r, 5v, 'Pippo dant.o dachalcinara' (for honey and rice); fo. 35r, 'Domenicho di mariano da san ghallo' (for honey).

35. J.-L. Flandrin and O. Redon, 'Les livres de cuisine italiens des XIVe et XVe siècles', *Archeologia medievale*, 8 (1981), 393–408: 403. Messisbugo, *op. cit.* (note 32), 39, suggests that honey could be used as a cheap substitute for sugar, 'se fosse etiamdio alcuno, a cui gravasse la spesa del zuccaro nelle compositioni, nelle quali è bisognevole, deve sapere che si potria fare ancho con mele'.

36. E878, the value of spices in the inventory in descending order, out of a total value of 4,379 soldi: ginger 46% (114 lbs valued at 1,998 soldi), pepper 30% (39 lbs valued at 1,326 soldi), cinnamon 13% (14 lbs valued at 584 soldi), cloves 5% (12 lbs valued at 210 soldi), saffron 4% (1 lb valued at 154 soldi), 'fine spices' 2% (2 lbs valued at 80 soldi) and insignificant quantities of nutmeg, 'camelline spices', coriander and cumin.

37. E541, the value of spices bought wholesale in the sample period, out of a total annual average of 11,403 soldi: pepper 58% (annual average 210 lbs for 6,642 soldi), saffron 16% (annual average 14 lbs for 1,808 soldi), ginger 13% (annual average 70 lbs for 1,467 soldi), cloves 6% (annual average 15 lbs for 699 soldi), cinnamon 5% (annual average 8 lbs for 467 soldi), nutmeg 3% (annual average 11 lbs for 297 soldi), and insignificant quantities of cardamom, galingale, coriander and cumin.

38. Ciasca, *op. cit.* (note 9), 495–8.

39. *Ibid.*, 539ff.

40. Archivio di Stato di Pistoia, Sapienza 389, '1426. Libro di Antonio Domenichi Speziale', fo. 15r for merchandise bought in Bologna and Venice in April–May 1428.

41. E882, fo. 113r, 'Ferrando di chastro spangniuolo lengniauolo', 29 October 1491 'per la vettura e la ghabella di [lbs 22.5] di bengui venne da vinegia di suo chonostre chose quando ando lorenzo nostro a vinegia cho lui'. See for example 29 October 1491, 16 lbs of clove stalks 'fusti digherofani', for an agreed price of 'ghrossi 3 per lb di vinegia dachordo', which was valued in the accounts at L13, equivalent to a price of s16.25 per lb.

42. C.H.H. Wake, 'The Volume of European Spice Imports at the Beginning and End of the Fifteenth Century', *Journal of European Economic History*, 15, 3 (1986), 621–35; *idem*, 'The Changing Patterns of Europe's Pepper and Spice Imports, ca. 1400–1700', in M.N. Pearson (ed.), *Spices in the Indian Ocean World* (Aldershot: Variorum, 1996) [1979]; E. Ashtor, 'The Volume of Mediaeval Spice Trade', *Journal of European Economic History*, 9, 3 (1980), 753–63; E. Ashtor, 'Spice Prices in the Near East in the 15th Century', in Pearson, *idem*; I. Naso, 'Sapori d'oriente alla corte sabauda: Le spezie in

cucina al tempo di Amedeo VIII', in R. Comba, A.M. Nada Padrone, and I. Naso (eds), *La mensa del principe: cucina e regimi alimentari nelle corti sabaude (XIII-XV secolo)* (Cuneo: Società studi storici di Cuneo, 1997), 130.

43. F.C. Lane, 'Pepper Prices before da Gama', in Pearson, *op. cit.* (note 42), 91–2.

44. This price hides significant differences according to quality. E878, fo. 14r, 5 oz of 'Gherofani sodi' valued at L1s10 (s72 per lb); fo. 14r, 6 lbs of 'Polvere di gherofani' valued at L1s4 (s4 per lb, which suggests the powder was stale); fo. 17r, 5 lbs 6 oz of 'Chappeletti digherofani' valued at L6s17d6 (s25 per lb).

45. This price hides significant differences according to quality. At the bottom end, the price of 'powder of cloves' was from 5 to 8 soldi per lb – see fo. 21r, 'Tommaso di Giovanni di Piero nostro prop[r]io', 29 October 1501; fo. 2v, 'Franc.o e ser piero di pagholo pinadori e chonpangni speziali ala pina', 14 December 1500). Clove heads cost 35 to 45 soldi per lb – see fo. 26r, 'Bernardo di pagholo', 4 January 1501 (m.f.); fo. 35v, 'Bernardo di pagholo', 10 November 1502; fo. 23v, 'Piero di giovanni derossi & chonpangni speziali a medici', 23 October 1501; fo. 21r, 'Tommaso di Giovanni di Piero nostro prop[r]io', 9 November 1501. Whole cloves cost 80 to 90 soldi per lb – see ff. 3r, 10v, 'Tommaso di Giovanni di Piero', 14 March 1499 (m.f.), 21 November 1500, 12 February 1500 (m.f.). Across the three-year sample, the majority of spending was on 'clove heads' (1109 soldi for 24.83 lbs), closely followed by the more expensive whole cloves (935 soldi for 10.96 lbs), while the powder was insignificant in terms of spending, though not volume (52 soldi for 8.25 lbs).

46. The price of ginger varied according to variety. Ground *belledi* ginger retailed at s24 per lb - E882, fo. 350r, 'Fratti e monaci della badia di firenze', 4 September 1494, s6 for 3 oz 'giengiovo beledi pesto'. Fresh or green 'Damascene' ginger retailed at around s64 per lb – fo. 233v, 'Niccholo di charlo salamoni banchiere ala piaza del ghrano', 25 November 1493, s4 for ¾ oz of 'giengiavo verde domaschino' (s64 per lb); fo. 120r, 'Giovanni Salamancha spangniuolo in chasa andrea lapi', 13 December 1493, s8d4 for 1¾ oz of 'giengavo verde domaschino' (s57.1 per lb). On these varieties, see Naso, *op. cit.* (note 42), 126; Ciasca, *op. cit.* (note 9), 388–90. The Giglio records suggest that otherwise unidentified varieties of 'ground ginger' retailed at around 40 to 50 soldi per lb, eg. fo. 311v, 'Munistero e donne di san nicholo dela via del chochomero', 2 May 1494, L1s10 for 1 lb of 'pepe sodo' and ½ oz of 'giengovo pesto', if we assume a pepper price of s28 per lb, ginger was s48 per lb.

47. Whole cloves retailed for s72 per lb – see E882, fo. 338r, 'messer Bartolomeo di [BLANK] schala', 7 January 1495 (m.f.); fo. 329r, 'Frati e monaci della

badia di firenze', 11 June 1494. Ground cloves retailed for s80 per lb – fo. 61r, 'Manfredi inbasciadore di ferrara', 2 October 1493, 3 November 1493.

48. M.N. Pearson, 'Introduction', in Pearson, *op. cit.* (note 42), xx; Wake, 'Changing Patterns', *op. cit.* (note 42), 148.

49. E882, fo. 97r, 'Guliano di bartolomeo dalancisa speziale', 20 December 1496, L4s10 for 5 lbs of 'pepe di portoghallo' (s18 per lb); fo. 255r, 'Tommaxo di giovanni di piero nostro', 13 May 1494, s1 for ½ oz of 'pepe pesto' (s24 per lb), 18 February 1493 (m.f.), s2 for 1 oz of 'pepe pesto' (s24 per lb), 11 April 1494, s2 for 1 oz of 'pepe pesto' (s24 per lb); fo. 331v, 'Antonio diachopo nostro gharzone pestatore', 15 March 1494 (m.f.), s2d4 for 1 oz of 'pepe pesto' (s28 per lb); fo. 34r, 'Tommaxo di Giovanni di piero nostro', 28 August 1493, s2d4 for 1 oz of 'pepe pesto' (s28 per lb); fo. 79v, 'Fratti e monaci della badia di firenze', 31 October 1493, L1s8 for 1 lb of 'pepe pesto' (s28 per lb); fo. 341r, 'Niccholo di giovanni s[er]nigi', 29 December 1494, s9d4 for 4 oz of 'pepe sodo' (s28 per lb); fo. 97v, 'Franc.o di pagholo pinadori e chonpangni', 2 January 1494 (m.f.), L9s13d6 for 9 lbs of 'pepe sodo', with an 'agreed' price of s21.5 per lb.

50. Ashtor, 'Spice Prices', *op. cit.* (note 42), 78; Wake, 'Changing Patterns' (note 42), 172; B. Laurioux, *Manger au moyen âge : pratiques et discours alimentaires en Europe aux XIVe et XVe siècles* (Paris: Hachette, 2002), 36; M. Balard, 'Épices et condiments dans quelques livres de cuisine allemands (XIVe–XVIe siècles)', in C. Lambert (ed.), *Du manuscrit à la table: essais sur la cuisine au Moyen Age et repertoire des manuscrits medievaux contenant des recettes culinaires* (Montreal: Les presses de l'Université de Montreal, 1992), 197.

51. 35 out of 515 active clients (7%) bought pepper during the sample year. Compare to n. 31 for sugar.

52. Excluding corporate clients, clients with surnames accounted for 30% of individual consumption of pepper (153 out of 515 soldi); this was much lower than their proportion for all products (58%). Clients with occupational titles accounted for 58% of individual consumption of pepper (301 out of 515 soldi); this was much higher than their proportion for all products (31%).

53. E541, fo. 27r, 'Pierfranc.o di michele seragli', 23 October 1501, 'disse esere di sua richolta di valdelsa'; Ciasca, *op. cit.* (note 9), 395, 582.

54. Average retail price for saffron was s287.52 per lb. E882, fo. 5r, 'Lorenzo di Tommasso di Giovanni nostro', 2 January 1493 (m.f.), s3 for 1 dr of 'zaferano nostrale' (s288 per lb).

55. The largest sale was to another company of apothecaries. E882, fo. 99r, 'Ugholino di bartolomeo di chanbio e chonpangni speziali', 6 March 1493 (m.f.), s72 for ¼ lb of local saffron (s288 per lb).

56. 19 out of 515 active clients (4%) bought saffron during the sample year. Excluding corporate clients, clients with surnames accounted for 27% of individual consumption of saffron (47 out of 172 soldi); this was much lower than their proportion for all products (58%). Clients with occupational titles accounted for 61% of individual consumption of saffron (106 out of 515 soldi); this was much higher than their proportion for all products (31%).

57. E882, fo. 314v, 'Antonio di ciecie da verrazano', 22 May 1494, payment in the form of 4.5 oz of saffron, valued at L5s8 (s288 per lb).

58. Cinnamon was mostly sold as a fine powder (114 soldi). 26 out of 515 active clients (5%) bought cinnamon during the sample year. Excluding corporate clients, clients with surnames accounted for 52% of individual consumption of cinnamon (62 out of 118 soldi); this was slightly lower than their proportion for all products (58%). Clients with occupational titles accounted for 52% of individual consumption of cinnamon (62 out of 118 soldi); this was higher than their proportion for all products (31%).

59. Cloves were mostly sold as a powder (65 soldi). The relative unimportance of cloves raises questions about the affirmation in Ciasca, *op. cit.* (note 9), 385–6.

60. The price of ginger varied widely according to quality. The cheapest 'beledi' variety cost only s24 per lb, while 'green damascan ginger' cost around s64 per lb.

61. The only definitive purchase of coriander seeds was E882, fo. 130v, 'Munistero e donne di santo anbruogio', 19 October 1493, purchase of 4 oz of 'churiandoli netti', probably for medicinal purposes because sold alongside pills. From this transaction, the price can be estimated s3 per lb. For cumin, fo. 61r, 'Manfredi inbasciadore di ferrara', 16 November 1493, lists an undefined quantity of 'chomino pesto', worth around 1 soldo; fo. 315v, 'Alamanno di [BLANK] rinuccini', 4 June 1494, 1 oz of 'chomino pesto' for 8 denari (s8 per lb).

62. C. Benporat, *Cucina italiano del quattrocento* (Florence: L.S. Olschki, 1996), 15, describes 'spezie fini' as a mix prepared from pepper, cinnamon, ginger, cloves and saffron, while 'spezie dolci' was a mix prepared from cloves, ginger, cinnamon and 'lauro indiano', especially to accompany fish.

63. BNF, Magl. XV.92, ff. 169r–169v, give a recipe for 'Spezie cammelino fine' containing cinnamon, ginger, malagueta, pepper, cloves, nutmeg, galanga, mace.

64. E882, fo. 67r, 'Domenicho di Lucha Marucielgli', 14 September 1493, 'noci moschade gherofani e pepe'; fo. 309v, 'Vespino di [BLANK] chalzaiuolo', 30 April 1494, 'zaferano pepe e spezie'.

65. E882, fo. 329r, 'Frati e monaci della badia di firenze', 10 June 1494, 'spezie fine' 'per la chucina'.

66. E882, fo. 119r, 'Fruosino di ciecie da verrazano', 10 December 1493, s8 for 1 oz of ground pepper, ½ oz of ground cinnamon and ¼ oz of ground cloves, 'per le noze dela sirochia'.
67. P. Hyman and M. Hyman, 'Table et sociabilité au XVIe siècle: l'example du sire de gouberville', *Revue d'Histoire Moderne et Contemporaine*, 31 (1984), 465–71: 469–70, reaches similar conclusions for sixteenth-century France, with spices bought in small quantities for special occasions, on an infrequent basis.
68. Clients mostly bought whole pepper (575 soldi in sample year), presumably for grinding at home, since it kept longer this way. Ground pepper (187 soldi in sample year) was also fairly significant. A small number of transactions refer just to 'pepper' (26 soldi in sample year).
69. Flandrin and Redon, *op. cit.* (note 35), find spices in around 75% of recipes examined.
70. Average monthly sales of 'fine spices' over the period March to August were 35 soldi per month, and over the period September to February 66 soldi per month.
71. 92% of sales of ginger took place in the four month period October–January.
72. Sales of pepper in October (119 soldi) and November (105 soldi) were significantly higher than the monthly average sales (66 soldi). This sales distribution is similar to that for pepper bread.
73. Sacchi, *op. cit.* (note 27), 181.
74. 81 out of 515 active clients (16%) bought spices during the sample year.
75. Corporate clients accounted for 43% of all consumption of spices (862 out of 2,008 soldi); this was significantly higher than their proportion for all products (18%). Most of this (76%) was accounted for by the Badia of Florence (see E882, ff. 34v, 79v, 220v, 257v, 309r, 329r, 342v, 350r), which spent 657 soldi on spices in the sample year, and the rest (22%) by the convent of San Niccolò (see ff. 68v, 311v, 'Munistero e donne di san nicholo dela via del chochomero'), which spent 190 soldi on spices in the sample year.
76. J.-P. Bénézet, *Pharmacie et médicament en Méditerranée occidentale: (XIIIe–XVIe siècles)* (Paris: H. Champion, 1999), 334.
77. Clients with sureties accounted for 2% of individual consumption of spices (19 out of 1,180 soldi); this was lower than their proportion for all products (7%). Clients with surnames accounted for 35% of individual consumption of spices (413 out of 1,180 soldi); this was much lower than their proportion for all products (58%). Clients with occupational titles accounted for 54% of individual consumption of spices (638 out of 1,180 soldi); this was much higher than their proportion for all products (31%). However, because the

total amount of spices retailed in the sample year is small, and the number of clients involved so low, this data must be regarded with caution.

78. E882, fo. 343r, 'Angniolo di lodovicho accaiuoli', 9 July 1494, L40 for 103 lbs of 'zuc[cher]o di madera' (s8 per lb).

79. There are a few one-off cases of purchases that may represent stop-gaps to meet demand when stocks were exhausted, e.g. E541, fo. 19r, 'Franc.o epulinari di Filippo di Salamone del charbo e chonpangni speziali', 18 March 1500 (m.f.), purchase of 21 soldi-worth of marzipan; fo. 3r, 23v, 'Piero di giovanni derossi & chonpangni speziali a medici', 27 January 1499 (m.f.), 17 June 1502, purchase of 12 soldi-worth of 'channella chonfetta' and 17 soldi-worth of 'semi chomuni chonfetti'.

80. Total sales of sweets in the sample year amounted to 11,658 soldi, 13% of the total. 221 out of 515 active clients (43%) bought sweets during the sample year.

81. E878, the value of sweets in the inventory in descending order, out of a total value of 1,666 soldi: comfits 82% (150 lbs valued at 1,369 soldi), quince *cotognato* 10% (19 lbs valued at 171 soldi), candied fruit 5% (10 lbs valued at 80 soldi), and insignificant quantities of marzipan, pennets and *savonia*.

82. Silberman, *op. cit.* (note 4), 21. By the seventeenth century, the distinction between candy-makers and apothecaries was widening, leading to guild disputes – see E.S. Cohen, ' Miscarriages of Apothecary Justice: Un-separate Spaces of Work and Family in Early Modern Rome', *Renaissance Studies*, 21, 4 (2007), 480-504.

83. Q. Augusti, *Lumen apothecariorum cum certis expositionibus* (Venice, 1495), ch. 13, fo. 35v, 'de artificio zucchari', contains 31 recipes for sweets, including 'savonia', 'manuschristi', 'pignocata', 'morsellata', 'zingiberata', 'penidiis', 'marzapanis', 'codognata', 'rancettis'.

84. Including *confetti* (sales of 4,738 soldi in 250 transactions), *inbrattati* (sales of 839 soldi in 78 transactions), *pizzichata* (sales of 64 soldi in 10 transactions), and *treggiea* (sales of 520 soldi in 24 transactions).

85. Sacchi, *op. cit.* (note 27), 157, on sugar, 'By melting it, we make almonds (softened and cleaned in water), pine nuts, hazelnuts, coriander, anise, cinnamon and many other things into sweets [*bellaria*]'

86. *Ricettario fiorentino*, (Florence: Compagnia del Drago, 1499), f.22, describes the 'hot' seeds as the 'semi chomuni maggiori, cioe pinocchi, ma'dorle & pistacchi, o nocciuole'. Another group were the 'cold' common seeds – *ibid.*, f.13 describes the 'minori' as 'lactugha, schariola, invidia, porcellana', and the 'maggiori' as 'Cedrioli, melloni, poponi, zuccha'.

87. 142 out of 515 active clients (28%) bought comfits (broadly defined – see n. 84)

88. Augusti, *op. cit.* (note 83), ch. 13, fo. 35v, 'Ad faciendum coriandros folios', 'Ad faciendum coriandros crispos'. The recipes include coriander seeds,

cinnamon, almonds, orange peel, clove, aniseed, pine-nuts, and hazelnuts. See also Suardo, *op. cit.* (note 19), fo. xxxiii.

89. *Inbrattati* are not listed in Augusti, *op. cit.* (note 83). However, they appear to have been an alternative form of 'smeared' comfits, only roughly coated in syrup. F. Castellani, *Quaternuccio e giornale B (1459–1485)*, Biblioteca Italiana, Università degli Studi di Roma 'La Sapienza', 2005. [Florence: L.S. Olschki, 1995], entry for 8 May 1460, 'E insin a dì detto on. 6 d'anici inbrattati e on. 6 di coriandoli d'una choverta: mandò per essi la Lena; recò Giovampiccino. lb.'

90. Ortensio Landi in E. Faccioli (ed.), *L'arte della cucina in Italia* (Turin: Einaudi, 1992), 278, describes 'piccicata' as a speciality of Foligno.

91. Augusti, *op. cit.* (note 83), ch.13, fo. 37, 'Ad faciendum marzapanum', gives a recipe containing 5 lbs of almonds and 5 lbs of sugar, with a small quantity of rose-water added. See also Suardo, *op. cit.* (note 19), fo. xxxiiii, (which appears to be copied from Augusti) and Benporat, *op. cit.* (note 62), 205–6.

92. The *torte* (cakes) typically weighed from 24 to 33 oz, ie. 0.68–0.93 kg, but were often cut into pieces for retail.

93. E882, *Pinochiati* typically weighed from 1.5 to 2.75 oz each, i.e. around 40–80 g. Augusti, *op. cit.* (note 83), ch.13, fo. 36, 'Ad faciendum pignochatam'. Sacchi, *op. cit.* (note 27), 177, on pine-nut cakes, 'Sugar is melted, and pine nuts are rolled in it with a scoop and made into the shape of a pastille [*pastilli*].'.

94. E882, fo. 119r, 'Fruosino di Cece da Verrazano', 10 December 1493 entries, 'per le noze dela sirochia'.

95. E882, fo. 119r, 12 December 1493 entries: L6s16 for 8 lbs 3 oz of fifty 'pinochiati bianchi' and a 'schatola', 4 lbs of 'mandorle e pinochi chonfetti'.

96. E882, fo. 338r, 'messer Bartolomeo di [BLANK] schala', 20 November 1494 entries 'per fare il desinare a franciosi'.

97. E882, fo. 333v, 'Franc.o di franc.o di lotto detto chapone', 7 June 1494, eight 'falchole bianche' weighing a total of 7 lbs 11 oz 'tolse lui detto quando si saghroorono lesua chongniate monache inchiarito'. Further entries on 7 June 1494 and 8 June 1494 were probably linked to these festivities.

98. E882, fo. 338r, 'messer Bartolomeo di [BLANK] schala', 14 January 1495 (m.f.), 9 lbs of 'pinochiati orati', 'tolse guliano suo figliuolo per le noze dela figliuola'. See other entries from 14 January 1495 (m.f.) to 26 January 1495 (m.f.) for a total of 17.17 lbs of other comfits and *pinochiati* linked to the celebration. On the wedding, see A. Brown, *Bartolomeo Scala, 1430-1497, Chancellor of Florence: The Humanist as Bureaucrat* (Princeton: Princeton University Press, 1979), 245–7.

99. E882, fo. 250r, 'Lorenzo di bartolomeo lanino nipote di bartolomeo di giovanni settecielgli', 22 January 1493 (m.f.), L4s2 for 5 lbs 7 oz of 'piu

ragioni chonfetti chon pinochiati orati' and a 'schatola nuova', 'per le noze sua'.

100. G. Rucellai, *Giovanni Rucellai ed il suo zibaldone*, A. Perosa (ed.), (London: Warburg Institute, 1960), 28, 'una chredenziera fornita d'arienti lavorati, molto richa.'

101. *Ibid.*, 'La quale cosa fu tenuto il più bello e 'l più gientile parato che si sia mai facto a ffesta di nozze'.

102. *Ibid.*, 'alle cholezzioni uscivano fuori in sul palchetto venti confettiere di pinocchiati e zuchata'.

103. P.L. Rubin, *Images and Identity in Fifteenth-Century Florence* (New Haven: Yale University Press, 2007), 229. Giannozzo di Antonio Pucci was Client 1633 'Giannozo dant.o pucci'.

104. *Ibid.*, 259–60.

105. I. Paccagnella, 'Cucina e ideologia alimentare nella Venezia del rinascimento', in A. Pertusi (ed.), *Civiltà della tavola dal medioevo al rinascimento* (Vicenza: Neri Pozza, 1983), 39, on Sanudo's diaries.

106. A. Brown, 'Lorenzo de' Medici's New Men and Their Mores: The Changing Lifestyle of Quattrocento Florence', *Renaissance Studies*, 16, 2 (2002), 113–42: 120.

107. E882, fo. 95r, 'Girolamo di maestro piero della barba nostro fattore', 1 November 1494, 2 lbs of 'pane inpepato' 'disse per donare a m.a ginevra'. See also fo. 249v, 'm.o Giovanni da raghugia', 11 February 1493 (m.f.), 2 lbs of 'torta marzapane' 'per mandare a domenicho mellini'.

108. E882, fo. 255r, 'Tommaso di giovanni di piero nostro', 26 March 1494, 27 March 1494, 'zibibo domaschino', 'marzapane' and 'anici inbrattati cho muscho', 'per mandare ale murate'.

109. Sacchi, *op. cit.* (note 27), 177, on pine-nut cakes, 'Gold leaf is added to these, for magnificence, I believe, and for pleasure.'

110. E882, fo. 254v, 'm.a Silvaggia donna fu di filippo strozzi', 14 September 1494, 6 lbs 9 oz (i.e. 2.29 kg) of 'pinochiato orato', 'per mandare a piero soderini'.

111. E882, fo. 104r, 'Lapo di pangnio da fiesole', 21 September 1493, 'schatola di chonfetto'.

112. E882, fo. 90r, 'Bartolomeo dapolonio lapi', 23 February 1493 (m.f.), 5 lbs 8 oz of 'piu ragioni chonfetti chon ciennamo' and a 'schatola nuova', 'per mandare a guliano orlandini'.

113. E882, fo. 44v, 'Antonio e franc.o di giano chalzaiuoli', 5 March 1493 (m.f.), 'schatola nuova' and 'piu ragioni chonfetti chon ciennamo orata'.

114. Mintz, *op. cit.* (note 26), 88–9.

115. A. Martini, *Manuale di metrologia ossia misure, pesi e monete in uso attulamente ed anticamente presso tutti i popoli* (Turin: Loescher, 1883), 206, 1 braccio fiorentino = 0.58 m.

116. L. Landucci, *Diario fiorentino*, Biblioteca Italiana, Università degli Studi di Roma 'La Sapienza', 2004. [Florence: Sansoni, 1985], 'E a dì 18 d'ottobre 1513, ci fu come el Re di Portogallo aveva mandato l'ubidienza al Papa e presentato queste cose: un Papa di zucchero con 12 Cardinali tutti di zucchero, grandi come uomini naturali, 300 torchi di zucchero di 3 braccia l'uno, 100 casse di zucchero e molte casse di spezierie sottili, di cannella, garofani e di tutte altre cose, uno cavallo bianco che passa tutti gli altri di bellezza; e più à mandato un moro, di quegli di Calicut, alto circa braccia 4, con molte gioie appiccate a gli orecchi e per tutto.'

117. D. Chambers and B. Pullan, *Venice: A Documentary History, 1450–1630* (Oxford: Blackwell, 1992), 179, for Venetian sumptuary law of 1562, 'collations must be provided in the rooms, on the tables, and not otherwise, and they must consist of modest confections, of the ordinary products of pastry cooks, and of simple fruits of any kind, according to the time of year.'

118. For comparison, the average for the year as a whole was 28 soldi per day. In the sample year, Carnival began on 7 January 1494, Lent began on 12 February 1494 (Ash Wednesday), and Easter Sunday was 30 March 1494.

119. G. Ciappelli, *Carnevale e quaresima: Comportamenti sociali e cultura a Firenze nel rinascimento* (Rome: Edizioni di storia e letteratura, 1997), 56–65.

120. Flandrin and Redon, *op. cit.* (note 35), 400; Naso, *op. cit.* (note 42), 123. Sacchi, *op. cit.* (note 27), 177, on pine-nut cakes, 'The nobler and richer eat these often in Lent at the first and last course.' – however there is no evidence that consumption of *pinochiati* was higher in Florence during Lent.

121. Bénézet, *op. cit.* (note 76), 333.

122. See above n. 72.

123. 22 out of 515 active clients (4%) bought pepper bread during the sample year.

124. Excluding corporate clients, clients with surnames accounted for 32% of individual consumption of pepper bread (165 out of 520 soldi); this was much lower than their proportion for all products (58%). Excluding corporate clients, clients with occupational titles accounted for 43% of individual consumption of pepper bread (225 out of 520 soldi); this was more than their proportion for all products (31%).

125. BNF, Magl. XV.92, ff. 69r, 121v, lists two almost identical recipes for 'Berrichuocholi sanesi fini': a mix of cinnamon, white ginger, black pepper, cloves, nutmeg, mace, galingale, honey, citron, flour, red sandalwood and 'salina'.

126. Archivio di Stato di Siena, Scala 859, fo. 46r, 23 July 1473, the expenses of the speziaria of the hospital of the Scala include items 'i[n] zuche per libirichuo[co]li... per achattatura della chaldaia per fare la cotta debirichuocoli e per fogli reali per legare birichuocoli...'; Scala 898, fo.110v, lists purchase of 'pepe sodo conprato per fare di birichuocholi per lisavi...'

The manufacture of these sweets by the hospital was partly related to festive functions.

127. E. Diana, 'Medici, speziali e barbieri nella Firenze della prima metà del '500', *Rivista di storia della medicina*, 4, 2 (1994), 13–27: 19, suggests that feast days presented great money-making opportunities for apothecaries, both for sweets and wax products, but the Giglio records do not support this conclusion.

128. E882, fo. 176v, 'Niccholaio di girolamo lapi', 26 October 1493 entries for a total of 624 soldi on sweets, mostly *confetti*. These included, for example, L20s9d4 on 24 lbs of 'piu ragioni chonfetti' and 5 'schatole nuove'; L8 on 10 lbs of 'anici chonfetti'; L2s6d8 on 12 pinochiati 'chevene fu vi orati', weighing 2 lbs 2 oz altogether.

129. E882, fo. 196r, 'ser Bastiano di [BLANK] notaio al arte de maestri', 20 April 1494, L9s9 for 23.5 lbs of 100 pieces of pinochiati, of which 've ne fu otto pezi orati', and a 'schatolone'. These products were sold at a significant discount (about half price), perhaps as a favour to the Guild on a special occasion. On the presentation of spices and sweets to honour guild consuls, see Ciasca, *op. cit.* (note 9), 382.

130. E882, fo. 177r, 'Niccholaio di girolamo lapi', 29 October 1493, return of 4 lbs 2 oz of 'piu ragioni chonfetti' and 1 'schatola nuova'.

131. E882, fo. 60r, 'Piero di Giorgio santo e giorgio suo padre', 25 August 1493, L3s4 for 4 lbs of 'piu ragioni chonfetti'; 26 August 1493, the client returned a quarter of these comfits (1 lb) to the shop, valued at s16. See also fo. 146v, 'Giovanni di tedicie delglialbizi', 29 August 1494, L2s16 for 4 lbs of 'anici inbrattati'; 2 September 1494, the client returned 3 lbs 4 oz to the shop for L2s6d8 – in both cases the price was s14 per lb.

132. E882, fo. 250r, 'Stagio di piero di stagio danuovoli', 18 January 1493 (m.f.), L2s14 for 3 lbs 7 oz of 'piu ragioni chonfetti' and a 'schatola nuova'; 1 February 1493 (m.f.), return of 1 lbs 10 oz of comfits and the box for L1s9d8.

133. Castellani, *op. cit.* (note 89), 'A lib. 3 di mandorle confette e lib. 2 di pinochi confetti a dì 12 di detto lb. s. d.', 'Rimandòsi allo speziale a dì 13 di detto lib. 2, on. 9 tra mandorle e pinochi avanzorono, portò Giovan Piccino.'

134. Only 158 soldi-worth of sweets were returned to the shop during the sample period, about 1.5% of total sales.

135. K. Park and J. Henderson, '"The First Hospital among Christians": The Ospedale di Santa Maria Nuova in Early Sixteenth-Century Florence', *Medical History*, 35 (1991), 181.

136. E882, fo. 32r, 'Antonio di giovanni del chaccia', 19 December 1493 entries list medicines and comfits bought together.

137. E882, fo. 314r, 'Alessandro di m.o ant.o di ghuido', 19 July 1494, 'disse per portare a sandro in villa per la donna aveva a partorire'.

138. Castellani, *op. cit.* (note 89), 'Ricordo che a dì 18 di novembre feci fare allo speziale della Palla uno gram pane di confetto per mandarlo alla mia sorella cugina Ginevra, donna di Giovanni di Cosmo de' Medici, ch'avea partorito un bel figlolo, che Dio gli guardi sano lungo tempo e facia valente homo come desidera.'

139. Archivio di Stato di Pistoia, Sapienza 414, fo. 68, entry for 25 August 1473, shows how the expenses of the doctor's visit, sweets and medicines were linked: 'a m.o agnolo medicho per medichare la do[n]na' s10, 'per manuschristi e confetti per la do[n]na cheramalata', s4, 'per lattovaro e unzione e confettioni' s18.

140. *Treggiea* were small comfits containing seeds or spices. E882, fo. 330r, 'Piero dandrea mazzi', 4 June 1494 to 4 July 1494 entries suggest that both 'treggiea' and 'pinochiati' were considered types of 'chonfetti'.

141. BNF, Magl. XV.92, fo. 92v, recipe for 'Treggiea da cchi fussi rotto di sotto', made with herbs, spices, gums and sugar.

142. Sacchi, *op. cit.* (note 27), 193, coriander, 'has great force to cool burning sensations. It should not be eaten alone on account of its innate harmfulness, but either with honey or raisins, or in our manner, which is more pleasant and healthful: prepared in vinegar and rolled in sugar.'

143. O. Redon, 'La réglementation des banquets par les lois somptuaires dans les villes d'Italie (XIIIe–Xve siècles)', in C. Lambert (ed.), *Du manuscrit à la table: essais sur la cuisine au Moyen Age et repertoire des manuscrits medievaux contenant des recettes culinaires* (Montreal: Les Presses de l'Université de Montreal, 1992), 116, n.34; Ciasca, *op. cit.* (note 9), 368, n.1, the fact that the Italian term *coriandoli* is synonymous with the English term confetti indicates the importance of coriander comfits in particular. Augusti, *op. cit.* (note 83), ch.13, fo. 35v, coriander comfits were the first products described in the sweets section.

144. Sacchi, *op. cit.* (note 27), 193, on use of coriander with sugar, honey or raisins, 'We use it better in the third course, to repress vapors seeking the head with that astringent quality with which it is especially endowed.'

145. *Ibid.*, 123, 'There is an order to be observed in taking food...'

146. Albala, *op. cit.* (note 27), 13; Sacchi, *op. cit.* (note 27), 127, 'we were ordered by our ancestors to eat melons on an empty stomach...'

147. Flandrin and Redon, *op. cit.* (note 35), 400; M. Ficino, *Three Books on Life*, C.V. Kaske and J.R. Clark (trans.), (Binghampton: Medieval & Renaissance Texts & Studies, 1989), 143, 'When the head is swimming with rheums [*destillationibus*] because of phlegm... after eating, we will control the fumes of the food with coriander and quinces.' Sacchi, *op. cit.* (note 27), 129, on the other hand recommended eating quince at the start of the meal, 'They are eaten as a first course, especially the Neapolitan, which are valued, since,

with anise and raisins or with pure wine or clarified honey, they do not harm the stomach much.'

148. Augusti, *op. cit.* (note 83), ch.13, fo. 37, 'Ad faciendum codignata[m].'

149. J.-L. Flandrin, 'Médecine et habitudes alimentaires anciennes', in J.-C. Margolin and R. Sauzet (eds), *Pratiques et discours alimentaires à la Renaissance. Actes du Colloque de Tours de mars 1979* (Paris: G.-P. Maisonneuve & Larose, 1982), 85–96, 87-88.

150. The average price of raisins was 3.2 soldi per lb.

151. E541, fo. 23v, 'Piero di giovanni derossi & chonpangni speziali a medici', 7 April 1502, purchase of 1 lb of 'uve di choranto', gives wholesale price of s5 per lb. E882, fo. 315r, 'Simone di bernardo di simone del nero', 24 April 1494; fo. 89r, 'Chino di christofano a zini', 5 June 1494; fo. 252v, 'Bernardo di piero del palagio', 4 June 1494, for an average retail price of s6.5 per lb. Fo. 255r, 'Tommaso di giovanni di piero nostro', 27 March 1494, s3 for ½ lb of 'zibibo domaschino' (s6 per lb). Mattioli refers to *zibibo* in his discussion of currants, where he states his preference for 'la Damaschina, che noi chimiamo zibibo'.

152. Sacchi, *op. cit.* (note 27), 123, suggests that 'certain sweets which we call *bellaria*, seasoned with spices and pine nuts, or honey, or sugar' (ie. comfits) were appropriate in the first course, but he does not offer a justification for this in terms of humoral theory. See above n. 120.

153. Messisbugo, *op. cit.* (note 32), 39, 'Dove è da sapere che se fosse alcuno Gentil'huomo mezzano, che facesse il convito, potrebbe egli fare col Terzo meno de zucchari & spiciarie'.

154. P. Fumerton, 'Consuming the Void: Jacobean Banquets and Masques', in *Cultural Aesthetics: Renaissance Literature and the Practice of Social Ornament* (Chicago: University of Chicago Press, 1991), 112.

155. F. Ambrosini, 'Ceremonie, feste, lusso', in A. Tenenti and U. Tucci (eds), *Storia di Venezia, Vol.V, Il rinascimento. Società ed economia* (Rome: Istituto della Enciclopedia Italiana, 1996). On Venetian banquets, see above n. 117.

156. Albala, *op. cit.* (note 27), 112.

157. Fumerton, *op. cit.* (note 154), 133–4.

158. RF, *op. cit.* (note 86), f.149, lists manuscristi as 'CONFECTIONI CORDIALI MAGISTRALI', ie. cordial confections.

159. *Ibid.*, f.149, 'La prima co'fectione si fa di zucchero & acqua rosa, et chiamasi manuschristo'; Augusti, *op. cit.* (note 83), ch.13, fo. 36v, gives a recipe made with sugar and rose-water.

160. E882, fo. 34v, 'Fratti e monaci della badia di firenze', 16 February 1492 (m.f.), 2.5 oz of 'manuschristo' for s5.

161. Augusti, *op. cit.* (note 83), ch.13, fo. 35v, and Suardo, *op. cit.* (note 19), fo. xxxiiii, list the same four varieties, including roses, violets, pearls and gemstones – 'rosati', 'violati', 'perlati' and 'cum frangmentis'.

162. RF, *op. cit.* (note 86), f.149, 'ALCHUNI aggiunghono Cennamo [sc] i'.
163. E882, fo. 160r, 'Marcho di [BLANK] santini da chalcinaia', 16 October 1493, 2 oz of 'manuschristo chon choralli' for s5d4. This variety was also known as *Diacorallo*, *ibid.*, f.149, 'ALChuni coralli: Verbi gratia. Zucchero fine [oz] iiii / Coralli rossi [dr] ii / Co' acqua rosa si fa panellino, & chiamasi Dyacorallo.'
164. E882, fo. 248v, 'Ant.o di giovanni del chaccia', 10 January 1493 (m.f.), 3.5 oz of 'manuschristo orato' for s7 (s24 per lb). However, fo. 59v, 'Jachopo dinuccio solosmei', 30 August 1493; fo. 31r, 'Giovanni di bona raghugieo alosteria deghuanti', 27 July 1493, suggest a price of around s32.
165. E882, fo. 349r, 'Bartolomeo di tomaso settecielgli e fratelgli', 15 August 1496, 6 dr of 'manuschristo perlato' for s3; fo. 350r, 'Fratti e monaci della badia di firenze', 9 August 1494, 3.5 oz of 'manuschristo perlato' for s14; fo. 139v, 'Franc.o di bartolomeo oste a santo andrea', 17 May 1495, 3.25 oz of 'manuschristo perlato orato' for s13; fo. 207v, 'Gannozo dant.o pucci', 3 February 1493 (m.f.), 3.25 oz of 'manuschristo perlato e orato' for s14, 4 February 1493 (m.f.), 2.5 oz of 'manuschristo perlato orato' for s10. RF, *op. cit.* (note 86), f.149, 'ALCHUNI aggiunghono perle non forate'. Augusti, *op. cit.* (note 83), ch.13, fo. 36v, the recipe lists 1 lb of clarified sugar, 5 lbs of rose-water and 5 dr of 'margarite subtilissime pulverizate'. On the use of pearls, see also G. Silini, *Umori e farmaci: terapia medica tardo-medievale* (Gandino: Servitium, 2001), 384; J. Castle, 'Treatments & Medicines between 1400 & 1600', Doctoral Thesis, DHMSA (1999), 13–14.
166. E882, fo. 315r, 'Jachopo di bartolomeo da girone linaiuolo', 28 February 1494 (m.f.), 4.5 oz of 'manuschristo chon p'le e frumenti preziosi' for approximately s18d4. RF, *op. cit.* (note 86), f.149, describes a precious version with powdered gemstones (pearl, coral, jacinth, garnet, sapphire, beryl, emerald, plus sanders).
167. Faccioli, *op. cit.* (note 90), 292, n.14; Augusti, *op. cit.* (note 83), ch.13, fo. 36v, the recipe lists 1 lb of clarified sugar, 4 dr of rose-water, 4 dr of starch. Suardo, *op. cit.* (note 19), fo. xxxiiii, gives two alternative recipes, one identical to Augusti, and another simpler 'Venetian' version.
168. E882, fo. 319v, 'Fruosino di ciecie da verrazano', 28 June 1494, s18 for 9 oz of 'savonia fatta chome chomune mandorle amido e chondita chonolio di mandorle dolci' for his sister Caterina, a nun in the convent of Sant'Ambrogio.
169. E882, fo. 220r, 'Pedone di domenicho pedoni', 18 November 1493, L1s2 for 11 oz of 'savonia fatta chon zuc.o fine arotovi sugho di regholizia pistachi semi di chotongnie e altre chose', and see the entry for 23 November 1493, which describes this as 'latt.o usato dela savonia'.
170. E882, fo. 295r, 'Rede di giovanni daghostino ritalgliatiore', 22 December 1494, s6 for 3 oz of 'savonia chon ispezie di diedraghante'.

171. Ciasca, *op. cit.* (note 9), 394; Silini, *op. cit.* (note 165), 385. Augusti, *op. cit.* (note 83), ch.13, fo. 36v, 'Ad faciendum penidios.' *Liber Pandectarum*, (Vicenza: 1480), cap. ccccccxx, 'Zucarum' quotes Serapione on pennets: 'Penidie sunt ca. et hu. in i gradu molliunt ventre': et sunt grossiores zucaro.'

172. 41 out of 515 active clients (8%) bought pennets during the sample year. Excluding corporate clients, clients with surnames accounted for 36% of individual consumption of pennets (68 out of 190 soldi); this was much lower than their proportion for all products (58%). Excluding corporate clients, clients with occupational titles accounted for 49% of individual consumption of pennets (93 out of 190 soldi); this was much higher than their proportion for all products (31%).

173. E882, ff. 311r, 321r, 'Munistero e donne di santo anbruogio', 2 May 1494, 22 May 1494; fo. 146v, 'Charlo di bartolomeo chalzaiuolo fratello di franc.o da santo andrea', 20 November 1493; fo. 135r, 'Jachopo di viviano da ccholle e chonpangni speziali', 16 October 1493; fo. 36v, 'Giovanbatista di [BLANK] stamaiuolo', 4 August 1493; fo. 55r, 'Giovanni dalancisa chalzolaio', 23 August 1493. RF, *op. cit.* (note 86), f.47, gives a recipe for 'dyapennidion' including pennets, pine-nuts, almonds, poppy-seeds, spices, gums, starch, syrups and camphor, boiled up with water of violets and violet flowers.

174. Mintz, *op. cit.* (note 26), 83–4.

175. 222 out of 515 active clients (43%) bought sweets during the sample year. Clients with surnames accounted for 49% of individual consumption of sweets (4,413 out of 8,943 soldi); this was lower than their proportion for all products (58%). Clients with occupational titles accounted for 29% of individual consumption of sweets (2,613 out of 8,943 soldi); this was only slightly lower than their proportion for all products (31%).

176. This can be seen if we accept that the people who required sureties to obtain credit were 'poor'. Clients with sureties accounted for 5% of individual consumption of sweets (475 out of 8,943 soldi); this was lower than their proportion for all products (7%). This trend is again most strongly seen with comfits: clients with sureties accounted for 3% of individual consumption of comfits (125 out of 3,821 soldi).

177. Laurioux, *op. cit.* (note 50), 37; Flandrin and Redon, *op. cit.* (note 35), 403, suggests that the taste for sweetness was not constant but rather 'discovered' in the course of the fifteenth century as the price of sugar fell.

178. E882, ff. 206r, 295r, 'Rede di giovanni daghostino ritalgliatore' treats the shop as a spicer's and sweetshop only.

179. Albala, *op. cit.* (note 27), 66, 78, 179.

180. *Ibid.*, 66.

181. Savonarola, *op. cit.* (note 11), ch.18, 'Zova al stomego, in el quale non se genera colera, il perché facilmente in quella se converte, absterze e mundificalo dal flegma e spetialiter l'antiquo e dà maiore nutrimento del

mele. Lenifica el ventre, lenisse il petto e rimove l'asperità dela canna, fa il cibo più delectevole, dico a multi, il perché comuniter i colerici amano il garbo. Conferisse al dolore dele rene e dila vesica, mundifica la obscurità dilo ochio e apre le opilatione.' These comments are echoed in the compilation of medical tradition, the *Liber Pandectarum, op. cit.* (note 171), cap. cccccccxx, 'Zucarum', which regarded sugar as being 'drying', 'cleansing' and 'resolving', and particularly effective for removing blockages and clearing out the pathways, comforting the kidneys and bladder. It had a gentle action, being warm and humid in the first degree.

182. Albala, *op. cit.* (note 27), 176–8.

183. *Ibid.*, 179; Savonarola, *op. cit.* (note 11), ch.18, 'È il suo nocumento ch'el fa sete e in colera se converte, dove chi per sanità cussì usar el volesse, il voria manzar cum pomi granati o cum prugne'

184. Albala, *op. cit.* (note 27), 212.

185. *Ibid.*, 275.

186. Quoted in O. Temkin, *Galenism: Rise and Fall of a Medical Philosophy* (Ithaca: Cornell University Press, 1973), 126.

187. F. Guicciardini, 'Ricordanze', in C. Grayson (ed.), *Selected Writings* (New York: Harper & Row, 1965), 125–70: 142.

188. B. Machiavelli, *Libro di ricordi*, Biblioteca Italiana, Università degli Studi di Roma 'La Sapienza', 2004. [Florence: Le Monnier, 1954], 'perchè non avessi a spendere.'

189. L. Martines, *Scourge and Fire: Savonarola and Renaissance Italy* (London: Jonathan Cape, 2006), 36.

190. J.-L. Flandrin, 'Prix et statut gastronomique des viandes: réflexions sur quelques exemples des XVIe, XVIIe et XVIIIe siècles', in S. Cavaciocchi (ed.), *Alimentazione e nutrizione secc. XIII–XVIII: atti della ventottesima settimana di studi, 22–27 aprile 1996* (Florence: Le Monnier, 1997), 603.

191. J.-L. Flandrin, M. Hyman, and P. Hyman, *Le Cuisinier François*, D. Roche (ed.), (Paris: Montalba, 1982), 19.

8

Medicines

If the Giglio was a shop where many of its clients popped in to buy candies for pleasure and festivities, and a small number came in to rent or buy the goods they needed to bury and remember the dead, its central purpose was as a retail outlet for the sale of medicines. The apothecary worked closely with the physician to create the right pills, syrups and other products that would prove therapeutic for a specific individual at a particular point in their life. As discussed in Chapter 2, this meant carefully analysing the humoral condition of the person in question before making a prescription. The medicines that resulted were usually either of the doctor's own devising or, more often, drawn from the long-standing manuals which had been inherited from the Graeco-Arabic tradition.

Fifteenth-century pharmacology was rooted in the classical text *De materia medica*, written around 65AD by the Greek physician, Pedanius Dioscorides.[1] His approach had been essentially empirical, limiting himself to describing the form and properties of medicinal simples, but his work was subsequently incorporated into the model of humours.[2] Building on Dioscorides' descriptions, theorists created a complex model where each simple was characterised in terms of two primary qualities (from hot, dry, cold, humid) ranked on a scale of intensity from one to four; for example, the herb nigella was 'hot and dry in the third degree'.[3] Each simple also had secondary and tertiary qualities – nigella had a 'diuretic virtue' and was 'dissolving and consuming'.[4] In order to balance the primary qualities of these simples, and to compensate for their side effects, they were not normally used alone but mixed together in compounds. Although relatively simple combinations might be prepared at home using basic kitchen equipment, the manufacture of these kind of elaborate compound medications was regarded as a difficult task requiring particular skill, care and honesty – an ill-trained or unscrupulous apothecary could be potentially fatal for patients. The preparation of such drugs was therefore the preserve of professional apothecaries, subject to city and guild regulation.

In practice, this translated into a 'recipe book' approach to pharmacy, where specific drug recipes provided tried and tested solutions for specific ailments. Rather than experimenting freely on their patients, doctors and apothecaries alike relied on a synthesis of Greek and Arab pharmacological

Image 8.1

Ricettario fiorentino di nuovo illustrato, *Marescotti, Florence, 1597,*
Courtesy: Wellcome Library, London.

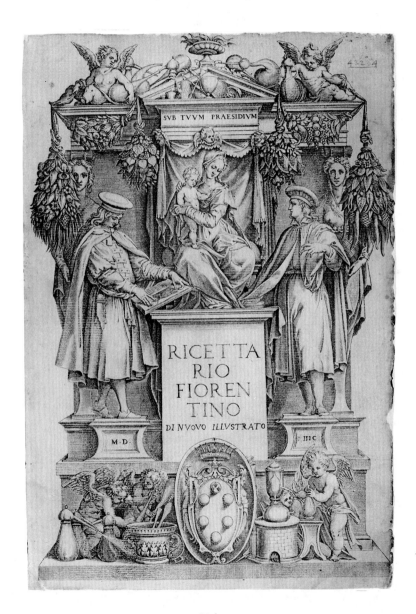

science received through the Latin editions of the Middle Ages, especially the medical school of Salerno.[5] The *Antidotarium Nicolai*, compiled between the late twelfth and the early thirteenth centuries, was the basis of most subsequent recipe-books of the later Middle Ages,[6] such as the *Compendium Aromatariorum* (1447), a specialist trade manual for apothecaries.[7] The *Ricettario fiorentino* (1499), intended to establish definitive recipes for the use of the city's apothecaries, was solidly rooted in this medieval tradition.[8] The debt was acknowledged in the first pages, where the *Antidotarium Nicolai* is listed as one of the fundamental texts that every good apothecary should own and have read, along with other medieval Arab and Christian texts.[9] Among the books owned by the Giglio were a 'Mesue' and a 'Serapione', for example.[10]

These sorts of manuals contained only limited information on the therapeutic functions of drugs, since apothecaries were supposed to know how to manufacture rather than to prescribe them. The *Ricettario fiorentino* simply provides recipes, with no indication as to how the drugs should be used – this sort of information was simply not relevant for apothecaries. This was symptomatic of a developing professional specialisation, in which apothecaries were forbidden to prescribe drugs or give medical advice.[11] It is clear from the accounts that the recipes for medicinal preparations were copied from doctors' prescriptions, since they almost always record *who* the medicine was for, and sometimes also further instructions, as in a purge that was 'to be used as the *maestro* stated'.[12] The Giglio appears to have had a particularly close working relationship with one doctor in particular, Mengo Bianchelli, although probably not an exclusive one (see Chapter 2).

This professional literature was generally written in Latin, a choice that helped to safeguard the 'secrets' of the trade.[13] Yet parallel to this specialist literature was a developing popular market for health manuals, which usually also included much advice on regimen in general. These were often intended to make learned medical theory simpler and more accessible, as with the thirteenth-century manual *Thesaurus pauperum*, aimed at provincial doctors serving the poor.[14] Although this was written in simplified Latin, it was followed by vulgar editions aimed at a broader public, such as the Tuscan manual *Libro che Ypochras mandò a Ccesare* [*sic*].[15] Similarly, a mid-thirteenth-century treatise by Aldobrandino da Siena was written in French and translated into Tuscan in 1310.[16] Such manuals catered to and helped construct a popular medicial culture, one where remedies were linked to specific conditions without going into the theoretical detail of how the cure functioned.

In addition, hospitals, doctors, apothecaries and educated consumers assembled their own collections of recipes, copying them from books or doctor's prescriptions, exchanging them with friends and relatives, writing down oral traditions or describing practices they had observed:[17] for example, the record book of Francesco Castellani contains three recipes for children suspected of 'worms'.[18] Such compilations could derive from a great variety of sources, as in the recipe book kept by the hospital of Santa Maria Nuova in Florence – known from a manuscript copy made in 1515 – which combines elements from both the learned and popular tradition as well as the practice of contemporary doctors, some of whom were employed at the hospital.[19] Such recipe books are particularly interesting because they present a point where the learned texts for an educated public intersected with the popular tradition and daily medical practice. This sort of recipe book approach was probably closer to ordinary practice than the rarefied academic texts of the Salerno school.[20]

One of the fundamental problems in the history of medicine is to bridge the gap between written works of theory and the reality of daily practice. John Riddle has argued that the pharmacological theory of the later Middle Ages was so complex that it was 'unworkable' in practice.[21] But is this really so? The accounts of the Giglio are particularly interesting in this regard, since they tell us not only which were the most widely used drugs and simples in the 1490s, but also how much they cost. The study of the retail market therefore sheds light on a key aspect of the relationship between medical theory and practice, and places this in social context. Medicinal products were the most important category of goods sold retail, constituting at least forty-two per cent of the market and providing the sustained baseline demand that kept customers coming to the shop throughout the year (see Table 6.1).[22] A vast range of individual products was retailed to customers, and space does not permit to discuss them all. This chapter will therefore focus on identifiable groups of medicinal products that were particularly important in terms of sales. By far the most important of these products were purges, which constituted at least thirteen per cent of all sales.[23] Following these, other ingested products of particular importance will be discussed, such as clysters, sweet electuaries, bitter electuaries and pills. The medicinal syrups that were important supplements to a purge, and frequently sold alongside, will be examined. The other leading products retailed were external therapies – epithems, fomentations, baths, ointments, plasters and cerates – and these will be handled separately. Throughout, the analysis will examine the extent to which these products were standardised 'official' products that were made up in advance and kept in store, and the extent to which they were 'magisterial' products made up according to a doctor's prescription for the individual patient.

Table 8.1

Price Distribution of Purges

Total Number	Minimum	Median	Maximum	Mean
560	3 soldi	10.33 soldi	243 soldi	19 soldi

Purges

A purge (*medicina*) consisted of a combination of simples and other ingredients made up for the patient according to a doctor's prescription.[24] A typical example was made from an ounce of pudding pipe 'tempered' in water of endive.[25] The great majority of purges (eighty-one per cent of the total) came in this 'liquid' form,[26] where the active ingredients were 'tempered' with a liquid, usually distilled waters made from herbal extracts.[27] The inventory lists five ladles that were specifically used 'for tempering medicines'.[28] These liquid purges were usually served in a small *bicchiere* (drinking glass).[29] The main alternative was a solid form, where the ingredients were combined with sugar in the form of a 'date', known elsewhere as a bolus.[30] Here, the ingredients were 'incorporated' in sugar to make a sort of medicinal candy,[31] as when an ounce and a quarter of pudding pipe were 'made into a date with sugar'.[32]

Both these examples were cheap preparations, costing seven and nine soldi respectively, about as much as an unskilled labourer could earn in a day.[33] Yet the composition and price of purges could also vary considerably (see Table 8.1). At the bottom end of the market were purges costing three or four soldi,[34] typically made from coralline (a vermifuge), 'worm powder' or purgatives such as pudding pipe. However, these products were relatively little used, probably because they were of specialist application.[35] At the top end of the market were products retailing at around a hundred soldi or more,[36] up to an absolute maximum of 243 soldi.[37] Within this range, the median price of just over ten soldi gives a good idea of what was typical. In fact, eighty-five per cent of all purges sold cost twenty soldi or less, well within the reach of the humblest clients, such as carters, labourers and maidservants.

The price of purges varied principally in relation to their ingredients. The most common was pudding pipe (also known as 'cassia solutiva', or 'cassia fistula'),[38] which appears in over half the purges sold.[39] Pudding pipe was also an ingredient in many of the standard compound drugs used in purges, such as *diacatholicon* and *diacassia*.[40] Its popularity is confirmed by Mattioli's comment that it was 'in common and most frequent use by all

Chart 8.1

Retail Sales of Cassia Pulp, 1493–4

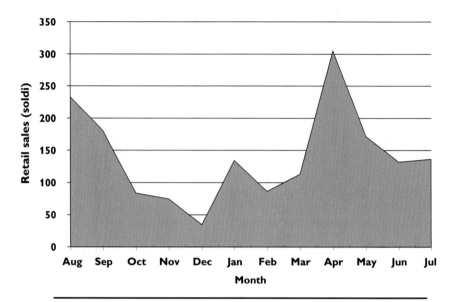

doctors to soften the body'.[41] However, the fact that his comments are buried away – within an entry on cinnamon – was symptomatic of how this commodity came to be neglected by medical scholarship in the sixteenth century. As the pudding pipe did not appear in Dioscorides – it came through the Arab medical tradition of the Middle Ages – it fell out of favour with humanist scholars like Mattioli. The 'cassia of the Arabs' was subsequently to fade from popularity, increasingly regarded as a corruption of 'pure' Greek medicine.[42]

Although pudding pipe was an 'exotic' commodity, originating in the Middle East and imported from Egypt, it was not particularly expensive, and was generally associated with cheaper purges.[43] The wholesale price was about fifteen soldi per lb – around fifty per cent higher than sugar[44] – and the retail price can be estimated at seventy-two soldi per lb.[45] Although pudding pipe required some processing for use (removing the pulp from the pods, careful weighing and mixing with other ingredients), labour costs were relatively cheap in Renaissance Florence and these figures suggest a considerable profit margin, far greater than was possible on wax products.

Pudding pipe was a cheap purgative with a wide customer base and broad social participation, similar to the profile for sweets.[46] Across the

Chart 8.2

Burials in Florence, 1493–4

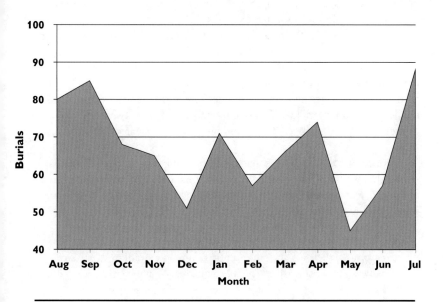

sample year (see Chart 8.1), consumption was higher during the summer (April to September), with marked peaks in August–September 1493 and April 1494. By contrast, consumption was lower in the winter (October to March), with a particularly strong dip in December, and a minor surge in January. The data for related products such as receptacles – mostly drinking glasses used to serve purges – show similar patterns. These figures correspond closely to the annual pattern of customer flow at the Giglio (see Chart 6.1) – a baseline popular demand with seasonal variations that corresponds to the underlying pattern of higher sickness in Florence during the summer and early spring.[47] Comparison with the available figures for burials in Florence in the same period (see Chart 8.2), shows a marked coincidence of the peaks in August–September, January and April and the trough of December 1493, even though the fit is not perfect – note May and July 1494. The particularly high peak of sales in April is likely to be related to the prevalence of fevers in the spring, which were not always mortal.[48]

Some customers bought pudding pipe by itself, rather than as part of a purge.[49] In such cases the cassia was usually still in the pods, so it would keep for longer, as when Albizzo da Fortuna bought nearly three ounces of 'cassia in pods',[50] or when Luigi Mormorai bought three ounces of 'best cassia in the cane' for his son.[51] This practice mirrors the advice that Morelli recorded in his memoirs in the early fifteenth century: 'Some mornings you should eat an ounce of cassia, still in the pods, and give some to the children: keep some in the house, fresh, and also sugar, rose water and julep.'[52] There is evidence, therefore, that some clients bought simples as described by Morelli, probably for self-medication without a doctor's prescription. This was a cheaper option, since the retail price of cassia 'in the pods' was only about twenty-four soldi per lb.[53] Despite this possibility, most consumers preferred to take their pudding pipe in the form of purges that were prescribed by a doctor and tempered to their individual complexion. In the sample year, the shop retailed over nineteen lbs of cassia in pods, and over twenty-six lbs of extracted pulp – mostly incorporated in purges – a far more expensive form.[54]

In contrast to cheap purges made with pudding pipe, at the other end of the market we find more complex preparations, such as a liquid purge that combined ready-made drugs like *diamanna* with simples such as pudding pipe, agaric and rhubarb.

> [F]or a purge… containing 6 drams of extract of pudding pipe, 1 dram of *diamanna*, 4 scruples of fine rhubarb placed in infusion with spike in water of endive and trebbiano wine, 4 scruples of fine agaric infused with rock salt and ginger in oxymel and water of celery, and the purge tempered with decoction of cordial flowers, follicles of senna, epithyme and other things made in water of endive and water of bugloss… 5 lire.[55]

This was relatively cheap compared to the most expensive purge in the sample, which cost more than twelve lire.

> [F]or a purge… containing 1 dram of fine rhubarb, and 1½ ounces of fine manna; the rhubarb placed in infusion in water of endive and trebbiano wine, and the manna tempered with fresh and cordial decoction… 12 lire 3 soldi 4 denari.[56]

In this case the recipe was simpler, but the large quantity of manna made the product much more expensive. The high price of the most expensive purges was primarily due to their incorporation of particular simples, especially rhubarb and manna. Raw materials determined the price, rather than the complexity of the manufacturing process.

Medicinal rhubarb – not to be confused with the English variety we know today[57] – was imported from China in the form of dried roots.[58] It was regarded as a mild purgative that was useful for treating dysentery, fevers etc., with the advantage that it had no harmful side effects and so could be given to children and pregnant women.[59] A Florentine herbal of the fifteenth

Image 8.2

Medicinal Rhubarb,
from P.A. Mattioli, I discorsi... nelli sei libri di Pedacio Dioscoride
Anazarbeo della materia medicinale...*(Venice: V. Valgrisi, 1568).*
Courtesy: Wellcome Library, London.

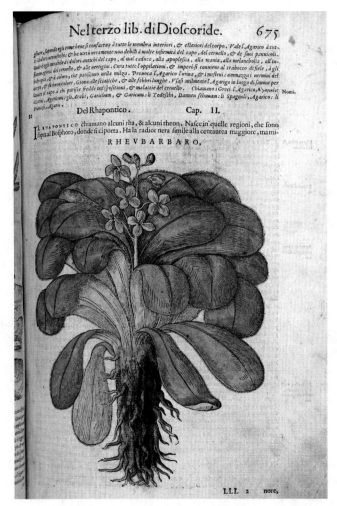

century describes how rhubarb was useful at all stages of an illness: as a
stimulant and strengthener at the early stage, as a mild laxative in the critical
stage, and as a purgative at times of crisis, noting in particular that:

[F]or purging this rhubarb is the best herb of all other purgatives, and so it is found in many of the apothecaries' and doctors' purgative electuaries... it is the flower of every purge.[60]

Giovanni Morelli also recommended rhubarb for children: 'use an electuary that the doctors have made for you from rhubarb: give some to the children, for it kills worms.'[61] Mattioli noted how its effects could be complemented by combining it with other substances, such as water of endive, or spikenard, and aromatic white wine could be added to help clear blockages.[62] At the Giglio, rhubarb was indeed often combined with endive water and trebbiano wine, and spikenard was an additional ingredient in many purges.

Mattioli notes how rhubarb was very expensive, being 'worth its weight in gold', and therefore normally regarded as a medicine of last resort.[63] The Giglio accounts show that the wholesale price was around six hundred soldi per lb,[64] and the retail price around six thousand soldi per lb or more.[65] Although the dosage required was typically very small, about one dram on average (ie. four grams),[66] rhubarb purges were therefore extremely expensive – even one dram of rhubarb cost around seventy soldi. Although therefore limited to an élite minority of clients,[67] the high price and margins of rhubarb gave it considerable commercial importance, with total sales exceeding those of pudding pipe.[68] Indeed, the price was so high that clients sometimes supplied their own rhubarb for inclusion in purges. Jacopo Galli, who bought a purge for his mother, kept the price down by providing his own rhubarb.[69] Similarly, Lando Tanagli supplied a tiny amount of his own rhubarb – two scruples, ie. about two grams – for addition to a simple purge made with cassia pulp and water of fennel.[70] Commodities like rhubarb, with a particularly high value relative to bulk, could be obtained through private links to those involved in long-distance trade. The consumption of rhubarb among shop clients was therefore higher than the sales figures suggest.

Manna was another costly medicinal simple. It had very strong biblical associations – Mandeville described it as the 'bread of angels', a 'dew of heaven' that was found in the 'land of Job',[71] but combined this with medical observations, describing how it could be used to 'purge evil blood'. What Mandeville described as a kind of dew was, in fact, the sap forming on the leaves of a type of ash, found mostly in Calabria.[72] Like rhubarb, manna was renowned as an effective purgative without unpleasant side effects. In his chapter on purges, Marsilio Ficino, whose father had been doctor to Cosimo de' Medici and whose brothers ran an apothecary shop in Florence,[73] recommended the use of pudding pipe, although he thought manna was even better.[74] Mattioli referred to it as 'a medication most noble and pleasant, prince among all the others [...] after taking a dose of two and a half ounces, it moves the body most well time and time again'.[75] It was less expensive than

Table 8.2

Comparison of Giglio and Santa Maria Nuova

	S. Maria Nuova, c.1500 (estimated purchases)	Estimated Doses	Giglio, 1493–4 (total sales)	Estimated Doses[76]	Ratio	Estimated Retail Price (Giglio data) soldi per lb[77]
Pudding Pipe	2,000 lbs	28,235	24.44 lbs	345	82:1	c.72
Rhubarb	20 lbs	1,846	0.65 lbs	60	31:1	c.5760
Manna	12 lbs	182	2.24 lbs	34	5:1	c.840

rhubarb, costing around 250 soldi per lb wholesale, and retailing for around 840 soldi per lb,[78] but because greater quantities were required (the average dose was three quarters of an ounce,[79] purges made with manna were extremely expensive and purchased only by a social élite.[80]

When the Florentine hospital of Santa Maria Nuova estimated the annual needs of its pharmacy, around 1500, it specifically listed these three key simples – pudding pipe, rhubarb and manna – along with other staples – sugar, honey and wax.[81] These rough estimates can be compared with annual sales at the Giglio.

Pudding pipe was heavily used at the hospital, with estimated annual consumption of two thousand lbs. This was enough for over twenty-eight thousand doses, assuming it was all used in this way.[82] By comparison, annual retail sales of pudding pipe at the shop amounted to just under twenty-five lbs.[83] The hospital used over eighty times as much as the Giglio, which was probably one of the middling retailers of the city. Rhubarb, by comparison, was prescribed for a more limited number of patients, reflecting its high cost. Estimated annual consumption of twenty lbs would have been sufficient for around 1,850 doses.[84] Again, this dwarfed sales at the shop, which were less than a pound in the sample year.[85] However, the shop accounts underestimate the importance of rhubarb in the private market because to some extent clients supplied their own. Finally, in the case of manna, the hospital's estimated consumption was twelve lbs, sufficient for just over 180 doses,[86] much closer to consumption at the Giglio.

This suggests that, relative to the hospital, the shop used a higher proportion of the most costly ingredients. Pudding pipe was the best seller in terms of number of consumers, but it did not dominate therapy to the overwhelming extent that it did at the hospital. Although both institutions covered the same *range* of treatments, their businesses focused on different social strata. The sick poor were more likely to go to hospital – where treatment was free – than spend money on shop medicines.[87] Renaissance Florentines had a range of alternatives to choose from, both inside and outside the shop. Apothecaries offered a range of products to suit the requirements of urban consumers of all social ranks. For the rich, costly purges could be created with the finest ingredients, but for ordinary folk, simple 'dates' made of pudding pipe and sugar were often sufficient. This is not to suggest, however, that the élite scorned the most simple preparations. Antonio Del Caccia, who was able to afford more than seventy lbs of wax for his mother-in-law's funeral, indicating a fairly high social level,[88] sometimes bought extremely expensive purges, such as one costing over three lire for his mother-in-law,[89] but also cheap examples costing only seven soldi.[90] The different products were not exclusively linked to different social groups in a simplistic fashion: instead, the degree of choice enjoyed by consumers varied in accordance with their access to credit.

Purges often combined key simples with compound drugs. These drugs, the kind of products whose recipes are listed in the *Ricettario fiorentino*, were only occasionally retailed direct to the public. Instead they were manufactured in advance of requirements and subsequently combined with other drugs and simples for specific patients according to a doctor's prescription. Furthermore, only a small proportion of the many drugs listed in the *Ricettario* were much used in practice. The *Ricettario* itself gives some basic indication of contemporary practice, often noting whether a particular drug was 'used' – or not – in 1490s Florence. The Giglio data permit more detailed analysis, and as Table 8.3 shows, the vast majority of drugs sold fell into two specific categories:[91] 'sweet electuaries' and purgatives, including Sugho Rosato[92]. The top five drugs – diacatholicon, diaphœnicon, diasenna, dieradon abbatis and electuary of juice of roses – form a distinct group in terms of sales, and almost entirely belong to the former category.

Diacatholicon was the best-selling drug at the Giglio, and especially common in liquid purges.[93] There was nothing particularly complex about it – it was basically a laxative that made people 'go'. This sort of purging was considered useful for most conditions, and the many therapeutic applications of the drug were reflected in its being called 'catholic'.[94] It was also fairly simple to make: the ingredients consisted of a number of exotic 'purgative' ingredients – senna, pudding pipe, tamarinds and rhubarb – mixed with other herbs and spices, ground in a mortar, boiled with water to a reduction, strained and then mixed with sugar.[95] Diaphœnicon was the second most important, found particularly in solid purges. It was made from dates marinaded in vinegar, combined with other purgatives like scammony and turpeth, and was used to treat an excess of 'choler' or 'phlegm', as well

Table 8.3

Top Ten Drugs, 1493–4

No. of Sales	Value (soldi)	English	Giglio	Category of electuary	Approx Price (soldi per lb)
171	1,192	Diacatholicon	Diechattolichon	Purgatives	120–8
141	355	Diaphœnicon	Diefinichon	Purgatives	120
126	735	Diasenna	Diasena	Purgatives	96
115	500	Diarrhodon Abbatis	Dieradon abat[is]	Sweet Electuaries	48
101	133	Electuary of Juice of Roses	Sugho Rosato	Purgatives	96
61	280	Electuary of Psyllium	Latt[ovar]o di Silio	Purgatives	132
45	234	Diamanna	Diamanna	Purgatives	288–384
41	200	Diatrion -santalon	Latt[ovar]o di Triasandoli	Sweet Electuaries	48
41	169	Rosata novella	Rosata novella	Sweet Electuaries	48
40	145	Aromatic Roset	Aromatico Rosato	Sweet Electuaries	48

as stomach problems and fevers.[96] Diasenna was the third most important drug sold at the Giglio. The main active ingredient was senna leaves,[97] and the drug was a common treatment for purging the 'melancholic' humour.[98]

Part of the function of the sugar, honey and spices found so abundantly in these products was to increase their shelf life.[99] For most electuaries this was two years, although products such as mithridate might last up to thirty.[100] This allowed large quantities to be made in advance and stockpiled. Comparing these quantities to average dosages (see Table 8.4, overleaf) shows that the shop had, for example, about two years' supply of diacatholicon in stock, assuming that sales in 1504 remained at 1490s levels. Apothecaries manufactured large stocks of standard drugs in advance of their use, taking them from store for combination with other ingredients to make products for retail to the consumer.

Table 8.4

Stocks of Key Compound Drugs

Commodity	Quantity in stock, 1504	Average Dosage	Doses in stock, 1504	Sales in sample year, 1493–4
Diacatholicon	18 lbs	0.61 oz	354	171
Diaphoenic	11.8 lbs[101]	0.22 oz	644	141
Diasenna	17.5 lbs[102]	0.72 oz	292	126

The other main component of every purge was a vehicle of some sort, allowing doctors to further 'temper' the mixture of drugs and simples according to the patient's needs. Most purges were in 'liquid' form and the majority (sixty per cent) of these vehicles were simple distilled 'waters' made from plant extracts,[103] generally local herbs such as fumitory, endive, fennel and scabious (see Table 8.5), all of which were associated with cheap purges.[104] Trebbiano wine was also sometimes used – always in combination with water of endive – and was associated with the more expensive purges containing rhubarb and/or manna.[105] Since distilled waters had a shelf life of one year they could be stored in large quantities, and large stocks appear in the inventory.[106] The wholesale price of these products was typically a little over one soldo per lb for the most common varieties, but higher for special varieties such as waters made from roses or maidenhair (both around three soldi per lb).[107]

Table 8.5

Top Ten 'Waters' Used in Liquid Purges, 1493–4

Number	Product	Proportion[108]
46	Water of Fumitory	11.6%
42	Water of Endive	10.6%
38	Water of Fennel	9.6%
36	Water of Scabious	9.1%
27	Water of Endive and Trebbiano wine	6.8%
25	Water of Borrage	6.3%
21	Water of Wormwood	5.3%
19	Distilled Water	4.8%
18	Water of Hops	4.5%
15	Water of Couch Grass	3.8%

An alternative form of liquid vehicle were decoctions (forty per cent of the total).[109] These had to be made to order as they could not be stored, and this would have involved significant waiting times for clients.[110] They are typically associated with more expensive purges.[111] Decoctions were made by boiling a mixture of simples in water and then straining the product.[112] In most cases – over two thirds – these were standard preparations whose recipes appear in the *Ricettario*, such as the 'pectoral', 'fresh', 'cordial' and 'common' decoctions.[113] For example, the 'fresh' decoction was made from prunes, tamarinds, violets, barley and various 'cool' seeds – melon, watermelon, cucumber and pumpkin.[114] Decoctions could also be found in combination – the best-selling variety was actually a mixture of the 'fresh' and 'cordial' types (nineteen per cent).[115] In addition to these standard types, decoctions might also be made to order, according to the doctor's prescription. In these cases the full recipe appears in the account book, as in a decoction of liquorice, currants, maidenhair, senna leaves, epithyme, and saffron boiled in distilled water,[116] or a 'decoction of red chickpeas in which parsley roots have been cooked'.[117] Doctors not only prescribed the precise mix of simples and compound drugs, but also the vehicles used to 'temper' them, all of which could be tailored to the individual needs of the patient. Purges were unique products.

Clysters, electuaries and pills

The personalisation of medicines is also found with other types of medicinal products. A means of 'opening' the body, often as preparation for a purge, was to administer *archomenti* (clysters), liquid medicines that were inserted into the rectum with a syringe.[118] At the Giglio, most clysters were made from pudding pipe and aromatic honey infused with violets or roses.[119] They were also usually combined with red sugar, a cheaper and less-refined variety whose applications were limited to medicine.[120] The basic ingredients correspond to the recipes in the medical literature, which combined pudding pipe and honey with flowers such as violet and mallow.[121] Yet, as with purges, clysters could be modified to suit the needs of the individual patient. Additions might include 'carminative substances' (herbs and flowers that encouraged the expulsion of wind, such as senna, camomile, aniseed or epithyme);[122] oil of violets, roses or camomile;[123] turpentine (which had purgative effects);[124] and 'solutive' compound drugs such as *diasenna, hiera pigra*, or *benedetta*.[125] The average price of around six soldi per clyster, therefore, masks a considerable variance, from two soldi for the simplest varieties,[126] to four soldi for clysters with added oil or camomile flowers,[127] to eight soldi for clysters with several types of oils and carminative substances,[128] and over twenty soldi for a bespoke preparation containing carminative substances, colocynth, oils of costmary and rue, compound drugs, red sugar,

Table 8.6

Price Distribution of Composite Electuaries

Total Number	Minimum	Median	Maximum	Mean
253	**2.33 soldi**	**8.67 soldi**	**68 soldi**	**11 soldi**

honey roset and turpentine.[129] Despite the existence of cheap alternatives, the data suggest that they were mostly consumed by a social élite.[130]

'Sweet electuaries' or 'aromatic confections' were a particular category of drugs that typically consisted of a mixture of red roses with honey or syrup, combined with other spices and simples.[131] *Dieradon Abbatis*, the bestseller at the Giglio, consisted of sandalwood, red roses and sugar candy, ground up in a mortar along with a whole range of gums, spices, seeds, sugar, pearls, camphor and musk, and then combined with a syrup of red roses to make a thick and sticky electuary.[132] Although occasionally retailed direct to consumers, these sorts of 'electuaries'[133] were typically retailed in combination with other ingredients, in particular aromatic sugars or honeys that were infused with flower essences – principally roses, violets, citron, bugloss and borage – or sometimes with thicker syrups called locs.[134] In particular, most sweet electuaries were combined with something called 'cordial mixture', supposedly very good for 'acute and pestilential fevers', which was made from flowers of borage and bugloss ground up with sugar, and then combined with ingredients such as pearls, coral, sandalwood, powdered gemstones, gold and silver.[135]

Like purges therefore, these 'electuaries' typically consisted of combinations of storeshelf drugs that were then mixed with other ingredients, in this case aromatic sugars and syrups. Like purges, the median price was around nine to ten soldi. At the bottom end of the market were products such as a combination of three different drugs, made in a such tiny quantity that it cost only around two soldi.[136] At the other end of the scale was a 'cordial electuary' costing sixty-eight soldi, which contained five different sweet electuaries – some made from gems and pearls – combined with a conserve of citron vinegar and coated in gold leaf.[137] Analysis shows that the price of the most expensive 'cordial' electuaries was due to ingredients such as gems, gold leaf, ivory, pearls, and musk. The most expensive purges, on the other hand, contained things such as manna and rhubarb.

'Electuaries' could also be produced in the more palatable form of *morselletti* – 'little morsels' of drugs and sugar, which typically cost around forty-eight soldi per lb, and weighed about ¼ oz (about seven grams, much bigger than pills).[138] The best-selling variety was made with *aromatico rosato*, a 'sweet electuary' containing red roses, syrups, various gums and spices,[139] and the recipe could be varied by adding other ingredients such as powdered gemstones,[140] or chicken pannicles.[141] Chicken was favoured as an easily-digestible and nourishing food for invalids, and occasionally more elaborate confections were sold, such as a 'confected chicken made with fine sugar and rose water, the flesh of the capon washed several times in rose water, made with 'common seeds' and almonds and pine-nuts',[142] covered with powdered gems and spices and packaged in a 'gilded box'.[143] Such products were extremely expensive – this example cost over three lire.[144]

Seemingly 'bizarre', such confections were part of the Arab medical tradition of costly ingredients, considered particularly effective in treating the heart, and appear to have been particularly fashionable in the late fifteenth century – similar recipes appear in Marsilio Ficino's *On Life*.[145] Such ingredients were extremely expensive but usually such tiny amounts were used that the final product was often quite cheap – a cordial electuary containing half a dram of powdered gemstones in a gilded albarello cost only fifteen soldi and was bought by a doublet-maker.[146] Yet, despite the fact that composite electuaries were not always particularly expensive, on the whole they were used by a restricted group of higher-status clients.[147] The social profile of demand for medicines was not simply detemined by price, but instead reflected the consumption practices established among determined social groups. Certain categories of products were regarded as supplementary to the principal therapy, or linked to problems that were considered less urgent in terms of health, such as pains caused by phlegm in the chest.[148]

'Bitter electuaries' were another distinct category of drugs, but one that was little used in practice. The only varieties retailed in the sample year were theriac and mithridate. These were to become the most famous drugs of the early modern period, notorious for the number and variety of their ingredients. However, they were only really to come into fashion in the sixteenth century, as advances in botany and philology held out the prospect of discovering the 'true' theriac.[149] In the fifteenth century, doctors recognised that theriac had many functions, but it was no panacea.[150] The Giglio data shows that theriac was a drug of moderate popularity, with thirty-nine sales in the sample year amounting to 141 soldi, falling just outside the top ten (see Table 8.3).[151] Despite its complex recipe, it was relatively cheap, retailing at around forty soldi per lb,[152] around half the price of more popular drugs such as diacatholicon.[153] Mithridate on the other hand was hardly used at all, with only one sale in the sample period, and retailing at only sixty-four soldi per lb, despite the extreme complexity of the recipe – it contained around a hundred different ingredients.[154] Theriac and mithridate are often taken as prime examples of the polypharmacy of the period, but in practice, just like the other drugs of the time, they were storeshelf products that were retailed in combination with other drugs and simples rather than separately. In one composite electuary, theriac was mixed with three other electuaries.[155] In another example, a 'capital electuary' was made from a mixture of three drugs – theriac, mithridate and diamoschum – but cost only just over fourteen soldi.[156] It was the use of simples such as rhubarb, manna, gold, gemstones, coral, musk and pearls that was the key factor in determining price, not the complexity of the manufacturing process.

A similar pattern of personalisation is found with pills, which were considered a particularly effective way of getting unpleasant medicines into the body, being coated with sugar or wax.[157] They were believed to transmit their effects to the body more effectively since they remained in the stomach for longer.[158] Since they were more potent, however, the literature also expresses some reserve about their use.[159] The Giglio accounts show that pills had a fairly large customer base, being bought by just under a third of clients.[160] Pills were one of the most standardised forms of medicines and, unlike other drugs, the standard varieties listed in the *Ricettario* were often retailed direct to the public. The best-selling variety – six per cent of sales of pills – were a standard purgative type called *sine quibus*, which contained scammony, rhubarb, agaric, and senna.[161] Other standard varieties that sold fairly well were pills known as *aggregative, auree*, fumitory and *bicicche*.[162] Clients usually bought these in small quantities as needed, with the exception of Don Domenico, a monk at the Badia, who bought nearly one hundred pills of agaric in a single transaction, perhaps to stock the abbey dispensary.[163] Bespoke compositions typically involved mixing different standard types of pill together and 'reforming' them in new composite varieties.[164] In one prescription, standard pills of rhubarb were combined with a dysentery powder and reformed into pills.[165] In another, 'fetid pills' were combined with trochisks of agaric and *sugo rosato*, and formed anew into pills.[166] Compared to other products, however, pills shows a much more limited degree of personalisation, with standard varieties retailed either singly or in combination.[167]

Standard varieties of pills typically cost only four denari each, but since they were extremely small – weighing only half a scruple, just over half a gram[168] – this corresponds to a high price, around 192 soldi per lb, more than most compound drugs. If gilded, they typically cost twice as much (eight denari each).[169] Bespoke varieties tended to cost more – a composition of agaric trochisks and 'aggregative' pills cost eight denari each.[170] Nevertheless, gilding (which involved only tiny amounts of gold) and bespoke composition (where the main cost was in cheap labour) had little impact on price by comparison to the inclusion of really expensive ingredients like rhubarb. Standard pills with rhubarb cost eight denari each,[171] or twelve denari each when gilded,[172] and a special variety of rhubarb pills 'for blockages', which presumably owed their laxative effect to even higher doses of rhubarb, cost even more: sixteen denari per pill, equivalent to s768 per lb.[173] This was cheap compared to the pills bought by a silk merchant, which cost around a hundred denari each.[174] The pills were gilded and made up specially for him, but it was the quantity of rhubarb (one and a half drams) that made them so expensive. However, such expensive variants were rare,[175] and although pills were fairly widely used they represented only a limited proportion of spending on medicines overall.[176]

Supplementary products: syrups

Certain products were supplements to a cure. In addition to sweets (Chapter 7), the clearest case is that of syrups, typically prescribed to be taken daily for a week after taking a purge. Michele Strozzi bought a purge for his daughter on 28 June 1493, which was followed by two doses of syrup on 30 June (along with coriander comfits), and a further dose of syrup on 2 July.[177] Similarly, the maidservant, Mona Mattea, bought a purge made with pudding pipe on 12 April 1494, and this was followed by daily doses of syrup.[178] On 18 April, around a week later, she was prescribed a different kind of purge, and a clyster, which was followed on 22 April by an electuary.[179] This was a fairly common pattern whereby a purge was followed by syrups taken daily for around a week, and then a second purge, at which point the doctor often modified the therapy rather than repeat the prescription. The vast majority of these syrups consisted simply of distilled water and sugar, which retailed at four soldi for a standard dose of two ounces (ie. 57g).[180] Specialist varieties could also be made with things such as violets, poppies, mint,[181] or currants,[182] and more complex recipes could be made to order,[183] but these were quite rare. Syrups had a wide customer base, roughly equivalent to that of cassia pulp,[184] and show similar patterns of consumption across the year, with a pronounced peak in April 1494, suggesting that consumption of syrups was strongly linked to that of purges.

Doctors often prescribed that syrups be used at particular times of day, such as the morning or evening.[185] This was often linked to mealtimes, as with a dose of 'syrup with sugar and decoction of currants' that was specifically 'for the evening after dinner',[186] while a combination of syrup of mint and rosato colato was 'to take before meals'.[187] Lucrezia Rinucci was prescribed various syrups 'to use when she is at table',[188] and on another occasion was instructed to take two spoonfuls of syrup 'before eating'.[189] Many of these syrups were supposed to be consumed with chicken broth,[190] a practice that Michele Savonarola, court physician at Ferrara, described as a 'singular medicine'.[191] The convent of Sant'Ambrogio bought four oz of 'syrup with sugar', enough for 'four doses with chicken broth',[192] and one client bought a dose of syrup that was 'to take in the morning with chicken *peverada*',[193] a kind of spicy meat sauce.[194] Chicken broth was traditionally given to the sick,[195] a practice implemented on the grand scale at the hospital of Santa Maria Nuova.[196] This suggests that the syrups were intended to provide the body with nourishing foods, easy to digest, so building up the strength of the patient between purges.

External therapies: epithems, fomentations, baths

The most important external therapies retailed at the Giglio were epithems. These were made from 'spices' (ie. drugs in powdered form),[197] which were mixed with a liquid and then applied to the body with a cloth or sponge.[198] The most common epithem was a 'cordial' variety containing musk and amber and used to treat heart complaints.[199] Many variations existed on this base recipe, adding ingredients such as malmsey wine,[200] vinegar roset,[201] sanders,[202] 'cordial flowers' (such as roses, violets and nymphæa),[203] violets,[204] and vinegar.[205] These ingredients were frequently red (roses, red sandalwood, saffron, coral and kermes), since the colour was linked to function (a cure for the heart) – and they were often also applied with a scarlet cloth.[206] The hospital receptary indicates the logic behind such variations, which allowed the doctor to adjust the composition to suit the patient:[207] for example, to make a 'hotter' epithem the quantity of sanders was reduced, and small quantities of amber and musk were added.[208] A little musk or aromatic wine might be added where the fever was weaker and the patient less hardy.[209] Epithems for other body areas (such as the liver or stomach) appear less frequently at the Giglio, but show a similar pattern of variations.[210] For an 'acute fever', for example, the doctor might add camphor to the basic recipe for an epithem for the liver, but in this case the recipe should also be 'tempered' with water of violets.[211] Epithems were fairly expensive, with an average price of about twenty-two soldi,[212] restricting their use to a minority of high status clients.[213] Nevertheless, because they were regularly used by that minority, epithems represented a fairly high proportion of medical spending (four per cent overall).[214]

Fomentations could also be retailed separately, without the addition of powdered drugs, for application to the skin with a cloth or sponge (the latter, sometimes described as 'fine' or 'Venetian' sponges, could also be bought from the shop).[215] The most common variety was a 'stomachic fomentation with various herbs and flowers'.[216] Commonly, the recipe was varied according to the patient, and the sorts of ingredients listed include aromatic herbs, spices and flowers, such as one fomentation for the stomach made with 'wormwood, dill, roses and camomile flowers, coriander, linseed and fenugreek'.[217] Fomentations were usually specific to particular areas of the body: in addition to the 'stomachic' varieties, we find a 'pectoral fomentation' for the chest,[218] a fomentation for the pubic and urinary areas,[219] and another for the spleen.[220] Of very similar nature to fomentations, were 'baths' – mixtures of dried flowers and herbs bought in the shop and added to hot water at home or in bath-houses.[221] Unlike fomentations, 'baths' were not specific to body area, suggesting that the patient's body was fully immersed in the water. Many of these were referred to as 'somniferous fomentations' – containing poppy heads, they were intended to relax the body.[222] Overall, the evidence for the retail of epithems, fomentations and baths reveals a remarkable range of composition and function that went far beyond the limited indications of the recipe books, showing how specialist products were available to suit a multitude of different therapeutic purposes and conditions of patients.

External therapies: ointments, plasters, cerates

A higher degree of standardisation is found with ointments,[223] plasters,[224] and cerates (a stiff variety made with wax or spread on strips of leather).[225] The most important ointment in terms of sales (eighteen per cent) was specifically for the stomach, and contained wax, various oils (wormwood, mastic, spike), flowers and spices.[226] Like epithems, these were specific to bodily area, as in a 'fresh' ointment that was 'to anoint the kidneys'.[227] Similarly, the most common type of 'sandalwood' cerate,[228] was often specifically described as being for the liver.[229] Other types of cerates were specifically made for the spleen,[230] kidneys,[231] head,[232] chest[233] or feet,[234] ranging in size from an *ostia* (communion wafer)[235] to a *tagliere* (chopping board).[236] In most cases the recipes for these products are to be found in the *Ricettario*, but there are also a number of 'magisterial' products specially made for clients. These included, for example, simple mixtures of the standard ointments, such as mixture of stomach and sandalwood ointments,[237] or more complex bespoke preparations, such as a particularly unusual 'magisterial' kidney ointment for the wife of a silk merchant, which contained 'turtle's blood, dragon's blood, bole armeniac, terra sigillata and other things'.[238] Despite the existence of a range of specialised standard products linked to specific bodily areas, doctors still often preferred to prescribe magisterial compositions suited to the particular condition of the patient. Part of this variation may have been related to season: the hospital receptary warns, for example, for one unguent 'if made during the summer then add less oil and vice versa this should be added during the winter'.[239] A recipe for a plaster for broken heads warned in dramatic terms: 'it must be winter and not summer because you would kill [the patient]'.[240] Climatic factors were probably factored in by doctors when making their prescriptions.

Packaging

Whether products were taken directly from the jars and boxes that lined the shelves and filled the cupboards and drawers of the shop, or whether they were made up for the client on the spot, they all needed to be packaged for retail, particularly since many consisted of liquids or syrups. Elsewhere, we have suggested how important the 'look' of the pharmacy was to consumer confidence, particularly in terms of the large number of storage jars that lined the shelves. This also applied to the presentation and packaging of the medicines sold retail. Customers had to pay for the vessels that they used, which are listed in the accounts as part of the bill, typically priced four denari. Where no vessel is mentioned, this suggests that customers were probably re-using vessels they had bought on other occasions. There are even instances where customers returned several vessels as part payment of their bill.[241] The shop sold its broken glass in turn to a firm of *bicchierai* (glass-makers).[242] *Bicchieri*, small drinking glasses, were used exclusively for liquid purges and were the most frequently appearing receptacles.[243] The term *albarello* is usually understood to refer to large ceramic storage jars, but smaller *albarelli* were used for retail, particularly for thick and sticky electuaries.[244] *Ampolle* (ampoules) were mostly used for medium volumes of liquid such as syrups or juleps, made from either glass or ceramic.[245] Larger volumes of liquid, such as those found in clysters and epithems, were generally supplied in a *pentola* (pot), probably made of terracotta.[246] For particularly special medicines, and especially for cordial electuaries containing powdered gemstones, pearls and gold, the packaging also might be gilded, as in the case of a gilded *albarello* used to serve an electuary containing ground pearls and gold leaf,[247] or the gilded boxes used to serve elaborate confections of chicken, gemstones and spices.[248]

Processing at home

The Giglio accounts show that there was some crossover between medicines that were ready-made or prepared in the shop, and those that were processed at home. Clients often purchased ingredients at the shop for final processing at home, although this was usually limited to simple operations such as boiling. One client bought honey, liquorice and currants 'to boil up at home to make a drink'.[249] Another client bought various flowers 'to boil up at home to make a long julep'.[250] Products such as decoctions and juleps had a limited shelf life, but in this way customers could buy dried ingredients to make up for use as needed. Epithems, in particular, were often sold 'dry', allowing clients to mix the powdered drugs with decoctions made at home,[251] as when a client bought 'dried herbs' to take home and 'boil in barley water and vinegar to make an epithem for the liver'.[252] This was probably according to a doctor's prescription, rather than being examples of self-medication.[253]

Clysters were also typically bought dried and made up at home immediately prior to use. One client bought four oz of 'electuary and sugar for clysters' along with four handfuls of camomile and melilot that were 'to boil up for the clyster'.[254] Another client bought red sugar and 'various herbs to boil for the clyster' as well as oil of spike and oil of camomile 'to put in the clyster'.[255] These events can be contrasted with the rare cases where clysters were made on the spot for clients: one entry notes that a 'fresh' clyster was 'made here in the shop'.[256] Another entry specifically describes how a clyster was 'made here in the shop and condited with oil and salt and with pudding pipe...', and then carried home in a pot by a maidservant.[257]

Clients could also save on costs by supplying their own ingredients, including not just everyday items but also imported exotica which circulated in the private market.[258] Some of these were probably left over from previous prescriptions, as when a client brought his own pills to the shop to be 'reformed' into a new compound.[259] Clients might also purchase drugs at the shop for combination with their own ingredients at home, as when a client bought diamanna, a decoction and spikenard for combination with 'his rhubarb and manna at home'.[260] In particular, syrups and drugs were sometimes prescribed to be boiled with chicken *peverada,* or other sauces that could easily be produced at home.[261] Other customers bought a cordial powder containing 'emeralds, red coral, cordial flowers and plantain seeds' that was specifically 'to put in the chicken' at home.[262] Clients could make their own decoctions for combination with shop-bought drugs and simples, as when a client purchased an infusion of rhubarb in water of endive and trebbiano wine, 'to add to his decoction at home'.[263] In some cases, clients bought ingredients at the shop to be mixed with electuaries that they had at home.[264] These were probably left-over drugs which clients thought to use again, rather than electuaries that had been manufactured at home. There is no evidence that clients purchased simples to make their own electuaries and drugs. Instead, the Giglio evidence suggests that they limited their operations to things like boiling or mixing, the final processing immediately before use. At most, there is some evidence that clients self-medicated by buying simples from the shop and consuming these without further processing, as we have seen with pudding pipe,[265] or with a client who bought 'finely ground camphor', 'for use at home'.[266]

The main savings in such cases regarded the cost of ingredients, rather than processing. It is difficult to obtain good evidence of processing costs, since this was not normally recorded. When one client supplied his own spices that the apothecary used to make an electuary, the accounts record a nominal price of five soldi 'for making it'.[267] In another case, where the client supplied his own rhubarb for incorporation in a pill bought from the shop, there was a charge of one soldo for 'reforming' the pill.[268] However, these were service charges applied where the apothecary processed ingredients that were provided entirely by the client, and cannot be used to represent real labour costs. In general, the evidence suggests that the price of products was primarily derived from the quantity of ingredients used. (In any case it should be remembered that these are nominal prices that served as a starting point for negotiations about payment). The primary motive for processing goods at home was to lengthen the shelf life of commodities or save on the cost of ingredients, rather than to reduce labour costs.

Conclusion

The Giglio records confirm the strong influence of the Arabic tradition in Renaissance medicine, in terms of the key medicinal simples (pudding pipe, rhubarb and manna, none of which were mentioned by Dioscorides) ,[269] product types (syrups, juleps, confections) and drug recipes (largely derived from authorities such as Nicholao and Mesue).[270] The retail accounts reveal a more nuanced and complex picture of the way that pharmacological theory was implemented in practice, casting new light on the composition of products for retail and their relationship to the standard drug preparations detailed in the theoretical literature. Although recipe books like the *Ricettario fiorentino* detail a vast number of drug recipes, only a limited range of these were much used in practice.[271] Only two of the main categories of drugs listed in the *Ricettario* were much used (purgatives and 'sweet electuaries'), and within those categories usage focused on a small selection of specific recipes (such as diacatholicon, diaphœnicon and diasenna, see Table 8.3).

Renaissance pharmacology, therefore, made use of only a limited range of drugs, but it used them in far more complex ways than the recipe books suggest. Standard drugs, such diacatholicon, were rarely used alone and instead were normally mixed with other compound drugs, simples, waters, decoctions and sugar, to create complex products that potentially combined hundreds of ingredients. Although the compound drugs listed in the recipe books were recognised as having multiple therapeutic applications, this did not make them universal panaceas that suited all patients and conditions – even drugs like theriac and mithridate still needed to be balanced with other drugs and simples to be effective. 'Universal' cures were to become increasingly popular in the sixteenth century, but their existence was not yet recognised in the 1490s.

Instead, the accounts show strong adherence to the Galenic theory that drugs should always be 'tempered' to the particular condition of the individual patient, taking into account characteristics such as constitution, age and sex, as well as external variables such as the season.[272] Rather than prescribing standard remedies for standard illnesses, doctors' prescriptions were *personalised* to a considerable extent. Key medicinal simples, such as pudding pipe, were sometimes bought for self-medication and used alone, but most clients accepted the prevailing wisdom that all drugs and simples could be dangerous when used in isolation and that their effects needed to be tempered by combination with other commodities. Patients may well have understood that they needed a certain type of product, such as a purge, or a particular simple, such as rhubarb, but the precise composition of that product was something best determined by a doctor. Even in the case of pills, one of the most highly standardised forms of drugs, doctors typically prescribed mixtures that had to be made up specially for the patient. Far more important than standard drug solutions was a 'magisterial' approach to drug therapy, whereby drugs were used in combination or adjusted to suit the complexion of the individual, or where bespoke recipes were created specifically for individual patients – as we have seen in particular for purges, clysters, confections and fomentations.[273] Doctors, therefore, employed a more limited range of standard products than was listed in the recipe books, but modified these extensively in practice in accordance with the condition of the patient. This emphasis on treating the *patient* rather than the disease was a factor that incidentally helped to protect the professional role of educated doctors.[274] Only in the sixteenth century did the shift towards standardised patent medicines come to threaten their position more seriously.

In this respect, the publication of the *Ricettario fiorentino* was an important step toward standardisation, establishing 'definitive' versions of drugs to be used in the city. Yet, while this extended greater regulatory control over apothecaries, at the same time it safeguarded the professional role of doctors, since the drugs still required tempering to suit the needs of individual patients.[275] A doctor's prescription was a *recipe* (as the contemporary Italian term *ricetta* suggests), designed for an individual, not just a list of standard products. The standardised solutions of the recipe books provided an important reference point and means of disciplining the apothecary practice, but coexisted with the freedom of doctors to adjust their cures. Within the relatively simple humoral model of explanation of disease that patients could themselves understand, there was much room for theoretical elaboration.[276] Rather than being 'unworkable', the complexity of medieval pharmacological theory actually created a space within which doctors could adopt their own approach, bringing their own experience into play in deciding which cures were appropriate.[277] Rather than a 'recipe-book' approach, where standard remedies were applied to standard illnesses, this evidence suggests that doctors knew and understood the properties of the different simples, drugs and vehicles, and were able to combine them according to the specific case. This principle was explicitly stated in the

257

Ricettario fiorentino, which recognised its inability to fully *describe* contemporary practice due to the discretion enjoyed by doctors:

> [M]any confections and cordial electuaries may be composed according to the fancy of the doctor, adding and removing [ingredients] at his discretion and according to the requirements of the patient for whom it is ordered: and similarly it is possible to make many and varied types of clysters, fomentations, plasters, unctions, epithems and such, which will not be included here due to the variety of practitioners and of their fancies....[278]

The approaches of different doctors varied considerably, rather than adhering rigidly to a fixed method. This belies the 'recipe book' approach to drug therapy identified in some of the literature, suggesting instead that doctors enjoyed considerable freedom to experiment within the broad explanatory framework provided by humoral theory, even if they did not do so in any very systematic fashion.

The Giglio evidence further shows that, rather than being restricted to an élite,[279] many medicinal products were actually quite cheap and accessible to the middling ranks of the urban population – artisans, shopkeepers and the like – a demand that was further boosted by the strong provision of consumer credit in this sector. Although it might be assumed that standard preparations tended to be used by poor clients and bespoke preparations by the rich, the primary determinant on price was not the cost of processing but the raw materials. A relatively simple purge containing rhubarb cost far more than a complex combination of drugs and pudding pipe made to order. One of the key differences between rich and poor consumption of medicines, therefore, regarded the kind of ingredients used in their manufacture, especially rhubarb, manna, musk, gold, coral and pearls. Costly purges could be created using rhubarb and manna, but pudding pipe and sugar were often sufficient for ordinary folk. The wealthy consumed pills coated in gold foil, but the less well-off could buy the same product without gold for half the price.[280] Similarly, for the medicinal sweets called *manuschristi*, the base recipe of sugar and rose water could be modified through the inclusion of expensive ingredients such as gold, coral, powdered gems and pearls, which cost up to twice as much. Doctors probably took these factors into consideration when making their prescriptions, adjusting the therapy according to the means as well as the complexion of the individual patient. The medical consumption of rich and poor can therefore be distinguished in broad terms by the quality of ingredients used in their medicines.

Furthermore, rich and poor also had access to a different *range* of products. The poor often limited their consumption to the purges considered essential for treating serious disorders, sometimes supplemented by courses of syrups, while the rich were able to afford more accessory products such as clysters, epithems, aromatic 'baths', and elaborate confections of 'sweet' electuaries and sugar, such as *morselletti*. Although such products were not particularly expensive compared to purges, they were not indispensable for a cure and therefore attracted lower demand from those who could not easily afford them. Whether particular medicines were considered 'luxuries' or 'necessities' was something that depended upon the means and opportunity of the patient. The Giglio evidence shows that even within the category of shop-bought medicines, there was a range of alternatives: the same basic types of medicines could be varied in terms of the cost of the ingredients, and the number and kinds of supplementary therapies employed.

This study, therefore, questions the idea of a clear divide between 'élite' shop-bought medicines and 'popular' remedies with regard to the urban population, since the city's shops and hospitals were able to cater to a wide range of consumers. Nevertheless, this opens up the possibility of such a gulf between the city and the countryside. Comparison of Giglio records with contemporary herbals suggests a divide between a local 'folk' tradition and the medicines retailed in the shops. Rosemary, for example, was a commonplace kitchen herb renowned for its myriad therapeutic virtues and commonly appearing in herbals, but it never appears in the Giglio records.[281] Peasants are entirely absent from the shop records and would have been forced to rely on country remedies - popular rhymes suggest that peasant identity may have partially formed around their exclusion from this market, forced to rely on substitutes for apothecary products – their 'pills' and 'syrups' were hens and wine from the cellar.[282] One way that the shop-based apothecary trade and learned doctors distinguished their trade from folk remedies was in placing the emphasis on the virtues of imported exotica rather than the 'spices of the poor' (things like mint, parsley, sage and rosemary).[283] This orientation was to be the focus of many critiques of the medical establishment in the sixteenth century, by figures such as Paracelsus. For example, Giovanni Battista Zapata in his book of 'marvellous secrets' (1577), criticised the traditional apothecary trade for being both costly and ineffective, consoling his readers with the thought that even if they could not afford 'gems, gold and precious stones', remedies based on these ingredients were, in fact, 'vain and of no benefit'.[284]

However, it should be noted that the blanket categorisation of therapeutic options according to a crude division between 'rich' and 'poor' obscures the choice that characterised the 'medical marketplace'.[285] The urban population had a range of alternatives to choose from, both at the shop and outside it. Although the doctors and apothecaries defined their identity through adherence to a particular 'school' of medical therapy, things were by no means so clear-cut from the point of view of consumers. The use of drugs, prescribed by doctors and bought at shops or administered by a hospital, did not preclude the use of alternative therapies at the same time. As many scholars have emphasised, prayer, pilgrimage, magic, herblore and learned medicine might all be combined in fighting disease. From the point of view of pharmacology, the exotica of the apothecary shop lived alongside local herbs and ingredients. Francesco Castellani made use of apothecary shop but his recipes against 'worms' used simple local ingredients, such as a clyster made with honey and goat's milk.[286] Exotic simples such as pudding pipe could be stocked at home, and used directly by consumers in their own recipes, perhaps with local herbs, or combined with shop-bought drugs. Similarly, the hospital of Santa Maria Nuova recorded recipes using simple local ingredients alongside those inherited from the learned medical tradition.[287] The identity of the city population was not defined through commitment to a single therapeutic approach, but through the greater choice they enjoyed.

Notes

1. J. Schönfeld, 'Pharmacy in the Medieval Arab World', in R. Pötzsch (ed.), *The Pharmacy: Windows on History* (Basel: Editiones Roche, 1996), 104.

2. G. Silini, *Umori e farmaci: terapia medica tardo-medievale* (Gandino: Servitium, 2001), 139–41; J.M. Riddle, *Dioscorides on Pharmacy and Medicine*, 1st edn (Austin: University of Texas Press, 1985), xix, 169–75; N.G. Siraisi, *Medieval & Early Renaissance Medicine: An Introduction to Knowledge and Practice* (Chicago: University of Chicago Press, 1990), 142.

3. J. Stannard, 'The Herbal as a Medical Document', *Bulletin of the History of Medicine*, 43 (1969), 212–20, reprinted in J. Stannard, *Herbs and Herbalism in the Middle Ages and Renaissance* (Aldershot: Ashgate, 1999), 219, quotes from the *Herbarius latinus* (1484).

4. *Ibid.*, 219.

5. J. Stannard, 'Dioscorides and Renaissance Materia Medica', in M. Florkin (ed.), *Materia Medica in the XVIth Century: Proceedings of a Symposium of the International Academy of the History of Medicine, held at the University of Basel, 7th September 1964* (Oxford: Pergamon Press, 1966), 7.

6. A. Corvi, 'Le pillole nel XVI secolo : la riforma proposta dal pilluarium di Pantaleone da Confienza', *Atti e memorie della accademia italiana di storia della farmacia*, 18, 1 (2001), 11–16: 12; D.L. Cowen and W.H. Helfand, *Pharmacy: An Illustrated History* (New York: Harry N. Abrams, 1988), 51; M.N. Pearson, 'Introduction', in M.N. Pearson (ed.), *Spices in the Indian Ocean World* (Aldershot: Variorum, 1996), xv–xvi.

7. M.A. Ciasca, *Speziali e farmacopee nell'Italia del secolo XV* (Amatrice, Rieti: Tip. Orfanotrofio Maschile, 1951), 37; A.M. Carmona-Cornet, A. Corvi,

and T. Huguet Termes, 'La farmacologia pratica nell'opera di Saladino
d'Ascoli e la sua ripercussione nella farmacopea europea', *Atti e memorie della
accademia italiana di storia della farmacia,* 12, 2 (1995), 132–6; Cowen and
Helfand, *op. cit.* (note 6), 68; E. Cingolani and L. Colapinto, *Dagli
antidotari alle moderne farmacopee* (Rome: Di Renzo, 2000), 22. Other
fifteenth-century apothecary manuals of this sort, circulating initially as
manuscripts and printed in the 1490s, included Manlius del Bosco,
Luminare majus, a sort of encyclopaedia of drugs (Pavia, 1494); Quiricus de
Augustis, *Lumen apothecariorum* (Turin, 1492); Paulus Suardus, *Thesaurus
aromatariorum* (Milan, 1496); and Nicole Prévost, *Dispensarium ad
aromaticus* (Lyon, 1478–88). On these, see H.C. Silberman, 'Les formulaires
des pharmaciens Manlius di Bosco Quiricus de Augustis et Paulus Suardus et
la place importante qu'y prennent les sucreries', *Atti e memorie della
accademia italiana di storia della farmacia,* 18, 1 (2001), 17–22; Cowen and
Helfand, *op. cit.* (note 6), 68; C. Masino, 'Interrogativi su Manlio di Bosco e
Paolo Suardo speziali', *Atti e memorie della accademia italiana di storia della
farmacia,* 5 (1988), 7–10.

8. R. Ciasca, *L'arte dei medici e speziali nella storia e nel commercio fiorentino dal
   secolo XII al XV* (Florence: Leo S. Olschki, 1927), 342–3.

9. *Ricettario fiorentino* (Florence: Compagnia del Drago, 1499) advised that
   'ogni diligente persona debbe havere questi libri, cioe uno semplicista, chome
   e Symon Genovese. Lepandette. Avicenna & li semplici suoi, & chosi
   Lalmansore. El quarto del servitore. Lo anthidotario di Mesue, &
   Lanthidotario di Nicholao'. On these authors see Cowen and Helfand,
   op. cit. (note 6), 42, 52; A. Corradi, *Le prime farmacopee italiane ed in
   particolare dei ricettari fiorentini* (Milan: Rechiedei, 1887).

10. The *Liber Serapionis aggregatus in medicinis simplicibus* was a Latin edition of
    an Arab manual of simples by Ibn Sarabiyun (latinised as Johannes Serapion
    the Younger). It was translated into Latin in 1292, and first printed in Milan
    in 1473. See Antonius Guarnerinus de Padua, *Herbe pincte,* G. Silini (ed.),
    (Gorle: Iniziative Culturali, 2000), 103. Serapione was also the author of a
    breviarum, containing recipes, and the Giglio accounts may be referring to
    this instead. E882, fo. 160v, 'Ant.o di bartolomeo tessitore', 21 October
    1493, specifically refers to 'loccho di giovanni di serapione', and such
    references can also be found at the hospital of Santa Mariva Nuova – BNF,
    Magl. XV.92, fo. 134v, 'Polvere di Serapione nel suo breviario di
    provochatione mestruo'.

11. R. Ciasca (ed.), *Statuti dell'arte dei medici e speziali* (Florence: L.S. Olschki,
    1922), 46, 180; E. Cingolani, 'Il Ricettario fiorentino e le disposizioni
    relative alla professione farmaceutica', *Atti e memorie della accademia italiana
    di storia della farmacia,* 16, 3 (1999), 122–32: 126.

12. E882, fo. 352v, 'Bernardo di piero del palagio', 8 August 1494, 'per usare chome disse il m.o'. Other instructions regard the time of day: fo. 119r, 'Fruosino di Cece da Verrazano', 25 October 1493, 20 'p'le supilative magistrali per pilgliare i.a per mattina'; fo. 320r, 'Niccholo di [BLANK] dacingniano', 17 May 1494, 'armaticho rosato' and 'zuc.o rosato', 'per usare ongni mattina'. Similar advice is found in the hospital receptary, where the patient should 'take *armaticho rosato* at a good hour of the morning...' – see note 148 below.

13. *Ricettario fiorentino* (Florence, 1567) made greater allowance for editions in the vulgar, since although ideally 'Il Buono Speziale' should 'sapere tanto della lingua Latina, che egli possa leggere Dioscoride, Galeno, Plinio, Serapione, Mesuè, Avice[n]na, e gl'altri', it was sufficient to be 'instriuito da uno intelige[n]te maestro, & esercitarsi in leggere i moderni, i quali hanno tradotto, ò scritto di tal materia in lingua volgare.'

14. M.R. McVaugh, 'Medicine in the Latin Middle Ages', in I. Loudon (ed.), *Western Medicine: An Illustrated History* (Oxford: Oxford University Press, 1997), 59; Siraisi, *op. cit.* (note 2), 131–2; S. Guaraldi et al., 'Su un trattato inedito di terapia medica del XV secolo: il codice Palatino 1045 (969-21,3) della Biblioteca Nazionale Centrale di Firenze', *Rivista di storia della medicina*, 5, 1 (1995), 39–63: 42–3.

15. Guaraldi, *ibid.*

16. M.S. Elsheikh and E. Coturri, 'Medici e medicina a Firenze fino alla metà del secolo XIX', in M.S. Elsheikh (ed.), *Medicina e farmacologia nei manoscritti della Biblioteca Riccardiana di Firenze* (Manziana, Rome: Vecchiarelli, 1990), xxviii; Ciasca, *op. cit.* (note 8), 748.

17. P. Slack, 'Mirrors of Health and Treasures of Poor Men: The Uses of the Vernacular Medical Literature of Tudor England', in C. Webster (ed.), *Health, Medicine and Mortality in the Sixteenth Century* (Cambridge: Cambridge University Press, 1979).

18. F. Castellani, *Quaternuccio e giornale B (1459–1485)*, Biblioteca Italiana, Università degli Studi di Roma 'La Sapienza', 2005. [Florence: L.S. Olschki, 1995], 'Medicina provata a' fanciulli o ad altri che sentissi di bachi.'

19. BNF, Magl. XV.92.

20. Siraisi, *op. cit.* (note 2), 132.

21. J.M. Riddle, *Quid Pro Quo: Studies in the History of Drugs* (Aldershot: Variorum, 1992), 172.

22. This value can be taken as a minimum because where data is unavailable on prices this mostly regards the ingredients of complex medicines.

23. Out of total retail sales of 88,609 soldi in the sample year, 11,168 soldi were spent specifically on purges. S. Rosati, 'Benedetto di Tacco da Prato speziale, 1345-1392: Vita, attività, ambiente sociale ed economico', graduate thesis,

Facoltà di lettere e filosofia dell'Università di Firenze (1970–1), 163, for a similar practice in fourteenth-century Prato.

24. In the Giglio accounts, *medicina* was a term used specifically to refer to purges, rather than medicines in general. It is an indication of the centrality of purgation in medical practice that *medicina* was employed in such a specific way in Florence. E882, fo. 104r, 'Bartolomeo delvantaggio', 29 January 1493 (m.f.), the record originally stated 'per una medicina', but this was then struck out and replaced with 'cioe un latt.o in che ent.o' 'dierisse' and 'diachodion', electuaries that did not fall into the 'solutive' category. This kind of usage, which appears specific to Florence, can also be found in M. Ficino, *Three Books on Life*, C.V. Kaske and J.R. Clark (trans.), (Binghampton: Medieval and Renaissance Texts and Studies, 1989), 151–3, Book 1, Chapter 21, 'On liquid medicine' [*De medicina liquida*], which might be better translated 'On the liquid purge'.

25. E882, fo. 2v, 'messer Michele di [BLANK] Strozzi', 3 July 1493, 'E adi detto p[er] una medicina p[er] la figliuola in che ent[ran]o [oncie] i di polpa di chas[s]ia st[enperat]a in aqua d'indivia porto franc[esc]o e [uno] b[icchiere]… [soldi] 7 [denari] 4'.

26. Of the total of 781 purges in the (extended) sample, 635 were in liquid form (81%), and 140 in solid form (18%), with a further 6 of unspecified type.

27. In most cases E882 gives uses the abbreviation 'st.a' for *stenperata*. Silini, *op. cit.* (note 2), 191–2, a liquid purge was referred to as a 'potion' in Gandino. T. Scully, 'Tempering Medieval Food', in M.W. Adamson (ed.), *Food in the Middle Ages: A Book of Essays* (New York: Garland Pub., 1995), on tempering.

28. E878, fo. 20r, '5 schodelle dastenperare medicine +[ii] di rame'.

29. J.-P. Bénézet, *Pharmacie et médicament en Méditerranée occidentale: (XIIIe–XVIe siècles)* (Paris: H. Champion, 1999), 244–5, in Arles, medicinal purges were administered in a decorated goblet, usually made of metal.

30. One of the other of the two formulae 'in forma soda' and 'fatto datt.o con zuc.o' were usually used to show this was medicine in solid form, though the two expressions were equivalent. The two expressions were occasionally found together – see E882, fo. 120r, 'Giovanni Salamancha spangniuolo in chasa andrea lapi', 23 December 1493; fo. 189r, 'Domenicho di filippo sarto a santomaso', 17 December 1493, which both list 'una m[edicin]a in forma soda… fatto datt[er]o con zuc[cher]o'. The formula was usually abbreviated in the accounts but for an expanded version of the text see fo. 208r, 'Ant.o di christofano bandieraio', 16 February 1493 (m.f.), 'fato datero chon zuc[cher]o'. Silini, *op. cit.* (note 2), 194, in Gandino, a similar solid preparation was called a *bolus*. Rather than containing dates, the word 'date' described the form of the purge, perhaps a more elongated equivalent of a *bolus*. The form is also described in J. Mesue, *Opera* (Venice, 1497), fo. 57r.

31. E882, fo. 23v, 'Girolamo di pagholo federichi', 19 September 1493, the drugs were 'inchorporata chon zuc.o'.

32. E882, fo. 59v, 22 August 1493, 'Andrea dicharlo ghalighaio de dare adi 22 daghosto p[er] una m[edicin]a in forma soda p[er] lui in che ent[ran]o [oncie] 1¼ di polpa di chas[s]ia fatto datt[er]o chon zuc[cher]o porto e detto... [soldi] 9'.

33. S. Tognetti, 'Prezzi e salari nella Firenze tardomedievale: un profilo', *Archivio storico italiano*, 153, 2 (1995), 263–333: 331, gives daily wages for unskilled agricultural labourers as from 7 to 7.6 soldi in the period 1493–4, and for unskilled construction workers as 8.4 soldi. For skilled builders in the same period it was from 14 to 16.2 soldi per day.

34. E882, fo. 319v, 'Fruosino di ciecie da verrazano', 9 July 1494, s3 for a medicine in solid form, made with sugar violet and coralline (a vermifuge).

35. Only 25 out of 559 purges (4% of the total) from the sample cost less than 7 soldi.

36. E882, fo. 2v, 'Giovanni di messer charlo federichi', 2 August 1493, recipe containing 1 oz of manna, 0.5 oz of pudding pipe and 1 dr of rhubarb.

37. E882, fo. 309v, 'Nero di franc.o delnero', 14 April 1494, a medicine containing 1.5 oz of manna and 1 dr of rhubarb. See also fo. 310r, 'Rafaello di guliano bastiere da san chasciano', 3 May 1494, for the same preparation sold to a different client at the same price.

38. OED, 'Cassia': distinguishes *cassia lignea* and *cassia fistula*. In order to avoid confusion we have chosen to translate 'polpa di cassia' as 'pudding pipe', although 'cassia fistula' is an equivalent term. On the potential confusion see G. da Orta, 'Colloquies on the Simples and Drugs of India: Cinnamon, Cloves, Mace and Nutmeg, Pepper', in M.N. Pearson (ed.), *Spices in the Indian Ocean World* (Aldershot: Variorum, 1996), 1–2; F.B. Pegolotti, *La pratica della mercatura*, A. Evans (ed.), (Cambridge: The Medieval Academy of America, 1936), 415–16. For detailed discussion of its medicinal properties, see *Liber Pandectarum*, (Vicenza, 1480), cap. clxxi.

39. Of the total of 781 purges (liquid and solid), over half (55%) included pudding pipe as an ingredient. G. Carbonelli, 'I conti di Giacomo Carlo speziale in Biella (1494–1523)', *Bollettino storico subalpino*, 14 (1909), shows that the most common medicinal product sold in Biella was a purge based on pudding pipe. However, Silini, *op. cit.* (note 2), 191–2, finds pudding pipe was an ingredient in only 23 out of 320 preparations (only 7%) prescribed by one of the doctors at Gandino.

40. RF, *op. cit.* (note 9), fo. 60, 'Dyachattolicon', was made from senna leaves, pudding pipe ('polpa di cassia fistula'), tamarind and rhubarb. fo. 61, 'Dyacassia' was made principally of pudding pipe 'polpa di cassia tracta' and white sugar, combined with jujubes, prunes, tamarinds etc.

41. P.A. Mattioli, *I discorsi di M. Pietro Andrea Matthioli Sanese, Medico Cesareo, nei sei libri di Pedacio Dioscoride Anazarbeo della materia medicinale* (Venice, 1585), fo. 48–9, 'Ma perche nè Dioscoride, nè altro degli antichi Greci scrisse (che io sappia) della CASSIA SOLUTIVA, chiamata l'alcuni Siliqua Egittia, la quale è in commune, & frequentissimo uso di tutti i medici per lenire il corpo: accioche questi nostri discorsi non restino senza tanto nobile, tanto eccellente, & tanto necessario medicamento, ne dirò quì quel tanto, che n'ho tratto dagli Arabi, come primi inventori di così bel frutto.'

42. *Ricettario fiorentino* (Florence, 1567) distinguishes between 'Casia de Greci' and 'Cassia degli Arabi' in its listing of simples.

43. The average price of purges containing pudding pipe was s16 for liquid purges (382 examples containing pudding pipe) and s9 for solid purges (50 examples containing pudding pipe).

44. E541, wholesale price *c.*15 soldi per lb for 'cassia in bocchuoli' (i.e. still in the pods).

45. The retail price is difficult to calculate, since cassia pulp was typically retailed along with other ingredients, not all of which were always quantified. Some useful individual entries can be used to estimate the price however – E882, fo. 299v, 'Frati e chonvento di san girolamo da fiesole', 7 May 1494, 6 soldi for 1 oz (s72 per lb); fo. 64v, 'Franc.o di [BLANK] Ghalli', 30 January 1497 (m.f.), 5.5 soldi per 1 oz (s66 per lb); fo. 240v, 'Jachopo di giovanfranc.o orafo', 16 August 1494, 8 soldi for 10 drams (s76.8 per lb); fo. 241r, 'Lionardo d'livo righattiere', 27 August 1496, 8 soldi for 1 oz (s96 per lb).

46. 202 out of 515 active clients (39%) bought cassia pulp during the sample year. Total sales amounted to 2,168 soldi in the sample year. Excluding corporate clients, clients with surnames accounted for 57% of individual consumption of cassia pulp (998 out of 1,740 soldi); this was roughly equal to their proportion for all products (58%). Excluding corporate clients, clients with occupational titles accounted for 32% of individual consumption of cassia pulp (561 out of 1,740 soldi); this was roughly equal to their proportion for all products (31%).

47. A.G. Carmichael, *Plague and the Poor in Early Renaissance Florence* (Cambridge: Cambridge University Press, 1986), 55.

48. *Ibid.*, 40.

49. E882, fo. 240v, 'Jachopo di giovanfranc.o orafo', 16 August 1494, s8 for 10 drams of 'chasia' (s77 per lb).

50. E882, fo. 335r, 'Albizo di [BLANK] da fortuna', 27 May 1495, s5d6 for 2.75 oz of 'chasia in boccuoli' (s24 per lb).

51. E882, fo. 56v, 'Luigi di niccholo mormorai', 31 August 1493, s6 for 3 oz of 'chasia in channa scielta' (s24 per lb), 'per el filgliuolo'.

52. G. Morelli, *Ricordi*, Biblioteca Italiana, Università degli Studi di Roma 'La Sapienza', 2004. [Florence: Le Monnier, 1986]. 'Mangia alcuna volta la

mattina un'oncia di cassia, così ne' bucciuoli, e danne a' fanciulli: fa d'averne in casa, e fresca, e del zucchero e dell acquarosa e del giulebbo.'

53. E882, fo. 56r, 'Girolamo di franc.o dant.o dachalcinaia', 1 September 1493, s6 for 3 oz of 'chasia in canna' (s24 per lb).

54. During the sample year the shop retailed 19.125 lbs of cassia in pods and 26 lbs of cassia pulp.

55. E882, fo. 331r, 'Angniolo di lodovicho accaiuoli', 4 June 1494, 'p[er] una medicina p[er] lui in che ent[ran]o [dramme] vi di chas[s]ia tratta [dramme] i di diamanna [scrupoli] iiii di ribarbero fine mes[s]o infusione chon ispigho in aqua dindivia ettrebiano [scrupoli] iiii d'aghariqho fine infuso chon salgiemmo e giengiavo in osimele e aqua d'ap[p]io e st[enperat]a la medicina chon dichozione di fiori chordiali folicholicholi di sen[n]a pittamo e alt[re] chose fatta in aqua d'indivia e bughrossa porto bastiano nostro fattore... [lire] 5.'

56. E882, fo. 310r, 'Rafaello di guliano bastiere da san chasciano', 3 May 1494, 'p[er] una medicina p[er] la margherita in che ent[ran]o [dramme] i di ribarbero fine [oncie] 1½ di manna fine mes[s]o e[l] ribarbero infusione in aqua dindivia ettrebiano e st[enperat]a la manna chon dichozione frescha e chordiale porto rafaello e ii anp[oll]a... [lire] 12 [soldi] 3 [denari] 4.'

57. Siraisi, *op. cit.* (note 2), 143.

58. C.M. Foust, 'Mysteries of Rhubarb: Chinese Medicinal Rhubarb through the Ages', *Pharmacy in History*, 36, 4 (1994), 155–9; C.M. Foust, *Rhubarb: The Wondrous Drug* (Princeton: Princeton University Press, 1992).

59. Mattioli, *op. cit.* (note 41), fo. 444, 'È il Rheubarbaro caldo, & secco nel secondo grado... Non è nel Rheubarbaro nocumento alcuno apparente: & imperò dassi egli in ogni tempo, & in ogni età, di modo che si può agevolmente dare ai fanciulli, et alle donne gravide.'

60. S. Pezzella, *Gli ebari: I primi libri di medicina (Le virtù curative delle piante)* (Perugia: Grifo, 1993), 236, quotes from a Florentine herbal of 1430–49 (Biblioteca Medicea-Laurenziana, manoscritto Redi/165), 'per purghare questo reubarbero è lla migliore erre [erbe] di tutte l'altre purghationi, inpero ch'enne tra in molti lattovari purghativi, degli speciali et e medici, a purghare. Questo è llo fiore d'ongni medicina...'

61. Morelli, *op. cit.* (note 52), 'Usa d'un lattovaro che fanno fare i medici di ribarbero: danne a' fanciulli, ché uccide i vermini.'

62. Mattioli, *op. cit.* (note 41), f.444, 'Mettesi sempre nelle infusioni sue un poco di vino biano aromatico, & massime quando intendono i medici d'aprire le oppilationi.', 'Magnifica il siero delle capre le sue operationi, & similmente si gli aumentano infondendolo in acqua di endivia, & d'apio, ò nelle loro decottioni.', 'Costumasi di mettere sempre con esso il nardo, per esservi molto conveniente, ne ciò bisogna dimenticarsi'.

63. *Ibid.*, fo. 444, 'è nata questa vana opinione nella mente de gli huomini, percioche ne i tempi passati era il Rheubarbaro in molto prezzo, & vendevasi a peso d'altrettanto oro. Il che ha poscia fatto creder alla gente, che l'ultima medicina delle malattie sia il Rheubarbaro.'

64. The wholesale price of rhubarb was 21.25 florins for 5 lbs, ie. 595 soldi per lb at a conversion rate of 1 florin = L7 = s140. R.A. Goldthwaite, *The Building of Renaissance Florence: An Economic and Social History* (Baltimore: Johns Hopkins University Press, 1980), 301, on lira : florin conversion rates over time.

65. The retail price is hard to calculate precisely because rhubarb was usually sold in combination with other ingredients, not all of them precisely quantified. However, a number of individual transactions allow us to produce a reliable estimate. E882, fo. 127r, 'ser Pierfranc.o di ser luigi ghuidi', undated, client returns 2 drachme of 'ribarbero fine' to the shop and is credited 7 lire (s6720 per lb); fo. 212v, 'Rede di giovanni di pagholo federighi', 20 November 1493, 1 lire for a product containing 1 scruple of rhubarb in an infusion (s5760 per lb); fo. 58r, 'Rede dangniuolo diachopo tani', 25 August 1493, s90 soldi for product containing 1.5 drams of rhubarb (s5760 per lb).

66. Mean dosage of rhubarb in *medicine* was 0.132 oz, slightly more than 1 dram.

67. 35 out of 515 active clients (7%) bought rhubarb during the sample year. Excluding corporate clients, clients with surnames accounted for 72% of individual consumption of rhubarb (2,269 out of 3,139 soldi); this was higher than their proportion for all products (58%). Excluding corporate clients, clients with occupational titles accounted for 24% of individual consumption of rhubarb (751 out of 3,139 soldi); this was lower than their proportion for all products (31%).

68. Total sales of rhubarb amounted to 3,751 soldi in the sample year, while total sales of cassia pulp amounted to 2,168 soldi in the sample year.

69. E882, fo. 65v, 'Jachopo di Bartolomeo ghalli', 11 September 1493, a purge containing 3 drams of cassia pulp, 3 drams of diacatholicon, 1 dram of trochisks of agaric, 3 grains of spikenard, mixed with 'dichozione frescho e chordiale fatta in aqua st.a aggiuntovi anici finochio fiori chordiali', 'messo suo ribarbero infusione', for a cost of s16d8.

70. E882, fo. 207v, 'Lando di giovanni tanalgli', 2 January 1493 (m.f.), s4d4 for a purge containing ½ oz of cassia pulp mixed with 'aqua di finochio' and 2 scruples of 'ribarbero di suo', plus a 'bichiere'. Similarly, fo. 112v, 'Lorenzo di tomaxo benci', 2 October 1493, client brought 1½ drams of his own rhubarb to the shop for inclusion in a purge.

71. J. Mandeville, *The Foreign Travels of Sir John Mandeville* (Project Gutenberg, 1997) [Macmillan, 1900], ch. 17, 'In that land of Job there is no default of

no thing that is needful to man's body. There be hills, where men get great plenty of manna in greater abundance than in any other country. This manna is clept bread of angels. And it is a white thing that is full sweet and right delicious, and more sweet than honey or sugar. And it cometh of the dew of heaven that falleth upon the herbs in that country. And it congealeth and becometh all white and sweet. And men put it in medicines for rich men to make the womb lax, and to purge evil blood. For it cleanseth the blood and putteth out melancholy.'

72. G.G. Pontano, *Meteororum Liber*, Bayerische Staatsbibliothek [Vienna, 1517] http://daten.digitale-sammlungen.de/~db/bsb00005239/images/, Image 25, 'De pruina et rore et manna', verses 228–46, 'Quin etiam Calabris in saltibus ac per opacum labitur ingenti Crathis qua cerulus alveo quaque etiam Syriis silvae convallibus horrent, felices silvae, quarum de fronde liquescunt divini roris latices, quos sedula passim turba legit, gratum auxilium languentibus aegris...'

73. A. Astorri, 'Appunti sull'esercizio dello speziale a Firenze nel quattrocento', *Archivio storico italiano*, 147 (1989), 31–62.

74. Ficino, *op. cit.* (note 24), 151–3.

75. Mattioli, *op. cit.* (note 41), fo. 92, 'toltone il peso di due once, & meza, muove molto ben più, & più volte il corpo, cacciandone fuori spetialmente la cholera', 'medicamento così nobile, & piacevole, & che tiene il principato tra tutti gli altri...'.

76. Note the discrepancy between estimated doses and total transactions involving that commodity. This is produced by measuring average dosage only when the commodity is used in purges, rather than any sales of that commodity.

77. For price estimates, see notes 45, 65, and 78.

78. E882, fo. 125v, 'Piero di franc.o nacchianti', 18 June 1495, L23s12 for 6 lbs of 'pepe sodo', 4 oz of 'turbitti fini' and 4 oz of 'manna fine', which specifies a price for the manna at 840 soldi per lb; fo. 159v, 'Michele di chorso e chonpangni speziali ale cholonbe, 22 October 1494, 9 lire for 1.5 oz (s1440 per lb); fo. 341v, 'Bartololello di franc.o bartolegli', 25 June 1494, 85 soldi for 1 oz (s1020 per lb). Larger amounts were sold at something close to the wholesale price, e.g. fo. 40v, 'Filgliuoli e rede di pagholo di piero delglialbizzi', 18 March 1493 (m.f.) 16 lire for 11 oz (s350 per lb).

79. Mean dosage of manna in *medicine* was 0.790 oz, ie. just over 6 drams.

80. 15 out of 515 active clients (3%) bought manna during the sample year. Total sales amounted to 1,506 soldi in the sample year. Excluding corporate clients, clients with surnames accounted for 81% of individual consumption of manna (1,224 out of 1,506 soldi); this greatly exceeded their proportion for all products (58%). Excluding corporate clients, clients with occupational titles accounted for 17% of individual consumption of manna (256 out of

1,506 soldi); this was much lower than their proportion for all products (31%).

81. K. Park and J. Henderson, '"The First Hospital among Christians": The Ospedale di Santa Maria Nuova in Early Sixteenth-Century Florence', *Medical History*, 35 (1991), 182, 'Each year we consume 4,000 pounds of cane sugar and as much again of honey, 2,000 pounds of native wax, 800 pounds of white wax, 2,000 pounds of cassia, 20 pounds of rhubarb, 12 pounds of manna, and other things of this sort. The total cost comes to between 1,500 and 2,000 gold florins.'

82. Mean dosage of pudding pipe in *medicine* was 0.847 oz, just less than 7 drams. This means that 2,000 lbs of pudding pipe was equivalent to 28,235 doses. It is possible that these preparations were retailed to the public through the hospital dispensary, as well as being given to in-patients. The hospital may also have bought pudding pipe in order to manufacture drugs.

83. Total volume of pudding pipe sold in sample year was 24.44 lbs.

84. 20 lbs of rhubarb (240 oz) with an average dosage size of 0.132 oz gives 1846.15 doses.

85. Total volume of rhubarb sold in sample year was 0.65 lbs.

86. 12 lbs of manna (144 oz) with an average dosage size of 0.790 oz gives 182.28 doses.

87. On this option see K. Park, 'Healing the Poor: Hospitals and Medical Assistance in Renaissance Florence', in J. Barry and C. Jones (eds), *Medicine and Charity before the Welfare State* (London: Routledge, 1991); Park and Henderson, *op. cit.* (note 81).

88. E882, fo. 248v, 'Antonio di giovanni del chaccia', 14 January 1493 (m.f.) to 20 January 1493 (m.f.), total spending of 846.33 soldi, with total 70.83 lbs of wax. This one funeral accounted for over half of Antonio's total spending of almost 70 lire across a period of more than a year (from 27 July 1493 to 3 September 1494). S.T. Strocchia, *Death and Ritual in Renaissance Florence* (Baltimore: Johns Hopkins University Press, 1992), 128.

89. E882, fo. 32r, 'Ant.o di Giovanni delchaccia', 19 December 1493, L3s2d4 for a purge containing rhubarb, manna and pudding pipe.

90. E882, fo. 32r, 31 August 1493, s7 for a purge containing sugar and diasenna; 16 December 1493, s5d4 for a purge for his daughter containing coralline, pudding pipe and 'holy seed'.

91. RF, *op. cit.* (note 9), fo. 3, the contents page lists the categories used to classify the different commodities. These include, for example, 'Lactovari dolci' (sweet electuaries), 'Lactovari amari' (bitter electuaries), 'Lactovari oppiati' (opiate), and 'Medicine lenitive & solutive' ('lenitive and solutive purges' – see note 24 for this usage of *medicina*). The contents page goes on to list other categories: syrups, robs, trochisks, powders, pills etc.

92. This assumes that the 'sugho rosato' described in Giglio accounts corresponds to the 'Lactovaro di sugho di rose' described in RF, *op. cit.* (note 9), fo. 68.

93. It does not appear in BNF, Magl. XV.92 (the recipe book of Santa Maria Nuova), or in Silini, *op. cit.* (note 2).

94. OED, 'Diacatholicon': 'A laxative electuary; so called from its general usefulness: hence, a universal remedy. As prescribed by Nicolaus, it was made of senna leaves, pulp of cassia and tamarinds, roots of male fern, rhubarb, and liquorice, aniseed, sweet fennel, and sugar.'

95. RF, *op. cit.* (note 9), fo. 60, the recipe for 'DYACHATTOLICON', attributed to Niccolò Salernitano, lists 3 oz each of 'Foglie di sena netta, Polpa di cassia fistula, Tamerindi' and 1 oz each of 'Reubarbaro f[ine], Polipodio quercino, Anici, Vivole, Zucchero chandito, Penniti, Regolitia, Se[mi] comuni mondi'.

96. *Ibid.*, fo. 65, the recipe for 'DIAFINICON DELLE XII', attributed to Mesue, lists 100 dr of 'Dactili infusi in aceto per tre di & tre nocte', 50 dr of 'peniti', 30 dr of 'Ma'dorle purgate', 35 dr of 'Turbitti', 12 dr of 'Scamonea', and various other herbs and spices, mixed with honey 'qua'to basta, cioe [6 lbs]'. An alternative variety, 'Diafinicon Delle XXII' contained more scammony, and would have been a stronger purgative.

97. *Ibid.*, ff. 60–2, lists various recipes, all of which relied on senna leaves as the main purgative.

98. OED, 'Diasenna': 'A purgative electuary of which senna formed the base; the confection of senna.'

99. RF, *op. cit.* (note 9), f.21, 'e lactovari facti & composti con il mele durano piu tempo assai piu che composti con zucchero….'

100. *Ibid.*, ff.32–3.

101. 9.5 lbs of 'Diefinichon delle 12' and 2.3 lbs of 'Diefinichon'.

102. 5.5 lbs of 'Diasenna' and 12 lbs of 'Diasena sanza sena', presumably the base product.

103. 396 out of 656 liquid medicines (60.4%) used waters as the vehicle.

104. Bénézet, *op. cit.* (note 29), 561–2.

105. The average price of purges containing 'Water of Endive and Trebbiano wine' was 99 soldi.

106. RF, *op. cit.* (note 9), fo. 20, 'Puossi di tutte lherbe in comune farne acque, & durano uno anno, & fannosi a uno modo'.

107. E541. It is extremely difficult to calculate the retail price of these waters, since the accounts do not give a separate price or indicate the quantity involved, but it was no more than a soldo. Silini, *op. cit.* (note 2), 192, notes that doctors' prescriptions tended to state *quantum sufficit*, leaving this to the discretion of the apothecary, but the total amount of liquid was probably around 1½ oz.

108. Out of a total of 396 waters used as liquid vehicles during the sample year.

109. 260 out of 656 liquid medicines (39.6%) used decoctions as the vehicle. The sum of these figures exceeds the total of liquid medicines (635) because some medicines contained more than one liquid vehicle.

110. RF, *op. cit.* (note 9), fo. 22, 'Tutte le decoctioni durano tre dì o meno. Et per questo niuno spetiale non debbe tenere fatte in bottegha: anzi le debbe sempre co'porre quando il medicho le ordini, & quelle usare.'

111. Decoctions normally acted as vehicles in purges, but were occasionally sold alone, e.g. E882, fo. 335r, 'Amadore di [BLANK] oste al ficho', 20 April 1496, 1 dose of 'dichozione di sena chorosato cholato'. Purges containing decoctions had an average value of 30 soldi.

112. RF, *op. cit.* (note 9), fo. 89, the standard instructions for decoctions were 'Fa bollire in acqua comune & cola'.

113. 181 out of 260 decoctions used in liquid medicines were standard varieties listed in the *Ricettario fiorentino*. However some of the varieties listed, eg. 'carminative' and 'capital' decoctions, were extremely rare at the Giglio.

114. RF, *op. cit.* (note 9), fo. 89, 'DECOCTIONE Frescha magistrale', made from currants, various types of flowers, polypody, scolopendrium, aniseed, fennel, and epithyme.

115. 121 out of 260 decoctions used in liquid purges consisted of a mixture of the 'fresh' and 'cordial' decoctions. Decoctions might also be mixed with other standard preparations such as strained honey roset – see E882, fo. 262r, 'Giovanni salamancha spangniuolo in chasa andrea di berto lapi', 15 April 1494, 'dichozione chordiale chorosato cholato'.

116. E882, fo. 236r, 'Domenicho di messer charlo pandolfini', 4 December 1493, 'dichozione daqua st.a in che si bolli regholizia passule an' [oz 1/2] chapelvenero folglie di sena e pittamo zaferano e alt.o'.

117. E882, fo. 338r, 'messer Bartolomeo di [BLANK] schala', 9 May 1496, a medicine containing a solution of pudding pipe in 'dichozione di cieci rossi chottovi drento barbe di prezemoli'.

118. P. Suardo, *Thesaurus aromatariorum* (1536) [Milan, 1496], fo. 3, 'Cassia fistulatu' pro clisterib[us] magistralis' describes the effect as cleaning the blood and stomach, purging choler and phlegm, resolving abcesses and conferring heat. On clysters, see Bénézet, *op. cit.* (note 29), 245; Schönfeld, *op. cit.* (note 1), 110–11.

119. E882, fo. 118r, 'Lorenzo di tomaxo benci', 4 October 1493, 6 oz of 'latt.o e zuc.o darchomenti', 'per ii archomenti'. The typical dosage was 2–3 oz per clyster. The specific ingredients are not listed, beyond the reference to 'electuary and sugar', and they were usually combined with *miele violato* and *rosato colato* (honeys made with violets or roses).

120. E882, fo. 52v, 'Ghaleotto di Niccholo masi', 14 August 1493; fo. 60r, 'Guliano diberto dasingnia', 25 August 1493; fo. 45v, 'Andrea di domenicho buti', 13 August 1493, specifically refer to 'zuc.o rosso per archomenti'.

121. RF, *op. cit.* (note 9), fo. 70, recipe for 'CASSIA PER ARgomenti magistrale' [*sic*], lists the ingredients as pudding pipe, honey, violet, mallow, *marchorella* (mercurial), *bietola* (chard), *paritaria* (pellitory) and absinthe (wormwood). For similar recipes see Q. Augusti, *Lumen apothecariorum cum certis expositionibus* (Venice: 1495), fo. 13v and Suardo, *op. cit.* (note 118), fo. 3.

122. E882, fo. 134r, 'Piero di giovanni chavalchanti', 17 May 1494, 2 oz of 'latt.o e zuc.o darchomenti', and 3 manipuli of 'chose charminative', 'per i archomento'; fo. 117r, 'Madonna Girolama donna di messer puccio dant.o pucci', 7 October 1493, 2 oz of 'latt.o e zuc.o darchomenti', 1.5 oz of 'chose charminative' and 3 oz of 'olio di chamamila'. The ingredients were usually listed in terms of 'handfuls' rather than by weight, a practice adopted for very light goods like flowers. These herbs and flowers were boiled before adding the cassia and other drugs, as can be seen on fo. 237v, 'Franc.o di tingho dabrucianese', 6 December 1493, 'chose charminative per uno arghomento in che ent.o folglie di sena chamamilla anici e alt.o per bolire aguntovi diasena chasia e gierapighra an[a] [dr 3.5]'.

123. I. Ait, *Tra scienza e mercato: gli speziali a Roma nel tardo medioevo* (Rome: Istituto Nazionale di Studi Romani, 1996), 290, for clysters made from cassia pulp and oil of violets.

124. E882, fo. 343v, 'Domenicho di bono rinucci', 3 July 1494, clyster containing 'latt.o e zuc.o darchomenti', 'trementina' and 'olio di cheri e rosato'.

125. E882, fo. 247v, 'Ghaleotto di nicholo masi', 9 January 1493 (m.f.), 3 oz of 'diasena', 3 oz of 'giera', 3 oz of 'olio di piu ragioni', 3 oz of 'latt.o e zuc.o darchomenti', 3 handfuls of 'sena pittamo chamomilla e altre chose'. See also fo. 7r, 'Bartolo di [blank] Stadiere alleporti', 3 October 1493, s7d8 for 4 manipoli of 'chose charminative per bolire nelarchomento', 2 oz of 'trementina', 2 oz of 'rosato colato' and 1 oz of 'benedetta per larchomento', all served in a glass. RF, *op. cit.* (note 9), lists all of these as 'medicine lenitive et solutive' and fo. 63 notes in particular: 'Hyerapigra Galeni... usasi per argomenti & per boccha... Et nota che in questa ricepta entra ta'to mele quante spetie: perche no' si usa se non per argomenti...'.

126. E882, fo. 4v, 'Chantino di [blank] chavalchanti', 26 June 1494, s2 for 2 oz of 'Latt.e e zuc.o darchomenti'; fo. 60v, 'Guliano mastaccho da singnia sta chomona chaterina dipierant.o pitti', 25 August 1493, s2 for 2 oz of 'latt.o e zuc.o darchomenti per larchomento'.

127. E882, fo. 51r, 'ser Simone di [BLANK] filipepi', 14 August 1493, s4 for 2 oz of 'latt.e e zuc.o darchomenti' and 3 oz of 'olio violato', 'per i archomento'; fo. 51r, 'Lionardo di [BLANK] arzinchelgli', 17 August 1493, s4 for 3 oz of

'latt.e e zuc.o darchomenti' and 1 manipolo of 'fiori di chamamilla'.

128. E882, fo. 46v, 'Franc.o di Giovanni dinofridalterrio', 14 August 1493, s8d4 for 3 oz of 'olio rosato e di chamomilla', 4 oz 2 dr of 'latt.o e zuc.o darchomenti', 1 manipolo of 'chose charminative' and an ampoule.

129. E882, fo. 124v, 'Ruffino di [BLANK] oste alaporta alachrocie', 21 October 1493, L1s5d8 for 7 oz of 'chose charminative e piu erbe e fiori', 3 dr of 'choloquintida', 10 dr of 'gera lochodion e gera pighra', 3 oz of 'olio di chosto e di ruta', 1 oz of 'zuc.o rosso', 1 oz of 'rosato cholato', 1 oz of 'ttrementina'. The price included s4 for syrup and d8 for two ampoules.

130. Clients with surnames accounted for approximately 72% of individual consumption of clysters and clyster products (1,209 out of 1,689 soldi); this was much higher than their proportion for all products (58%). Clients with occupational titles accounted for 18% of individual consumption of clysters (299 out of 1,689 soldi); this was much lower than their proportion for all products (31%). This was despite a fairly wide customer base – 121 out of 515 active clients (23%) bought clysters and clyster products over the sample year, roughly equivalent to the figure for pills.

131. RF, *op. cit.* (note 9), fo. 3, the contents page lists these as 'lactovari dolci'. In Augusti, *op. cit.* (note 121), the same drugs are referred to as 'aromatic confections'.

132. RF, *op. cit.* (note 9), ff. 36–7, 'Dyaradon Abatis', 'Questo lactovaro è posto da Nicholao: & è quello si usa comunemente'.

133. These complex combinations were also called 'lattovari' (electuaries) in the Giglio accounts. This is potentially confusing since 'electuary' was the standard term for all standard compound drugs in this period.

134. RF, *op. cit.* (note 9), fo. 72, 'ZUCCHERo rosato', 'MELE Rosato', and fo. 74 on locs 'sono piu teneri che lactovari & piu sodi che li sciroppi...'

135. *Ibid.*, fo. 149, classes this as a 'cordial confection', 'ALChuni con le medesime pietre pretiose fa'no lactovaro, et puossi chiamare Mixtura cordiale: la quale nelle febre acute & pestilentiali usando giova assai…'. The conserves of bugloss and borage were known respectively as *diabuglossato* and *diaborraginato*.

136. E882, fo. 253v, 'Piero di maso dalarena', 3 February 1493 (m.f.), s2d4 for an electuary composed of 1 dr of *diamargeriton* (containing pearls, spices, trochisks, musk, amber, camphor and honey roset), 0.5 dr of *dianbra* (containing spices, amber, musk, syrup and water of roses) and 0.5 dr of *diaradon abbatis*. For another example, see fo. 17v, 'Frati e chonvento di san franc.o da saminiato', 16 March 1494 (m.f.), 2 ounces of an electuary for the chest: 'Latt.e pettorale chon diechoridionne e spezie di diedraghanti', costing s4.

137. E882, fo. 239r, 'ser Zanobi diachopo di borgianni', 16 December 1493, L3s8 for a 'latt.o chordiale' containing 1 ½ oz each of 'latt.o chordiale',

'rosata novella', 'latt.o letifichans almansoris', 'chonserva dacietosita di ciederno', 1 oz of 'latt.o di giemme' and 2 oz of 'latt.o darre perlati dischrezione di misue', 'fatto mist.a orata' and served in an *albarello*. See also fo. 82v, 'Angniolo di lodovicho accaiuoli', 22 May 1494, L2s6d8 for 5.5dr of powdered gems and pearls, half of which were mixed with drugs to make a 'cordial electuary', the other half being mixed with sugar to make a 'panellino', which was then gilded.

138. The Giglio evidence makes it clear that these should be considered medicinal products rather than sweets, because they were made to order rather than to a standard recipe, and because they almost always contained compound drugs from the class of 'sweet electuaries'. E882, fo. 254v, 'm.a Silvaggia donna fu di filippo strozi', 21 August 1494, s4 for 4 morselletti weighing 1 oz altogether.

139. RF, *op. cit.* (note 9), fo. 37, 'Aromatico Rosato... Puossi fare & usasi in morselli.'

140. E882, fo. 331r, 'Angniolo di lodovicho accaiuoli', 14 June 1494, 'morselletti fatti chon ispezie di dieradonne abate frumenti preziosi channella fine zuc.o chiarito chon aqua rosa e altre chose.'

141. E882, fo. 305v, 'm.a Angniola de girolami', 20 February 1496 (m.f.), L1s4 for 6 oz of 'morselletti fatti chon zuc.o fine pannicholi di pollo preparati ciennamo fine pinochi mondi e lavati e altre chose fatto morselletti orati' (s48 per lb).

142. E882, fo. 110r, 'Madonna Girolama donna di messer puccio dant.o pucci.' 26 September 1493, 'pollo chonfetto fatto chon zuc.o fine e aqua rosa lavata le polpe delchapone piu volte in aqua rosa fatto chon semi chomuni e mandorle e pinochi'. This appears to be an enriched version of a recipe listed at Santa Maria Nuova: BNF, Magl. XV.92, fo. 83r, 'Lattovaro di pollo fine', chicken flesh was pounded with spices, pine-nuts, almonds, currants, sebesten, hazelnuts, various seeds, salt and sugar, to make a thick paste of similar consistency to marzipan, 'fane lattovario in quella forma et modo che ssi fa ne il marzapene'.

143. E882, fo. 110r, 26 September 1493, 1 dr of 'frumenti preziosi', 1 dr of 'choralli macinati chon cienamo fine chroci e sandareli', and 1 'schatola orata'.

144. E882, fo. 110r, 26 September 1493, total cost L3s3d4. Estimating the cost of the box at s6, the price of the chicken confection was s57d4. For further examples, see fo. 229r, 'ser Zanobi di jachopo borgianni', 18 November 1493; fo. 49v, 'Lorenzo di salvetto becchaio a sanfriano', 12 August 1493; fo. 237r, 'Munistero e donne di santo anbruogio', 10 January 1493 (m.f.); fo. 247r, 'Bernardo di piero del palagio', 5 January 1493 (m.f.).

145. Ficino, *op. cit.* (note 24), 141, 149, 155; K. Albala, *Eating Right in the Renaissance* (Berkeley: University of California Press, 2002), 249–50.

146. E882, fo. 26v, 'Michele dichante farsettaio', 6 August 1493, s15d8 for a cordial electuary containing only 0.5 dr of powdered gems, served in a gilded *albarello*. For another cheap example, see fo. 53r, 'Indacho raghugieo', 17 August 1493.

147. 109 out of 515 active clients (21%) bought composite electuaries in the sample year. Clients with surnames accounted for approximately 74% of individual consumption of composite electuaries (1,560 out of 2,105 soldi); this was much higher than their proportion for all products (58%). Clients with occupational titles accounted for 17% of individual consumption of composite electuaries (367 out of 2,105 soldi); this was much lower than their proportion for all products (31%). Religious corporations were particularly prominent in consumption, with the convent of Sant'Ambrogio (client 304) consuming 24 electuaries in the sample year. Similarly, clients with surnames accounted for approximately 72% of individual consumption of *morselletti* (322 out of 449 soldi); this was much higher than their proportion for all products (58%). Clients with occupational titles accounted for 20% of individual consumption of *morselletti* (91 out of 449 soldi); this was much lower than their proportion for all products (31%).

148. The hospital receptary indicates *armaticho rosato* for pains in the chest or stomach caused by phlegm – BNF, Magl. XV.92, fo. 61r, 'A cchi fusse flematicho avendo pena nel petto overo nel petto o nella boccha dello istomacho abbi a usare la mattina a buona ora armaticho rosato et per volta tanto quanto una buona fava et digiunarlo ò una ò dua ore et questo e ne provato.'

149. R. Palmer, 'Pharmacy in the Republic of Venice in the Sixteenth Century', in A. Wear, R.K. French, and I.M. Lonie (eds), *The Medical Renaissance of the Sixteenth Century* (Cambridge: Cambridge University Press, 1985), 108–9; M. Beretta, *The Treasure of Health. From the Omnipotence of Medicinal Herbs to the Atomization of Drugs*, A. Brierley (trans.), (Florence: Giunti, 1997), 16.

150. Mesue, *op. cit.* (note 30), fo. 50v; Suardo, *op. cit.* (note 118), fo. xxvi; Ficino, *op. cit.* (note 24), 139. There is no evidence at the Giglio for the sort of regular use of theriac that Ficino advises for melancholics. This contradicts the position in Slack, *op. cit.* (note 17), 264–5.

151. Silini, *op. cit.* (note 2), 207, notes that theriac was also rarely prescribed in Gandino.

152. E882, fo. 51v, 'Davitte di landino fornaio', 17 September 1493; fo. 7r, 'Bartolo di [blank] Stadiere alleporti', 2 October 1493, both suggest theriac retailed at s40 per lb.

153. The retail price of diacatholicon was around 72 to 96 soldi per lb.

154. E882, fo. 124r, 'Lorenzo di buonachorso pitti', 3 February 1494 (m.f.), suggests mithridate cost s2 for 3 dr (s64 per lb); fo. 124v, 'Ruffino di

[BLANK] oste alaporta alachrocie', 21 October 1493, confirms that this is about right, if we estimate that diemuscho cost s72 per lb.

155. E882, fo. 169v, 'Ruffino di [BLANK] oste alla porta ala [croce]', 25 April 1494, s6d8 for a composite electuary containing 1.5 oz of 'latt.o di brettonicha', 1.5 oz of 'latt.o diachori', 0.5 oz of 'latt.o di stichadosso' and 2 drams of 'triacha fine', served in an ampoule.

156. E882, fo. 124v, 'Ruffino di [BLANK] oste alaporta alachrocie', 21 October 1493, s14d8 for a 'latt.o chapitale' containing 1 oz of 'triacha fine', 1 oz of mithridate and 1 oz of 'diemuscho', served in an *albarello*.

157. Corvi, *op. cit.* (note 6), 11.

158. Mesue, *op. cit.* (note 30), fo. 74r. See also the quotes from Arnoldo di Villanova in Corvi, *ibid.*, 12, 'sono esse rotonde per girare in tutto lo stomaco e impregnarlo di sostanze medicamentose, senza concentrare in un punto la loro eventuale tossicità. Saranno più grosse le pillole che devono arrivare nei distretti organici più distanti (come la testa), medie quelle dirette al fegato, più piccole quelle destinate agli organi vicini'.

159. Mesue, *ibid.*; Ficino, *op. cit.* (note 24), 141, 'Drugs against Phlegm', describes various pills for putting up a 'strong fight' against an excess of phlegm, and then warns 'But we altogether denounce all strong and sudden flux and purgation, for it weakens the stomach and the heart, it drains away many spirits, and it brings the humors into confusion and with the black fumes of the humors darkens those spirits which remain.'

160. 147 out of 515 active clients (29%) bought pills during the sample year.

161. RF, *op. cit.* (note 9), fo. 103, 'PILLOLE Sine quibus', the ingredients included scammony, myrobalans, rhubarb, mastic, senna, agaric. Ficino, *op. cit.* (note 24), 141, 'If along with phlegm all the other humors are acting up, it will be fitting to purge them with the rhubarb-pills of Mesue,... or with pills which are called by moderns "sine quibus".'

162. In terms of number of transactions in the sample year, the most important varieties of pills were all standard varieties: *sine quibus* (10%), fumitory (7%), *bichicche* (6%), *aggregative* (6%), and *auree* (5%)

163. E882, fo. 136v, 'don Domenicho monacho in badia di firenze', 20 April 1494, L1s8d4 for 2 oz of 'torcisci dagharigho fatto p'le' – this was probably around 96 pills, nearly 6% of all sales of pills in the sample year. Trochisks were dried tablets of drugs, larger than pills, which enabled ingredients to be stored for a long time. RF, *op. cit.* (note 9), fo. 94, 'TROCISci di agarico di Mesue', for a recipe containing agaric, rock salt, and ginger mixed with oxymel (a syrup of honey and vinegar). Mesue, *op. cit.* (note 30), fo. 70v, Cristoforo degli Onesti described them as being either a round disc like a lupin bean, or in elongated form, like a chess pawn. They could be pulverised as required and the powder used in bespoke preparations, usually combined with other ingredients to make purges or pills. Suardo, *op. cit.*

(note 118), fo. xxvi and *Liber Pandectarum, op. cit.* (note 38), cap. xxii, on the purgative effects of agaric trochisks.

164. E882, fo. 252v, 'Niccholo di marchionne del m.o ridolfo nostro gharzone', 4 March 1493 (m.f.), 4 'p'le aghreghative' combined with 1 'p'la chozia', and then 'riformate orate'. Ait, *op. cit.* (note 123), 288, describes similar combinations at Rome, 'Pillularum sine quibus, agarici trociscati, ana scrupoli 2, diagridii quantum satis, reformentur cum syropo de sticados fiat pillule'. Corvi, *op. cit.* (note 6), 13–14, discusses one doctor's view of the need to 'adapt pills to the constitution of the patient'.

165. E882, fo. 130v, 'Munistero e donne di santo anbruogio', 9 October 1493, 'p'le di ribarbero di misue' combined with 'polvere strettiva da pondi', 'fatto p'le no. xii'.

166. E882, fo. 119r, 'Fruosino di Cece da Verrazano', 16 October 1493, 0.5 dr of 'p'le fetide', 0.5 dr of 'turcisci dagharigho' and 6 gr of 'sugho rosato', combined and 'fatto p'le'.

167. Silini, *op. cit.* (note 2), 199–200.

168. About 0.59 g. See E882, fo. 272r, 'Tommaxo di [BLANK] delgli alesandri', 26 March 1494; fo. 331r, 'Angniolo di lodovicho accaiuoli', 20 June 1494; fo. 67v, 'Indacho Raghugieo', 20 September 1493; fo. 235v, 'Rede di giovanni di pagholo federighi', 9 December 1493. However, with such limited data it should be noted that the dosage might also vary according to the doctor's prescription. BNF, Magl. XV.92, fo. 152v, 'la presa di queste pillole sie da due scrupoli insino inn una drachma secondo la natura della persona', which suggest that pills could be bigger than those found at the Giglio.

169. E882, fo. 272r, 'Tommaxo di [BLANK] delgli alesandri', 26 March 1494, 0.5 dr of 'p'le asezerette riformate p'le n.o iii orati' for s2 (s384 per lb, or d8 per pill). The standard variety of these sort of pills cost half that amount – see fo. 321r, 'Munistero e donne di santo anbruogio', 26 May 1494, s4 for 10 'p'le asezerette' weighing 2dr (s192 per lb, or d4.8 per pill). A similar pattern is found with 'chozie' pills, where the standard variety were half the price – fo. 62r, 'Simone di bernardo niccholini', 13 October 1493, 2 'p'le chozie orat.e' for s1d4 (d8 per pill); fo. 237r, 'Munistero e donne di santo anbruogio', 1 February 1493 (m.f.), s2 for 1 dr of 'p'le chozie' (s192 per lb). Other transactions – fo. 316v, 'Nicholo di bernardo di simone del nero', 6 May 1494, 1 dr of 'p'le aghreghative avre e luci orate' for s3 (s288 per lb); fo. 331r, 'Angniolo di lodovicho accaiuoli', 20 June 1494, 1 scruple of 2 'p'le aghreghative cioe [sc 1] orate' for s1d5 (s408 per lb); fo. 67v, 'Indacho Raghugieo', 20 September 1493, 1 dr of 'torcisci di rose fattone p'le n.o vi orat.e' for s3 (s288 per lb).

170. E882, fo. 235v, 'Rede di giovanni di pagholo federighi', 9 December 1493, 4 'p'le in che ent.o [sc 1] di torcisci dagharigho e [sc 1] di p'le aghreghative' for s2d8 (d8 per pill or s384 per lb).

171. E882, fo. 299v, 'Frati e chonvento di san girolamo da fiesole', 30 May 1494, 6 'p'le di ribarbero di misue' for s4 (d8 per pill). For the recipe, see *RF, op. cit.* (note 9), fo.104, 'PILLOLe di reubarbero di Mesue, & usasi'.

172. E882, fo. 104v, 'm.a Silvaggia donna fu di filippo strozzi', 28 November 1493, 3 'p'le di riberbero orate' for s3.

173. E882, fo. 342v, 'Frati e monaci della badia di firenze', 30 June 1494 entries, purchase of 1 dr of 'p'le reub[er]berate daopilazione' for s8; fo. 329r, 24 June 1494, 0.5 dr of 3 'p'le reub[er]berate daopilazione' for s4; fo. 329r, 21 June 1494, 0.5 dr of 'p'le reuberberate daupilate di m.o mingho' for s4.

174. E882, fo. 316r, 'Piero di franc.o di bettino', 29 November 1496, 'p'le in che ent.o [dr 1.5] di ribarbero fine eletto riformato p'le n.o [9] orate' for L3s15.

175. 92% of sales of pills were for five soldi or less. The median value of transactions involving pills was only two soldi.

176. Total sales of pills in the sample year amounted to 1202 soldi, around 3% of the total spending on medicines.

177. E882, fo. 2v, 'messer Michele di [BLANK] Strozzi', 30 June 1493 to 2 July 1493.

178. E882, fo. 306r, 'm.a Mattea di [BLANK] serva dalamanno rinuccini', 12 April 1494, purge for s7d4, and entries from 14 April 1494 to 18 April 1494.

179. E882, fo. 306r, 20 April 1494 to 22 April 1494.

180. In the sample year, 84% of all syrups retailed were simple varieties, variously described as 'syrup with sugar and distilled water' (75% of transactions), 'syrup with sugar' (7%) and 'syrup' (2%). The price of such syrups can be calculated at 24 soldi per lb, which allows us to estimate the typical dosage to be 2 oz. In the case of the typical mixture of 'syrup with sugar and distilled water', E882, fo. 254v, 'Domenicho di filippo sarto a san tomaso', 12 May 1494 shows that half the value was constituted by distilled water (d2) and half by the syrup (d2).

181. Transactions in the sample year, syrup of violets (2%), syrup of poppies (1%), syrup of mint (1%). The price of each was twenty-four soldi per lb.

182. E882, fo. 342r, 'Luigi di [BLANK] partini', 30 June 1494, L2 for 5 oz of 's.o di ribesse domaschino' (s96 per lb).

183. E882, fo. 229r, 'ser Zanobi di jachopo borgianni', 26 November 1493, 's[ciropp]o usato' is a reference to entry for 25 November 1493, 's.o chon zuc.o e aque st.a in che ent.o [dr 17] di s.o dupatorio dasenzio e dipomi e [oz 2.5] di aquest.a', but with the further addition of 'torcisci di rose edupatorio per meta', i.e. ½ dr each. See also fo. 212v, 'Rede di giovanni di pagholo federighi', 25 November 1493, L1s7 for 1 dose of 's.o chon zuc.o e dichozione di passule fatta in aqua st.a', with addition of 1 sc of 'ribarbero fine' and 1 sc of 'torcisci dagharigho' and entry for 14 November 1493, s10 for 2 doses of 's.o chon zuc.o e dichozione di pasule fatta in aqua di chapelvenero i[n]divia ed asenzio'.

278

184. 223 out of 515 active clients (43%) bought syrups during the sample year.
185. E882, fo. 55r, 'Giovanni dalancisa chalzolaio', 23 August 1493, 4 oz of 's.o di papaveri' (totalling 3 doses) 'per la sera' and 2 doses of 's.o chon zuc.o e aque st.a... per la mattina'. See also fo. 149r, 'ser Benedetto di [BLANK] dalascharperia', 20 April 1495, syrups 'per la sera' and 'per la mattina'.
186. E882, fo. 30v, 'Pagholo di ser giovanni salvetti', 28 July 1493, 's.o chon zuc.o e dichozione di pasule', 'per la sera dopo ciena'.
187. E882, fo. 187v, 'Matteo di toniello da chalcinaia', 18 December 1497, 'per pigliare ina[n]zi pasto'.
188. E882, fo. 352r, 'm.a Luchrezia donna fu di domenicho di bono rinucci', 23 July 1494, 'per usare quando va a tavola'.
189. E882, fo. 348v, 'm.a Luchrezia donna fu di domenicho di bono rinucci', 18 July 1494, s10 for 5 oz of 's.o chon zuc.o di piu ragioni', 'per pigliare dua chuchiai per volta inanzi mangiare'.
190. E882, fo. 44r, 'Franc.o di Giovanni dinofri dalterrio', 6 August 1493, 1 oz of 'zuc.o per bere cholla peverada del pollo'; fo. 131v, 'Lucha di paradiso botteghaio fuori della porta a sanpiero ghattolini', 17 November 1494, 1 oz of 'zuc.o rosso per pigliare cola peverada del pollo'. Syrups might also be prescribed to be drunk with barley water – see fo. 179v, 'Ghuido di maestro ant.o di ghuido', 20 April 1494; fo. 312r, 'Ghuido di maestro ant.o di ghuido', 22 April 1494, 22 April 1494; fo. 305r, 'Biagio di stefano malischalcho', 9 April 1494; fo. 320r, 'Niccholo di [BLANK] guntini', 3 February 1494 (m.f.).
191. M. Savonarola, *Libreto de tute le cosse che se manzano: un libro di dietetica di Michele Savonarola, medico padovano del secolo XV edizione critica basata sul Codice Casanatense 406*, J. Nystedt (ed.), (Stockholm: Almqvist & Wiksell International, 1988), 88, 'E con il zucaro beuto è singulari medicina, la qual è anco conveniente a tua Signoria....'
192. E882, fo. 344r, 'Munistero e donne di santo anbruogio', 16 August 1494, 4 oz of 's.o chon zuc.o', 'per iiii prese chol brodo del pollo'.
193. E882, fo. 36r, 'Nigi di ristoro da santa maria inpruneta', 30 July 1493, 3 oz of 's.o chon zuc.o', 'per pilgliare la mattina chon peverada di pollo' and 3 oz of 's.o chon zuc.o e aqua rosa', 'per la sera'. See also fo. 106r, 'Piero di franc.o di bettino setaiuolo', 20 April 1494, 's.o chon zuc.o', 'per la donna chon brodo di pollo'.
194. A.J. Grieco, ' From the Cookbook to the Table: A Florentine Table and Italian Recipes of the Fourteenth and Fifteenth Centuries', in C. Lambert (ed.), *Du manuscrit à la table: essais sur la cuisine au Moyen Age et repertoire des manuscrits medievaux contenant des recettes culinaires* (Montreal: Les presses de l'Université de Montreal, 1992), 36; Rosati, *op. cit.* (note 23), 147.
195. E882, fo. 345r, 'Giovanbatista di bernardo della tosa', 12 July 1494, 3 oz of 's.o di pomi e di fumo st.o', 'per dua prese chon peverada di pollo'. Chicken

was a traditional food for invalids – B. Laurioux, *Manger au moyen âge: pratiques et discours alimentaires en Europe aux XIVe et XVe siècles* (Paris: Hachette, 2002), 143; D. Romano, *Housecraft and Statecraft: Domestic Service in Renaissance Venice, 1400–1600* (Baltimore: Johns Hopkins University Press, 1996), 96.

196. Park and Henderson, *op. cit.* (note 81), 173–4.

197. Powdered drugs for use in epithems were typically referred to as *spezie* (spices) in both the Giglio accounts and in the *RF, op. cit.* (note 9), which on fo. 148, 'SPETIE DI PICTIMA Cordiale frescha', states, 'pound each item separately, then sieve, mix together and make into spices', suggesting that these were composite drugs in powder form (just as 'fine spices' meant a mix of powdered spices used at table). The descriptions in the accounts are inconsistent – sometimes referring to epithems, and sometimes to fomentations with added 'powders' or 'spices' – but essentially refer to the same thing: a combination of powdered drugs and a liquid fomentation that was applied to the stomach with a cloth or sponge.

198. BNF, Magl. XV.92, fo. 111v, suggests that epithems were applied with a cloth of linen, wool or felt – 'usa con panno lino ò vuolgli lano o feltrello'. Less commonly, the powdered drugs might be incorporated in a sacculus, that is, a small bag containing herbs and drugs for application to the skin, but these appear only rarely at the Giglio. E882, fo. 63r, 'Iachopo dilionardo mannelgli', 20 February 1493 (m.f.), 'spezie di pittima chordiale chomuscho e anbra per fare sacchetto alquore'. See also fo. 267v, 'Tommaxo di messer otto nicholini', 17 March 1493 (m.f.); fo. 106v, 'Angolino di lorenzo chapponi', 8 October 1493.

199. At least 44 out of 58 epithems (76%) in the sample year were 'cordial' varieties. E882, fo. 13v, 'Pagholo dimeo fabro atterrenzano', 20 July 1493, for a typical example 'per fare pittima al quore', containing 5 dr of 'spezie da pittima chordiale chomuscho e anbra' combined with 18 oz of 'aqua chordiale'.

200. E882, fo. 61v, 'Fratti e chonvento di san Girolamo dafiesole', 16 September 1493, an epithem containing an unspecified quantity of 'malvagia'.

201. E882, fo. 130v, 'Munistero e donne di santo anbruogio', 24 October 1493, an epithem where 3 oz of 'acieto rosato' were added to 25 oz of 'aque chordiale'.

202. E882, fo. 337r, 'Zanobi di lazero daenpoli', 18 June 1494, an epithem containing 1.5 dr of 'sandoli rossi bianchi eccitrini'; fo. 253v, 'Piero di maso dalarena', 3 February 1493 (m.f.), an epithem containing 3 dr of 'iii sandroli'.

203. E882, fo. 337r, 'Zanobi di lazero daenpoli', 18 June 1494, an epithem containing 3 handfuls of 'fiori chordiali rose e viole e fiori di neufarro'.

204. E882, fo. 258r, 'Bartolomeo di ser franc.o da anbra', 22 February 1493 (m.f.), L1s18d8 for an epithem containing 1 handful of 'viole seche' and 1dr of citron sandalwood.

205. E882, fo. 46v, 'Franc.o di Giovanni dinofridalterrio', 7 August 1493, L1s3d4 for an epithem containing 2 oz of 'aceto' and 3 oz of 'malviagia' added to the 18 oz of 'aqua chordiale', served in a 'fiaschetto'.

206. BNF, Magl. XV.92, fo.136r–136v, 'Pittima temperata da chuore', 'usa al chuore con panno iscarlatto'. this variant included similar ingredients but with the addition of spode of reeds, mace, crocus and camphor.

207. BNF, Magl. XV.92, fo. 95v, 'ongni cosa piu ò meno secondo pare al medicho bene experto et valente'. The 'heat' of the epithem could be adjusted by varying the ingredients – *idem*, fo. 136v, 'se voi che lla pittima sia fredda agiungni piu acqua rosa si che sia ve ne la meta et nelle dette ispezie agiungni cose fredde piu quantita'.

208. *RF, op. cit.* (note 9), fo. 148, Comparing the recipes for 'SPETIE DI PICTIMA Cordiale frescha' and 'SPETIE DI PICTIMA CORDIALE CALDA' shows that for a 'hot' cordial epithem, the quantity of sanders was reduced, and crocus (ie. saffron), cinnamon, cloves, aloe wood were added along with small quantities of amber and musk.

209. BNF, Magl. XV.92, fo .95v, 'secondo che pare al medico prudente secondo si conviene et secondo la febre grande ad uno huomo piu a cquelle fredde et difera in picchola febre et debilezza di virtu un pocho di muscho agiungniendo in questo caso un pocho di vino biancho odorifero.'

210. BNF, Magl. XV.92, fo. 111r, 'se vuoi che ssia calda metti piu delle cose chalde piu et meno delle fredde'; *idem*, fo. 137r, 'se vuoi che ssia fredda agiungni sandali bianchi et rossi et piu rose rosse et acqua rosata et un poco d'acieto et se vuoi che ssia piu calda agiungni le cose calde in piu quantita et delle fredde meno nella temperanzia.'

211. *RF, op. cit.* (note 9), fo. 148, 'SPETIE DI PICTIMA FRESCHA DA FEGHATO', 'Et nota che la canfora no' si agiugnie se non nelle febri acute & con epsa [*sic*] acqua di viole, o con altre acque secondo le intentione [sic] de medici.'

212. The mean value of the 58 epithems in the sample year was 25 soldi and the median 22 soldi.

213. 37 out of 515 active clients (7%) bought 58 epithems during the sample year. Excluding corporate clients, clients with surnames accounted for 67% of individual consumption of sweets (875 out of 1,313 soldi); this was higher than their proportion for all products (58%). Excluding corporate clients, clients with occupational titles accounted for 22% of individual consumption of sweets (284 out of 1,313 soldi); this was lower than their proportion for all products (31%).

214. Total spending on epithems in the sample year amounted to 1,442 soldi, ie. 4% of all spending on medicinal products.

215. E882, fo. 31r, 'Stagio di lorenzo barducci', 3 October 1493, 8.5 oz of 'fumentazione stomaticha chon piu erbe e fiori' and 2.5 oz of 2 'spungnie'; fo. 105r, 'ser Zanobi di iachopo borgianni', 14 November 1493, 14 oz of 'fumentazione stomaticha in che ent.o mortine rose quriandoli chose charminative e piu erbe e fiori' and 3.5 oz of 2 'spungnie ghrandi'. Sponges retailed at a uniform price of around 32 soldi per lb, although occasionaly 'thin sponges' were sold at a lower price – see fo. 75r, 'Munistero e donne di Santo anbruogio', 2 October 1493; fo. 53v, 'Andrea di Berto di michele lapi', 16 August 1493.

216. For example, E882, fo. 75r, 'Munistero e donne di Santo anbruogio', 1 October 1493, 'fumentazione stomaticha chon piu erbe e fiori'.

217. E882, fo. 110r, 'Madonna Girolama donna di messer puccio dant.o pucci', 25 September 1493, 'fumentazione stomaticha i' che ent.o asenzio aneto rose e fiori di chamamila churiandoli seme di lino e fieno ghrecho'. For other examples see fo. 105r, 'ser Zanobi di iachopo borgianni', 14 November 1493; fo. 61r, 'Manfredi inbasciadore di ferrara', 4 November 1493.

218. E882, fo. 160v, 'Ant.o di bartolomeo tessitore', 17 October 1493, 'fumentazione pettorale in che ent.o isapo timo miloloto chose charminative e piu erbe e fiori'.

219. E882, fo. 220r, 'Pedone di domenicho pedoni', 13 November 1493, 'fumentazione pel pettingnione e menbri orinali in che ent.o schorze di mandraghola churiandoli fienghregho chamamila e piu erbe e fiori'.

220. E882, fo. 353r, 'messer Michele di [BLANK] strozi', 24 July 1494, 'fumentazione per la milza in che ent.o barbe di malvavistio tamerigia fieno ghrecho e fiori di chamamilla'.

221. A number of fomentations were specifically described as being 'to make a bath'. For example, E882, fo. 315r, 'Simone di bernardo di simone del nero', 10 May 1494, 'fumentazione per fare bangnio'; fo. 258r, 'Bartolomeo di ser franc.o da anbra', 21 February 1493 (m.f.), 'fumentazione per fare bangnio in che ent.o fiori di neufarro viole rose s.e di papaveri s.e disquiamo schorze di papaveri'; fo. 307v, 'Bartolomeo di salvestro', 15 April 1494, 'fumentazione per fare bangniuolo in che ent.o rose e viole e piu erbe e fiori'.

222. E882, fo. 157r, 'ser Batista di [BLANK] chatenacci darezo', 17 February 1493 (m.f.), 'fumentazione sonifera in che ent.o fiori di neufarro viole rose chapi di papaveri e fiori di chamamilla per fare bangniuolo'. See also fo. 53r, 'Indacho raghugieo', 15 August 1493, 'fumentazione sonifera in che ent.o viole fiori di neufarro buccie di papaveri e altre chose'.

223. Products described in the accounts as *unguenti* (unguents) and an *unzioni* (unctions) have been considered together as 'ointments', since the terms

appear to be synonymous in the Giglio accounts. The *Ricettario fiorentino* employs only the term *unguento*, distinguishing this from *empiastro*.

224. Plaster were a stiffer variety of ointment made with gums and resins, but the similarity between them can be seen in *RF, op. cit.* (note 9), fo. 139, 'EMPIASTRO, o vero unguento del Conciliatore'. Although ointments and plasters formed separate sections of the *Ricettario fiorentino*, J. Mesue, *Opera* (Venice: 1497), lists these as the same category, 'de unguentis et emplastris'.

225. Cerates were not 'bandages' but were made from wax or applied to strips of leather. BNF, Magl. XV.92, fo. 51r, 'Cierotto da distendere in sul chuoio secondo maestro Aghostino'; *idem*, ff. 114v–15r, 'Cierotto da stomacho secondo comune', consisted of mastic spread hot on a strip of leather, 'spiced' with ladanum, red roses, cinnamon and cloves and 'made into a cerate' with colophony, to be applied hot to the skin. A *difensivo* ('defensive') was a similar sort of product made with wool, although rarely sold at the Giglio. In the sample year there is only a single example – E882, fo. 63v, 'Ponpeo delvantaggio', 29 August 1493, s5 for a 'difensivo per la testa'.

226. *RF, op. cit.* (note 9), fo. 122, 'UNGUENTO da stomacho magistrale, & usasi', consisting mostly of wax mixed with various oils (wormwood, mastic, spike), and aromatised with roses, coral, cloves, cinnamon, aloe wood, mastic, mint and squinant.

227. E882, fo. 343r, 'Angniolo di lodovicho accaiuoli', 12 July 1494, a mixture of 'unzione sandolino' and 'unzione infrigidans di ghalieno', 'fatta di frescho per ungniere le reni'; fo. 58v, 'Domenicho ditone', 20 August 1493, 'unzione populeo perungniere lereni'

228. For example, E882, fo. 348v, 'm.a Luchrezia donna fu di domenicho di bono rinucci', 18 July 1494 'cierotto sandolino'.

229. E882, fo. 51r, 'Lionardo di [BLANK] arzinchelgli', 12 August 1493, 'cierotto sandolino per ungniere el feghato'; fo. 237v, 'Franc.o di tingho dabrucianese', 6 December 1493, 'cierotto sandolino per feghato'. *RF, op. cit.* (note 9), fo. 126, 'UNGUENTO Sandalino, cioe Cerotto sandalino', made from red roses, three types of sanders, bole, spode of reeds, camphor, wax and oil roset. The wax was broken up in oil, washed in cold water, and then combined with powdered drugs. The Giglio accounts show that saffron and camphor were sometimes added – fo. 46r, 'Bartolomeo di nicholaio dallaquila', 6 August 1493, 7 August 1493, 'cierotto sandolino arotovi chanfera e zaferano'.

230. E882, fo. 58v, 'Nanni di [BLANK] fornaio chondavitte dilandino', 20 August 1493, 'cierotto dighome da milza ghrande'; fo. 273v, 'Matteo di [BLANK] squarcialupi', 31 July 1494, 'cierotto di ghome da milza'.

231. E882, fo. 23v, 'Girolamo di pagholo federichi', 3 August 1493, 'cierotto magistrale ghrande dareni'; fo. 340v, 'Vicho di [BLANK] cialdaio da monte varchi', 25 June 1494, 'cierotto da reni chonfortativo estiticho'; fo. 54r, 'm.o

Bartolomeo di [BLANK] dapisa medicho', 19 August 1493, 'cierotto da reni magistrale ghrande'.

232. E882, fo. 118r, 'Dionigi di bernardo chomi', 16 November 1493, 'cierotto rottoro disteso in sul quoio pel chapo'.

233. E882, fo. 64r, 'Giovanni di [BLANK] dalancisa chalzolaio', 30 August 1493, 'cierotto di sapo perungiere elpetto'.

234. E882, fo. 67r, 'Giovanfranc.o di me[ser]poggio', 16 September 1493, 'cierotto dosso chrozio e di laldano per pore alpie'.

235. E882, fo. 119r, 'Fruosino di Cece da Verrazano', 18 October 1493, 'cierotto chapitale in forma dostia fatto chon istoracie cienamo sandracha e altre chose'; fo. 75r, 'Munistero e donne di Santo anbruogio', 23 September 1493, 'cierotto chonfortativo e disechativo i' forma dostia dachapo in che ent.o masticie sandracha nocie moschade chubebe rose spodio e altre chose'.

236. E882, fo. 115v, 'Madonna Girolama donna di messer puccio dant.o pucci', 27 September 1493, 'cierotto ghrande a forma di talgliere in che ent.o masticie opoponacho ghalbano serapino incienso storacie liquida e altre pel chorpo'; fo. 51r, 'Lionardo di [BLANK] arzinchelgli', 11 August 1493, 'cierotto dighome i[n] forma ditalgliere dove ent[ran]o ghalbano opoponacho armoniacho lengnio aloe cienamo e altre chose'; fo. 343v, 'Domenicho di bono rinucci', 2 July 1494, 'cierotto di ghome in forma di talgliere in che entt.o ghalbano armoniacho delio lengnio aloe e altre chose'.

237. E882, fo. 25r, 'Rusticho dant.o rustichi', 13 September 1493, 1 oz of 'unzione dastomacho e sandolino'.

238. E882, fo. 316r, 'Piero di franc.o di bettino', 19 November 1496, s10 for 2.5 oz of 'unzione magistrale da reni in che ent.o sanghue di testugine sanghue di dragho bolo armeno terra sugielata e altre chose', 'per la donna'. Other examples include fo. 237v, 'Franc.o di tingho dabrucianese', 6 December 1493, 'unghuento populeo in che ent.o piu chose sonifere cioe chanfera oppio rose viole sandoli rossi', which was specifically 'per ungniere le tenpie e polsi'.

239. BNF, Magl. XV.92, fo. 97v, 'è fatto al tempo d'istate si vole mettere meno olio et cosi per contrario si vuole mettere al tempo di verno'.

240. *Ibid.*, fo. 38v, 'metti sopra la infrantura del capo ma vuole esse d'inverno ma non d'istate per che l'amazeresti'.

241. For example E882, fo. 59r, 'Lionardo di [BLANK] arzinghelgli', 21 August 1493, return of 4 *anpolle* and 5 *albarelli* for a total value of 3 soldi; fo. 252v, 'Bernardo di piero del palagio', 27 January 1493 (m.f.), return of 10 ampoules, 3 *bicchieri* and 8 *albarelli*; fo. 260r, 'Bartolomeo di ser franc.o da anbra', 28 February 1493 (m.f.), return of 12 ampoules, 1 *bicchiere* and 2 *albarelli* for a total value of 5 soldi; fo. 229v, 'Luigi di niccholo mormorai', 13 February 1493 (m.f.), return of 21 ampoules and 15 *albarelli* for a total value of 12 soldi; fo. 253r, 'Pedone di domenicho pedoni', 5 February 1493

(m.f.), return of 22 ampoules for a total value of s7d4; fo. 254r, 'Lando di giovanni tanalgli', 31 January 1493 (m.f.), return of 11 'anpolle e bichieri' and 1 *albarello* for a total value of s4; fo. 315r, 'Simone di bernardo di simone del nero', 5 May 1494, return of 8 ampoules for a total value ofs2d8. See also fo. 332v, 'Alamanno di filippo rinuccini', 19 June 1494; fo. 347r, 'Lionardo di [BLANK] arzinghelgli', 21 July 1494, 23 July 1494. The fact that most of these refer to ampoules and *albarelli* suggest that it was more common for customers to re-use *bicchieri* than sell them back to the shop. For all three kinds of receptacle the price was d4 each, whether being bought or sold.

242. E882, fo. 234v, 'Bartolomeo di niccholaio di ghino e chonpangni bichierai', 19 December 1493, sale of 94 lbs of 'vretto [*sic*] rotto' at an agreed price of d8 per lb. See also fo. 248r, 'Giovanni e ser girolamo di bartolomeo di nicholaio di ghino e chonpangni bichierai', 4 August 1494, sale of 41.5 lbs of 'vretto [*sic*] rotto' at an agreed price of d8 per lb.

243. Bicchieri were used only to supply *medicine* (purges). E882, fo. 325r, 'Angniolo di lodovicho acciaiuoli', 23 May 1494, refers specifically to 'bichieri da medinicine [*sic*]'.

244. *Albarelli* were sold along with at least 160 out of 253 composite electuaries (63%). Although the term is often considered as referring to the large storage jars in pharmacy shelves, these were clearly smaller versions for retail. ASF, Pupilli avanti il Principato 159 lists for example 'alberelli da 1/2 quarto in giu', 'alberelli da quarto dipinti'.

245. E882, fo. 344r, 'Munistero e donne di santo anbruogio', 2 July 1494, 'dua altre prese di s.o usato perche neruppe dua per la via'

246. E882, fo. 45r, 'Indacho raghugeo', 15 August 1493, a 'pentola' and an epithem. Epithems were generally mixed with around 2 lbs of liquid, making a larger vessel necessary.

247. E882, fo. 96v, 'Giovanbatista di benedetto dighoro', 19 September 1496.

248. See n.143.

249. E882, fo. 220r, 'Pedone di domenicho pedoni', 20 November 1493, 'mele' and 'regholizia e pasule', 'per bolire a chasa per fare bevanda'; fo. 237r, 'Munistero e donne di santo anbruogio', 11 December 1493, 'rose mortina balaustri e chamamilla', 'per bolire cholaqua ferata'.

250. E882, fo. 342r, 'Luigi di [BLANK] partini', 27 June 1494, 'fiori di borrana e di bughrossa e viole e fiori di neufarro', 'per bolire a chasa e fare gulebo lungho'.

251. E882, fo. 44r, 'Franc.o di Giovanni dinofri dalterrio', 5 August 1493, 'pittima secha pel feghato' containing 'spezie di triasandoli' and 'asenzio chapelvenero rose e altre chose'.

252. E882, fo. 335v, 'Domenicho di bono rinucci', 23 June 1494, s6 for 'piu erbe seche in che ent.o rose rosse squinanti asenzio eupatorio chapelvenero', 'per bolire in aqua dorzo e acieto per fare pittima al feghato'.

253. E882, fo. 237v, 'Franc.o di tingho dabrucianese', 6 December 1493, 'per bolire chomedisse il m.o per fare pittima al quore'.

254. E882, fo. 315r, 'Jachopo di bartolomeo da girone linaiuolo', 28 February 1494 (m.f.), specifies that the flowers are 'per bolire per larghomento', implying that this was to be done at home by the client.

255. E882, fo. 236r, 'Domenicho di messer charlo pandolfini', 5 December 1493, 1.5 oz of 'zuc.o rosso', 2 handfuls of 'piu erbe per bollire per larghomento' and 3 oz of 'olio di spigho e olio di chamamilla per meta', 'per metter nelarghomento'. See also fo. 220r, 'Pedone di domenicho pedoni', 21 November 1493, 'chonsolida seme dorticha e chartamo' and 'schorze dagharigho', 'per bollire per larghomento'. In the same transaction the customer also bought 'latt.o e zuc.o darchomenti' and 'olio daneto'.

256. E882, fo. 46r, 'Chancia spangniuolo in chasa andrea lapi', 7 August 1493, 'archomento frescho fatto qui i' bottegha dove ent.o chasia zuc.o rosso olio e sale'.

257. E882, fo. 305v, 'Franc.o di zanobi martini', 16 April 1494, lists a debt 'per uno arghomento fatto qui in bottegha e chondito chon olio e sale e chon chasia e altr.o', which was supplied in a 'pentola' and carried home by the female servant 'porto la serva'. The fact that the records took the bother to specify this detail implies that clients usually did this at home. For a similar case, see fo. 306r, 'messer Ghirighoro schovardo spangniuolo', 12 April 1494, 'per uno arghomento fatto qui in bottegha e chondito entrevi [oz 3] di latt.o e zuc.o darchomenti e piu chose charminative', and fo. 33v, 'Chostantino di marcho di ser tomme bracci', 31 July 1493, 'archomento fatto qui in bottegha'.

258. E882, fo. 257v, 'm.a Piera donna dandrea di berto lapi', 16 February 1493 (m.f.). For rhubarb, see notes 69 and 70.

259. E882, fo. 315v, 'ser Giovanni di domenicho patani daenpoli', 26 April 1494, 'per una chonposizione di sua p'le dachordo cholui', L1s16.

260. E882, fo. 258r, 'Bartolomeo di ser franc.o da anbra', 22 February 1493 (m.f.), 'per. istinquare manna e ribarbero suo a chasa'. Similarly, fo. 2v, 'Giovanbatista di [BLANK] stamaiuolo', 15 July 1493, the client bought red sugar and sugar roset 'per uno archomento chon olio di chasa'.

261. E882, fo. 131v, 'Lucha di paradiso botteghaio fuori della porta a sanpiero ghattolini', 17 November 1494, 2 dr of 'dicienamo per bolire chon peverada di pollo'. See also fo. 307v, 'Bartolomeo di salvestro', 16 April 1494, 's.o giugiolino e violato', 'per usare cholachocitura a fare achasa'.

262. E882, fo. 229v, 'Luigi di niccholo mormorai', 3 December 1493, s6 for 3.5 dr of 'polvere per mettere nel pollo in che ent.o smeraldi choralli rossi fiori

chordiali seme di piantagine'. This again appears similar to a 'fine cordial powder' listed in the hospital receptary – BNF, Magl. XV.92, fo. 135r, 'Polvere cordiale fina', 'fa polvere sottile et usala in sul pollo ò in sullo istillato ò in sul lattovario et se vuolgli un poco arromatizata ponvela a aromatizare'

263. E882, fo. 99r, 'Taddeo di romolo ducci', 19 September 1495, 1 dr of 'ribarbero fine mondo e netto messo infusione in aqua di indivia ettrebiano per fare spresione earogie auna sua dichozione achasa'

264. E882, fo. 2v, 'Giovanbatista di [BLANK] stamaiuolo', 17 July 1493, 1.5 oz of 'chonserva dacietosita diciederno', 'sarose a latt.o dachasa'; fo. 160v, 'Ant.o di bartolomeo tessitore', 19 October 1493, 1 oz of 'latt.o di farfero', 'aroto al suo latt.o'. Other examples fo. 288r, 'Tommaxo di messer otto niccholini', 25 March 1494, 'ventricholi di pollo' and 'gulebo rosato', 'per arogiere a suo latt.o'; fo. 307v, 'Bartolomeo di salvestro', 17 April 1494, 'ossimele semplice', 'per agungnie al gulebo da chasa', and 'latt.o daltea', 'per agungniere a latt.o dachasa'; fo. 120r, 'Giovanni Salamancha spangniuolo in chasa andrea lapi', 19 October 1493, 1 oz of 'savonia', 'agunto a latt.e da chasa'; fo. 305r, 'Giovanni di [BLANK] falchoni', 14 January 1496 (m.f.), 1 oz of 'savonia', 'aroto al suo latt.o'.

265. See above (notes 49, 50, 51 and 52).

266. E882, fo. 220r, 'Pedone di domenicho pedoni', 16 November 1493, 0.5 oz of 'chanfera pesta sottile', 'per adoperare a chasa'.

267. E882, fo. 250r, 'Diegho salamancha spangniuolo in chasa andrea di berto lapi', 9 February 1494 (m.f.), 'del quale gli faciemo un lattovaro chon sua spezie e per facitura [soldi] 5'.

268. E882, fo. 254r, 'Lando di giovanni tanalgli', 1 February 1493 (m.f.), of which d4 is for one 'p[illo]la aghreghativa' and s1 'per riformatura di p[illo]le chon suo ribarbero'.

269. Neither pudding pipe, rhubarb or manna were mentioned by Dioscorides, as Mattioli specifically noted in his translation. Mattioli, *op. cit.* (note 41), ff.48–9, 'nè Dioscoride, nè altro degli antichi Greci scrisse (che io sappia) della CASSIA SOLUTIVA...'; fo. 444, 'Non essendo del Rheubarbaro solutivo stata fatta mentione alcuna da Dioscoride, nè da quel si voglia altro degli antichi, nè narrerò quì l'historia sua, togliendone la maggior parte da Mesue....'; fo. 90, 'Ma poscia che la manna dell'incenso m'ha ridotto a memoria la manna solutiva, che scende dall'aria, non se ne facendo nel processo da Dioscoride altra mentione, acchioce si sodisfaccia ai lettori, ne dirò di mente degli Arabi quanto essi ne scrissero....'

270. RF, *op. cit.* (note 9), ff. 32–3. J. Henderson, *The Renaissance Hospital: Healing the Body and Healing the Soul* (New Haven: Yale University Press, 2006), 299–301, in the recipe book of Santa Maria Nuova, 69% of the

recipes came from Florentine practitioners, while only 31% of recipes were attributed to traditional medical authorities.

271. Riddle, *op. cit.* (note 21), 175; Slack, *op. cit.* (note 17), 257.
272. Riddle, *ibid.*, 172–3; J. Arrizabalaga, J. Henderson, and R.K. French, *The Great Pox. The French Disease in Renaissance Europe* (New Haven: Yale University Press, 1997), 258.
273. Bénézet, *op. cit.* (note 29), 488–9.
274. G. Silini, 'La cultura medica e farmaceutica', in G. Silini (ed.), *Herbe pincte* (Gorle: Iniziative Culturali, 2000), 21; Siraisi, *op. cit.* (note 2), 120–1.
275. Silini, *ibid.*, 23.
276. Bénézet, *op. cit.* (note 29), 697.
277. Silini, *op. cit.* (note 2), 220–1; Riddle, *op. cit.* (note 21), 172.
278. RF, *op. cit.* (note 9), ff. 149-50, 'Et nota che molte confectioni et lactovari cordiali si possono comporre secondo la phantasia del medico arrogendo & levando a sua discretione & secondo la necessita del paziente per chi si ordina: & chosi anchora si possono fare molti & varii argomenti, Fomentationi, Empiastri, Unctioni, Pictime & simili che non acchade a porle qui per la varieta delli operanti & loro phantasie: perche sarebbono superflue: et qualche ignorante & presumptuoso speziale si presummerebbe poter fare da se medesimo senza el medico perito: & seguiterebbene scandali infiniti: & pero in questo nostro presente riceptario non si e' posto cosa alchuna a che si sia appropriata: perche speriamo che chi l'ha adoperare lo sappia: & chi non lo sa, lo impari, et poi lo adoperi canonicamente: il perche porremo fine a questo secondo libro, & co'ladiutorio di Dio verremo al terzo libro.'
279. E. Diana, 'Medici, speziali e barbieri nella Firenze della prima metà del '500', *Rivista di storia della medicina*, 4, 2 (1994), 13–27: 18.
280. E882, fo. 272r, 'Tommaxo di [BLANK] delgli alesandri', 26 March 1494, 0.5 dr of 'p'le asezerette riformate p'le n.o iii orati' for s2 (s384 per lb, or d8 per pill). The standard variety of these sort of pills cost half that amount: d4 per pill. Similarly, fo. 62r, 'Simone di bernardo niccholini', 13 October 1493, 2 'p'le chozie orat.e' for s1d4 (d8 per pill). The standard variety of these sort of pills cost half that amount: d4 per pill.
281. R. Ciasca, 'La cultura di un farmacista del '400', in A.E. Vitolo (ed.), *Raccolta di scritti in onore di Giulio Conci* (Pisa: Arti Grafiche Pacini Mariotti, 1953), 127.
282. G.M. Nardi, 'La medicina popolare in Toscana', *Lares*, 6, 4 (1935), 272–82: 277, 'Sciroppo di cantina, pillole di gallina e buon mantello, manda il medico al bordello.'
283. M. Giagnacovo, 'Due "alimentazioni" del basso medioevo: la tavola dei mercanti e la tavola dei ceti subalterni', in S. Cavaciocchi (ed.), *Alimentazione e nutrizione secc. XIII–XVIII: atti della ventottesima settimana*

di studi, 22–27 aprile 1996 (Florence: Le Monnier, 1997), 827; P. Skinner, *Health and Medicine in Early Medieval Southern Italy* (Leiden: Brill, 1997), 105. Local herbs are also mostly absent from the supply records. There were no herb-women listed among the shop suppliers, as can be found for shops outside Florence, or in the lists of purchases by the dispensary of Santa Maria Nuova. Santa Maria Nuova 5080, fo. 19r, lists L1 owed to a woman for supplies of horehound 'a m.a Gostanza per lbs 30 di prasia'. G. Borghini, *et al., Una farmacia preindustriale in Valdelsa: la spezieria e lo spedale di Santa Fina nella città di San Gimignano secc. XIV–XVIII* (San Gimignano: Città di San Gimignano, 1981), 126, for payments to various herb-women.

284. G.B. Zapata, *Li maravigliosi secreti di medicina e chirurgia: nuovamente ritrovati, per guarire ogni sorte d'infirmita* [Rome, 1577] (Turin, 1580), the text was specifically addressed to the 'poor': 'se ben non havrete gemme, oro, e pietre pretiose, come i ricchi e potenti per discacciar detti mali (medicamenti che veramente sono vani, e di niun porfitto [*sic*]) havrete almeno rimedii facili, che la sagace natura ha fatto, e prodotto in util vostro'. W. Eamon, *Science and the Secrets of Nature: Books of Secrets in Medieval and Early Modern Europe* (Princeton: Princeton University Press, 1994), 135–7.

285. Siraisi, *op. cit.* (note 2), 189.

286. Castellani, *op. cit.* (note 18), 'Medicina provata a' fanciulli o ad altri che sentissi di bachi.' 'Poi per terza medicina, quando arai facto tutto dell'unzione e del beveragio detto di sopra, togli lacte di capra e on. tre di mèle, e fanne uno cristeo'.

287. BNF, Magl. XV.92.

9

Epilogue

The Shop and the Court

The previous chapters have captured a very specific moment in the history of the Speziale al Giglio, one where Florence was poised for enormous political, social and economic change. The city's transformations can be followed in the shifts in the Giglio's own records, and while this epilogue cannot cover the full story of its sixteenth-century evolution, a brief examination allows some conclusions about the continuities and changes, not only in the apothecary's business, but also in the nature of pharmacy more generally, its regulation and its relationship to new commercial and medical practices.[1]

In November 1494, with French troops nearing Tuscany, Piero de' Medici and his associates were finally forced to flee Florence. Despite numerous attempts to return, Piero remained in exile for the rest of his life. The city's interim government persuaded the invader, Charles VIII, to continue the Medici's banishment and the family's possessions were taken out of their house on Via Larga and put up for sale by auction in order to pay their numerous debts.[2] In the frenzied bidding, clothing, textiles, furniture and even the *desco da parto* given to Lorenzo de' Medici's mother to celebrate his birth were all sold to eager bidders. The bronze statues cast by Donatello for the Medici to celebrate their Florentine credentials, such as the *David* and the *Judith and Holofernes*, were moved from the family palace to the main square in front of the Palazzo Vecchio, signalling the revival of republicanism and moral values that the Dominican preacher Savonarola had encouraged. It is no coincidence that along with the reassertion of communal ideologies came the enhancement of communal authority. One aspect which has already been discussed at length was the publication of the *Ricettario fiorentino*, first printed in Florence in 1499 under the jurisdiction of the Guild of Doctors and Apothecaries.[3] The ostensible reason for its publication was the poor quality of the materials and ingredients being produced by the city's pharmacies; this was meant as a clear guide to accurate and effective practice but it was also an assertion of civic pride and standards. Yet as we have seen, while the *Ricettario* provided a set of commonly accepted recipes, it was not accompanied by any enforcement or oversight, something that would change in the 1560s. Moreover, the revival of traditional republican rule with a strong guild base proved equally short-lived. Savonarola was eventually burnt at the stake for his attacks on papal authority, and Piero Soderini was elected as Gonfaloniere di Giustizia for life in 1502. There would never be a new Florentine republic again and the relationship between the court, the commune and the guilds would remain contested.

There were considerable vicissitudes over the next two decades, but by 1537, wearied by internal and external struggle, senior figures in the city, including Francesco Guicciardini, invited an obscure seventeen-year-old member of a side-branch of the Medici family to take nominal authority over the city under their guidance. This was Cosimo I de' Medici, the son of Giovanni delle Bande Nere and Maria Salviati. Despite the assumptions that the young man would rule in name alone, he quickly transformed his position into one of real authority. More gradually, he changed Florence from a city dominated by republican symbols of communal power to one where he, his family, and his court were the central focus for civic authority. In 1539, Cosimo married Eleanora di Toledo, establishing a dynasty that, following their establishment as Grand Dukes of Tuscany in 1570, would remain in control of the region until the eighteenth century.

Although Cosimo himself did much to suggest that the transition was uncontested, the creation of a new principality had had very immediate economic as well as political consequences. These were not always unwelcome and local businesses often proved willing to adapt. The creation of a court centralised and eventually raised expenditure on just the types of products that apothecaries could supply. While the Medici court was initially modest in comparison with its counterparts elsewhere in Italy and Europe, its growth was significant. Salary rolls from 1540–3 show a very small number of servants but ten years later the number had almost doubled to eighty members of staff.[4] By 1587, the growth was exponential. Almost three hundred servants were employed, a figure that does not reflect the large number of guests and other associates who had to be fed, entertained and looked after when they were ill. The 'service' sector grew in line with the new court requirements and one of the interesting aspects of the apothecary's business was how this impacted on their structures of credit and supply. The court needed a steady supply of the speziale's products, from medicines, sugar and confectionery for its entertainments, to candles for illumination and ritual offerings. During special festivities, such as marriages, baptisms and funerals, the demand could soar as the city's pharmacies supplied the artists producing the ephemeral decorations with pigments, glues and other products along with the items needed for banquets and gifts. The economic importance of the right to maintain control over goods in demand, such as candles, were reflected in the changes to guild statues of 1536 which confirmed the apothecaries' exclusive rights over candle sales as well as the growing trade in illuminations and fireworks.[5]

The concentration of political authority in the new court structures also had an impact on medical care. In the fifteenth century, the Speziale al Giglio generally dealt with families and individuals who bought products for themselves, their immediate relatives and their servants. While consumption was already strongly polarised, with a minority of clients responsible for the majority of its profits, it was rare to have bulk purchases or a single, substantial client on whom the shop relied exclusively for its profits. But as well as candles, artists' supplies, spices and items for the kitchen, the Medici required medical treatments on a much larger scale, making the distinction between 'minor' clients and this very major client even more dramatic. The ducal family was expected to not only look after its own health but also that of a substantial number of servants, loyal followers and the deserving poor, such as nuns and monks who might petition for help. Indeed, requests multiplied as the court expanded, because the only thing that would not change over time was the considerable expense of falling ill. In 1544, for example, Agnolo Dovizi da Bibbiena wrote to the Medici master of the *guardaroba*, Pier Francesco Riccio:

> I have come to the house of ser Tommaso Berni in order to recover... It is impossible to sustain my expenses without getting into debt further, on top of what I have already had to pay for my previous illness and above that which I have to pay now to the doctor and for the medicines along with the two purges that I owe to Viviano speziale.[6]

The hope, of course, was that such a petition would result in the court taking on the costs of such medical care. This was certainly something that those in the service of the Duke and Duchess could expect. When one of Eleanora of Toledo's Spanish ladies-in-waiting fell ill, it was made abundantly clear to those in charge of expenditure that all her requirements from the speziale should be met.[7]

The creation of a single major client had other, perhaps less expected, impacts on businesses such as the Speziale al Giglio. Unlike his predecessors, the new Duke of Florence, Cosimo I de' Medici had a strong personal interest in alchemy and botany, a fascination that he passed onto his sons, Francesco and Ferdinando, who developed their own scientific laboratories and practices (see Image 9.1, overleaf). In 1561, the Venetian ambassador to Florence, Vincenzo Fedeli, described Cosimo as follows,

> I want to say something unusual about this prince, who understands and is skilled in such things that it seems to be his own profession. Above all he is

Image 9.1

Jan van der Straet (Giovanni Stradano), Alchemical experiments in the
Medici fondaco, *c.1580, fresco, Palazzo Pitti, Florence.
Courtesy: The Bridgeman Art Library.*

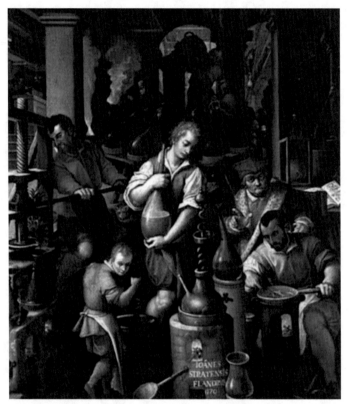

most knowledgeable in herbs and simples of which he has a great
understanding. He has a garden full of these and takes particular care and
pleasure in planning, caring and experimenting with them... and he
continually creates waters and oils by distillation in order to experiment on
diverse illnesses and wounds, and he has found remedies for the *punta del
fianco*, for the constriction of urine and for head wounds, which in Tuscany,
due to the subtlety of the air had all been fatal illnesses and are now all
curable. With great diligence, he makes *sopravvivo* and mithridates to such
perfection that can be seen in action and he makes antidotes to poisons...he
does all this in the place known as the Foundry of the Duke where he works
constantly with an infinite variety of kilns and stills.[8]

The ducal involvement in distillation and medical innovations meant that there was a constant requirement for ingredients of every type.[9] However, it is important to note that not all such items were acquired from Florentine apothecaries; many were ordered directly through agents from Venice using the offices of the Carnesecchi and Strozzi bank. In 1566, for example, a long list of goods was ordered for the ducal foundry directly from Venice, including cardamom, aloe, dragon's blood, manna, mastic and sugar.[10]

Nonetheless, the court did make local arrangements drawing on the resources of a range of apothecaries, rather than relying on a single supplier. Their choices had, however, diminished considerably by mid-century. The 1561 Florentine census, the *decima*, only listed forty-five apothecary shops in contrast to the over sixty-six that had existed almost a century earlier.[11] Their location was also more concentrated. Most apothecary shops (twenty-six or seventy-six per cent of the total) were clustered in the market centre of the neighbourhood of San Giovanni, with much smaller numbers in the other quarters of the city.[12]

This concentration seems to have meant that the businesses that did survive into the sixteenth century – when there was a rise in population in Florence and presumably growing demand from the court – were larger than their predecessors and often involved multiple partners and investors rather than simply being a family-run business. This may have simply been because the costs of entry into the profession were now much higher and credit arrangements may have been more complicated. This, however, is not new but a continuation of the trends already identified in the fifteenth century.

But other influences may have created new restrictions. Although there was still no requirement for a university degree, professional *speziali* had to increasingly argue their competency and standing against doctors and other university-educated professionals. This meant that of those recorded in the 1561 Catasto, thirty-one per cent of *speziale* shop-owners were patricians, although the latter accounted for only fourteen per cent of shopkeepers in total.[13] This was far closer to the numbers recorded for physicians than other associated trades, such as mercers, and the links became ever closer as the century drew to a close. Thus when Tommaso di Giovanni Guidi died in 1504, he left a reasonably prosperous business to his son-in-law, Lapino di Agnolo. Lapini ceded it, in turn, to his son, Lorenzo Lapini, who eventually died without heirs in 1568, leaving behind an even more successful business.

Did success in the sixteenth century mean something quite different from success in the fifteenth century? Certainly, family relationships rather than personal reputation remained key to entering and sustaining the business. Although Lapino di Agnolo already had a mercer's shop in the neighbourhood of San Lorenzo[14] he had no difficulty in taking over the speziale's role until his own sons, Lorenzo and Agnolo, were able to take on the Giglio, eventually running it in their own names after 1546.

But, if there was familial continuity, one major change is immediately obvious. From 1535 onwards, the Speziale al Giglio was not only a supplier to clients who came and went through the shop doors: it was also one of the most important suppliers of sweets, medicines and candles to the Medici court. Goods were provided to all members of the Medici household, and eventually, Lorenzo Lapini ended up creating a specific account book to manage this side of the business.[15] Another set of accounts, which ran from 1546 and 1568, was further sub-divided between provision listed as *medicinale, cere* and veterinary supplies to the stables.[16] Although the Giglio was not the only, nor even the main supplier to the court, the success of the relationship between the apothecary and the court can been seen in a request of December 1549 to send *manna vecchia* and pills made by Angelo Lapini to Bartolomeo de' Medici, who had fallen ill in Livorno.[17]

The Medici were not only good customers: they, and their appointed officials, had an increasingly dominant role in how business was managed and regulated. The 1550 version of the *Ricettario fiorentino* was published by the ducal printer at Cosimo I de' Medici's command, making it accessible not only to specialists but also to a wider public looking for reassurance about healthcare. By 1560, apothecaries could not operate unless they could demonstrate, through annual inspections, that they were following agreed precepts on practice and were obeying the rules set down, not only by their guild, but also by the *Magistrati della Sanità*. This is in distinct contrast to the rather loose institutional controls that allowed Lapini's predecessor to operate without even being enrolled in the apothecary's guild, or to trade, however discreetly, on feast days. In the Guild deliberations of the 1470s, concerns were raised when apothecaries were careless in filling prescriptions or when empirics wore the long gown and gold buckle that only university-trained doctors were supposed to wear; a century later the disputes and demarcations would be much fiercer, with physicians vying to control and dominate the dissemination of pharmaceutical products.

The *Ricettario*, which was issued to all apothecaries, joined an increasing number of more popular and academic treatises on medical products, a shift caused both by changes in the publishing industry, and by concern over diseases and cures, both new and old.

The half-century between the first and second publications of the *Ricettario* had seen not only political and social transformations but also dramatic innovations in pharmaceutical products on several fronts. The first half of the century had seen considerable investigation into Hellenistic and Roman medical treatises, with a renewed drive to identify the ingredients referred to by Galen. A comparison of the 1499 and 1567 *Ricettario fiorentino* reveals that the latest version contained almost half of the earlier recipes, 262 out of 489. While the majority of the earlier recorded treatments were drawn from the Arabic tradition, with over two-thirds taken from the Antidotarium of Mesue, the 1567 edition privileged modern and Greek recipes; only twenty-nine had their origins in Mesue.[18]

The inventory of the Speziale al Giglio taken at Lorenzo Lapini's death in 1568 hints at the impact these changes had on the family's business.[19] It had clearly prospered under the new regime. Lapini, like his grandfather, had a large number of devotional and secular art works, including a range of terracotta figures such as two *putti*, a David (a classic figure of Florentine pride), images of saints such as San Girolamo and San Francesco, and a gilt-framed image of the Virgin Mary.[20] In contrast to his grandfather, however, there were barely 'three bits of books to read' in the house, suggesting that he did not share the same lively intellectual interests.[21] The inventory also shows that the Giglio heirs had doubled the shop space at their disposal. Although it is not clear when the expansion took place, the Lapini eventually ran two sites, the *bottega* and the *bottega nuova,* adjacent to each other. While these do not seem to have been differentiated by the goods they sold, the latter had far more specialised facilities for the skilled preparation of their goods. In contrast to the old shop which only had a *cucina*, the *bottega nuova* not only had a kitchen but also housed a separate room for working in high-quality wax, the so-called *camera della cera bianca,* and an area for storage: the *palco delle cere* containing 478 lbs of new yellow torches, 145 lbs of white wax torches, 141 lbs of white candles and a further 145 lbs of white wax waiting to be processed. Additionally, there was a *stanza dei grassi,* a *camera de fogli* where paper goods were kept, a *stanza del' herbe*, and a site where goods designated for use in theriac were kept.

The inventory also suggests that this new shop was rather more elegant than its neighbour. The first item listed in the old shop inventory was the shop sign, the *insegna al Giglio;* this was immediately followed by a coat-of-arms, that of the Medici *palle,* which was displayed inside demonstrating both their loyalty to and patronage by the ruling family. The old shop was dominated by shelving, drawers and chests carrying bottles, painted boxes for sweets, two large bronze mortars and a marble version, which stood in the shop itself, scales and weights. One can suspect that these were versions of, or even the very same, items that Tommaso had used sixty years before. While the new shop was much the same, it was more elaborately decorated with a gesso Madonna and angels on its walls and substantial wooden cases with large numbers of *albarelli*. Nonetheless, the same products could be found in both stores. As in the fifteenth century, medical products were sold alongside an increasingly large numbers of candles, torches and wax, as well as sugar and confectionery. The funerary goods, however, had disappeared, at least from the inventory.

There were numerous waters and oils, but only a few medicinal products bearing 'brand' names, such as some 'pills of Maestro Franco Ruggieri'.[22] There was also a greater emphasis on items associated with the 'chemical medicine' promoted by Paracelsus, including the extraordinarily large amount of one hundred lbs of arsenic.[23] Nonetheless, of the drugs and spices listed, many would have been very familiar to the Lapini's grandfather: dragons-blood, manna, senna, aloe, mastic, rhubarb, pepper, nutmeg, cinnamon and other spices, and traditional Galenic cures. This suggests that the customers who came into both the old and new shops on the Canto del Giglio would have seen a very reassuring, familiar physical environment; only this time they would have had to choose which door to enter.

Holy Wood

Despite much that was traditional in the pills, elixirs and syrups on offer, the 1568 Giglio also sold some very innovative products. By weight, the most important ingredient sold in the shop, after wax and sugar, was a completely new item that would simply have been unavailable for sale in Europe earlier in the century. This was guaiac or *legno santo*, the resin of a New World tree that was used to treat the *mal francesce, morbo gallico* or syphilis.[24] Although its properties had been known since the late fifteenth century, there was considerable debate over its efficacy, and the Fugger merchants had held a monopoly on its sale until 1525. It is not surprising, therefore, that it is entirely absent from the 1504 inventory. But by 1568, there was almost 480 lbs of this New World ingredient at the Speziale al Giglio and a further 33 lbs waiting to be collected from the customs officials at the *dogana*. The guaiac cure was a very unpleasant experience. It involved remaining enclosed in a hot room for a month, eating lightly, undergoing purges and taking a decoction that was only to be prepared under a physician's supervision but was which often self-administered.[25] The wood was grated and then infused in twelve litres of water for twenty-four hours before being boiled and filtered; a second decoction was then put into a further twelve litres of water and reduced, while a final unction was created from the reduction. The patient was supposed to take the first decoction as the principle cure, drinking the second instead of wine with meals and using the ointment on ulcerated skin and lesions. *Legno vecchio* was meant for advanced stages of the disease while *legno nuovo* was used as an early intervention. The treatment, designed to replace the extremely painful mercury cures, was initially promoted in the early sixteenth century by Ulrich von Hutton, whose treatise on curing the *morbo gallico* was translated and extensively circulated across Europe. It was further promoted by key figures, such as

Girolamo Fracastoro, who sent a copy of his 1546 *De contagione et contagionis morbis* to Cosimo I de' Medici as soon as it was published.[26] Cosimo's reply was polite rather than enthusiastic, asking Pietro Camaiani to formally thank the doctor for the book which he said he intended to read in the future:

> We have received the little book that doctor Fracastoro has sent us, which we have seen and will read most willingly knowing that it cannot be but excellent as he is famed for his singular standing in his profession. Thank him on our part as is appropriate to the kindness that he has shown us and that is due to his good qualities and virtues.[27]

Just over twenty years later, however, Cosimo also turned to Fracastoro's recommendations when he suspected that he too had contracted the disease. His staff reported how, on 20 December 1572, the Duke had 'begun to take the wood' and was bearing up well under the treatment.[28]

The Giglio had a range of supplies of guaiac in different forms that were appropriate to the specific treatment that was recommended; although scholars have argued that the cure fell out of fashion by the mid-sixteenth century, the sheer quantity of holy wood in this and other pharmacies suggest that suffers were still willing to undergo this cure, along with other attempts to rid themselves of the painful and inevitably fatal disease.[29] Certainly, by this period, one of Cosimo's favourite court artists, the Flemish painter and engraver Giovanni Stradano included the guaiac cure as one of ten most important inventions of mankind in his series the 'Nova Reperta'. Standing alongside gunpowder, the water-wheel, windmill, distillation and silk weaving, the picture showed the treatment being administered under the direction of a physician while the wood itself was prepared within the home itself rather than in the pharmacy (see Image 9.2, overleaf).

Theriac

It is certainly possible that the large quantities of *legno santo* in the Giglio inventory were destined for hospital clients rather than individuals. In Rome, the Ospedale degli Incurabili treated almost five thousand patients and required large amounts of this expensive imported product. In addition to new commodities, there is some evidence that traditional products were being revised. Theriac was a well-known and long-standing cure-all made from multiple ingredients including viper's flesh which was designed to protect against poison, heal numerous illnesses and maintain overall good health, and which had been retailed in minor amounts at the Giglio in the previous century (see Chapter 8). The 1568 inventory, however, indicates greater attentiveness to theriac and its preparation, since the ingredients were stored separately and listed as being 'arranged for the theriac'.[30] This reflects

Image 9.2

Jan Galle after Jan van der Straet (Giovanni Stradano),
Nova Reperta: Treatment with Holy Wood, c. *1580.*
Engraving: Max-Planck-Institut für Wissenschaftgeschichte, Berlin.

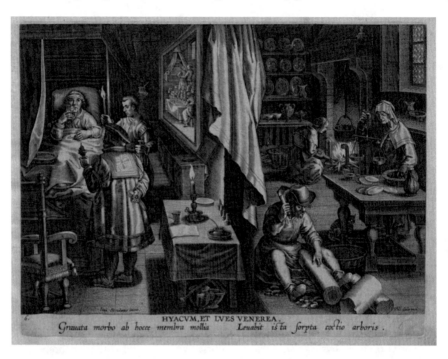

a more general tendency towards regulation of this product. In the sixteenth century, theriac became strongly associated with Venice – in England it was known as Venice treacle – where the government kept its manufacture under close observation. From the 1480s, the responsible magistracy, the *Giustizia Vecchia,* kept an *armadio delle teriache* in order to provide a set of standard ingredients against which others could be measured. The chest was, of course, not evidence that there was consensus over how theriac should be defined but a sign that oversight was required. This concern would only increase during the sixteenth century as apothecaries vied with each other to argue that they, and only they, had discovered ingredients which matched the original Galenic recipes. As apothecaries and others investigated New World botany and the herbs within their own gardens, they increasingly identified their discoveries with simples described by Galen and entered into lengthy arguments over accuracy and efficacy.[31] While the theriac ingredients listed in the Giglio's cabinets were not particularly unusual: storax, cardamom, cinnamon, gum Arabic, gentian etc., they were part of this attempt to demonstrate that one shop's 'theriac' was superior to another's. In the case of the Giglio, however, only the fact that almost fifty ingredients were listed and the inclusion of scorpions might be regarded as unusual. The snakes that were a key part of medication were present in the preserved form of 'viper trochisks'.[32] Interestingly, two theriac vases were kept in Agnolo's private chamber in his home.[33] It isn't clear if this was because the finished product was so valuable that he wanted to have greater oversight, or because it was for his personal use, or because the jars themselves were regarded as precious in their own right. Certainly, the two vases designed to hold theriac and another classical recipe, *mithridatum*, in the Getty Museum, Los Angeles, must have been a significant investment designed to demonstrate the sophistication of their owner (Images 9.3 and 9.4, overleaf).

While the image of the product was important, there were continued discussions about its content. Interestingly, less than a decade after the Lapini inventory was taken, the Florentine guild decided to change its official theriac recipe, using a new 'balsamo del'India', instead of a more standard, more easily accessible balsam. It was Cosimo's own doctor and biographer, Baccio Baldini, who ordered the change indicating that the Arte degli Speziale would not license any other form of theriac.[34] This was not a purely intellectual argument. Theriac was a very profitable product that could be marketed and branded both at home and abroad. In Bologna, for example, the famed naturalist, Ulisse Aldrovandi, one of the *protomedicati* responsible for supervising the city's speziali entered into a particularly bitter public dispute with the Collegio dei Medici and the city's apothecaries in the 1570s. Aldrovandi had publicly prepared a sample of his theriac using ingredients that were very difficult to obtain, but the local *speziali* contested his authority which threatened to damage their products. The latter publicly prepared their own version which Aldrovandi then tried to ban, accusing them of having used vipers which were pregnant in contravention of the recipe. In the disputes that followed, Aldrovandi lamented the confusion between those who were learned and those whom, he argued, were effectively simple grocers, claiming that:

> The majority of apothecaries who ought to be knowledgeable in this material are, nonetheless, completely ignorant and often barely know how to read. From time to time, they mistake one simple for its opposite with poisonous qualities as can be said of many. One can find apothecaries in Flanders, Bohemia and Germany who are more expert than in Italy. As a minimum they know Latin and make a knowledge of simples their profession rather

Image 9.3

Painted and Gilt Terracotta Jar for Theriac,
attributed to Annibale Fontana, c.1580,
J.P. Getty Museum, Los Angeles, 90.SC.42. Photo: The Getty Museum.

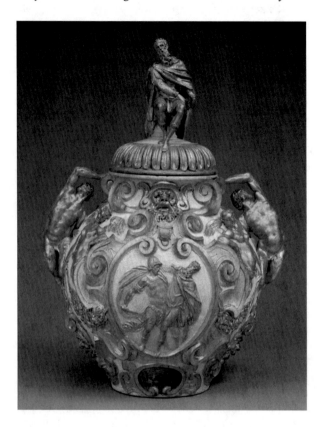

than selling groceries such as wax, oil, soap and a thousand other impertinent things as we do, but they sell medicines separately from other drugs.[35]

Lapini may indeed have been seen as one of these 'grocers' whom Aldrovandi lamented. Despite Aldrovandi's scathing portrayal, as indicated in the earlier chapters, the apothecary or *speziale* had to be both numerate and literate; figures such as Matteo Palmieri and Luca Landucci kept journals as well as account books and participated actively in the cultural and political life of the city; by the sixteenth century many were members of the patriciate. But as the city moved towards a more courtly environment, their

Image 9.4

Painted and Gilt Terracotta Jar for Mithridatum,
attributed to Annibale Fontana, c.1580,
J.P. Getty Museum, Los Angeles, 90.SC.42. Photo: The Getty Museum.

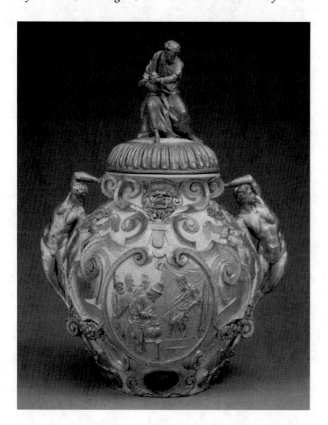

successors were able to retain this intellectual position by participating in serious arguments about botany and medicine and adapting the new techniques of dissemination to ensure that their arguments were heard. For example, the apothecary Antonio Francesco Grazzini was one of the founders of the Academia degli Umidi, with the pseudonym Il Lasca or 'The Roach' and went on to found the Accademia della Crusca, publishing a dictionary of 'pure' Tuscan words.[36] There were institutional investments taking place as well. By the mid-sixteenth century, many Italian cities had appointed university chairs in botany with the intention of reforming medical practice along Galenic lines. In Florence, Cosimo I de' Medici founded the 'Giardino dei Semplici' in 1556 which, along with the university of Pisa's botanical garden, was designed to support investigations into new discoveries and identifications of plants with medicinal and scientific properties. Initially, these posts were held by doctors but increasingly the city's apothecaries became involved. The final element of this epilogue focuses, therefore, on a figure who was responsible for evaluating the value of the Speziale al Giglio's stock in 1568, the neighbouring apothecary, Stefano di Romolo Rosselli.

Stefano Rosselli: selling secrets

The apothecary's shop which Rosselli managed, the Speziale al San Francesco, has left behind little in terms of financial records or accounts, in contrast to the Giglio. But in compensation, we have an inventory taken in 1570, along with three manuscripts which recorded the apothecary's collection of recipes and 'secrets'. Born in 1522, Stefano was a descendant of the painter Bernardo Rosselli. These connections may be important, for Stefano's grandfather Bernardo was a long-standing Giglio client during the period that Tommaso di Giovanni Guidi ran the shop; as we have seen, Bernardo's cousin, the artist Cosimo Rosselli, also had close connections with the Giglio. Whether or not these connections led to the Rosselli moving into the apothecary business is a matter for speculation; what is not is the fact that these were not simply neighbours – the two apothecaries could look back to several generations of interaction and contact between their families.

Interestingly, Stefano's father was neither a painter nor an apothecary. Stefano was the son of Romolo Rosselli, who had studied and then taught medicine at the university in Pisa, obtaining his medical degree in 1530.[37] Ten years earlier, he had matriculated as an apothecary and had already written a treatise in Latin on simples. While it isn't clear how many children he had, he was not determined that his sons should follow him into medicine. Most took Holy Orders, while Stefano trained as an apothecary and eventually rented a shop on the Via degli Speziali Grossi from 1554. His pharmaceutical connections may have given him access to the Medici court and he quickly became closely associated with the ducal family, collecting botanical specimens which he planted in Ferdinando de' Medici's villa of Quarata nell'Antella. Eventually, his involvement was formalised and between 1588 and 1595 Rosselli was on Ferdinando's official salary roll. He was paid three scudi a month and given a horse for the work that he did in developing the Giardino dei Semplici in Pisa.

But this court role did not prevent him from continuing with his own business. When he took over the shop on the Canto del Giglio opposite that of the Lapini on 5 April 1569, he did so in partnership with Jacopo di

Andrea Dori, whose son worked in Ferdinando de' Medici's alchemical laboratory in the Palazzo Pitti, while another member of the Dori family illustrated medicinal plants for Rosselli. It was Jacopo di Andrea Dori's death that prompted the creation of a lengthy inventory of the shops and their contents. The document demonstrates that, like the Giglio, the Speziale al San Francesco was also a 'double shop' with two adjacent *botteghe*. The product range was also remarkably similar – the main items were wax of all types, sugar and confectionery and spices, simples and metals that could be used in medicines, perfumes and cosmetics. As with the Giglio, the major new medical product was guaiac but San Francesco also held sarsaparilla, another New World root that was also recommended for the treatment of syphilis.

While today it might seem surprising to have two large shops carrying almost the same range of products and serving the same clientele standing opposite each other, this made sense in the sixteenth century. The proximity meant that customers knew exactly where to go when they wanted something. They would have found it easy to compare goods and credit arrangements. More importantly perhaps, it also allowed the apothecaries to share supplies and to work collaboratively to ensure their mutual survival in difficult economic periods. It is not surprising that the notary who took down the Giglio's contents turned to Rosselli for advice on the value of each product. The two men would have known each other well and would certainly have shared an understanding of their stock. As we have seen throughout this study of the Giglio, individuals benefitted from being embedded in a dense network of other operators.

Although the links between the Lapini and the Rosselli can only be surmised, the interconnections between commercial, court and university worlds can be seen clearly in the three manuscripts that Stefano Rosselli compiled towards the end of his life. One, begun in 1593, was described as:

> [A] purple book with metal bindings, in which shall be described various non-medicinal secrets, such as confections, azures, laquers, perfumery, cosmetics and other such, and a purple book for all the medicinal things and everything written will have been tested repeatedly.[38]

It contains a series of recipes for sweets, cakes and candies followed by perfumes and finally medical products. While the recipes themselves, if elaborate, are quite traditional, the care with which the manuscript was put together is unusual, particularly as it does not appear to have been designed for publication. Although this was a period in which 'books of secrets' were printed on a large scale in Florence, Venice and Rome for an avid audience of readers, Rosselli's three manuscripts seem to have been designed primarily for his sons. Carefully illustrated, they reveal a network of contacts and connections as well as mechanisms for advertising special products.

A substantial percentage of the recipes in all the manuscripts were for sugar and confectionery products, including instructions for how to make sugar shoes, sugar fans, sugar boxes and other novelties. There was also a selection of perfume and soap recipes. In one case, Rosselli noted that he had paid twenty scudi to Fabrizio Vismara Milanese for a perfumed water used by the Queen of Spain; in another case, he obtained the recipe for melon-scented soap that was the signature product of the Speziale del Melone from their mutual suppliers, the friars of San Michele in Boscho.

Along with these products, Rosselli noted a lengthy list of medicines or *medicinali*. These included an unguent for the French pox which was used by Paolo Banchelli in Rome. Rosselli carefully noted that the Roman had started his treatment on 9 November 1572 and seemed cured twenty-five days later. He also took down a 'pill of Maestro Meichel Fiamingo paracelsista' which he received from Ferdinando de' Medici and copied recipes for theriac and mithridate. Here, Rosselli noted that although Galen's theriac was well known through printed texts, he had received his from a noted scholar:

> A method of composing theriac, found in an ancient Greek text, written by hand and translated by the most excellent doctor messer Francesco del Gardo who made it for me in 1560. It is true that the texts of Galen have been printed but as this concerns a text translated by Garbo who had, in his time, no equal in letters and as I know it is good, I will write it down.[39]

He obtained information on distillation from the monastery where his brother served, numerous recipes from other pharmacists both in Florence and in Ferrara, while one, a tooth powder was inherited from his father. But the bulk of the 'secrets', both medical and non-medical, that he recorded came from members of the Medici court, with a substantial number given to him directly by the Grand Dukes Cosimo and Francesco themselves. Rosselli's pride at these connections meant that he not only noted connections in terms of the provenance of recipes – such as the hair dye recipe given to him by messer Carlo, the ducal barber – but also when other recipes, such as that for lemon confit – which he received from Coriolano Osio of Verona – had been used at court festivities including Ferdinando de' Medici's wedding in 1589. In a number of cases, Cosimo's daughter, Isabella de' Medici and her supposed lover, Troilo Orsini were credited with providing recipes. Isabella's name was attached to a face wash and to a wine infusion that she supposedly made for her father, providing the pharmacy with the instructions which Rosselli recorded.

In his *Treatise on Agriculture*, Agostino del Riccio wrote about Stefano Rosselli, 'The city of Florence owes a debt of gratitude to this noble man, because he has cured many citizens by the secret remedies which he compounded in his shop.'[40] While no such gratitude was recorded for Rosselli and Lapini's predecessors from the late fifteenth century, this is not because they were less important in the preparation and marketing of medicines; but with printing, came the potential both to promote generic products and to suggest secrets. But this change should not disguise the important continuities of practice that offered reassurance to Florentine citizens who sought out the apothecary at the Sign of the Lily in the sixteenth century. With its expensive fittings, ceramic and glass containers, bronze mortars, weights and scales, the reliability of a traditional setting may have been key in ensuring the apothecary's continued success.

Conclusion

Whether men and women became ill in either the fifteenth or sixteenth centuries, their responses were remarkably similar. They turned to as many potential solutions and sources of help as possible. Facing new diseases, such as syphilis, and long-standing epidemics such as the plague or common illnesses including fevers, stomach pains and ulcers, Florentine apothecaries were quick to respond to these new challenges. A comparison of the inventories taken of the Speziale al Giglio between 1504 and 1568 show very clearly that the discoveries of the New World were incorporated in a highly instrumental fashion. Unlike the better-known shop of Francesco Calzolari in Verona – who had a small museum of theriac ingredients on show – the Giglio and its neighbour only stocked ingredients from the Americas that they knew they could sell to a substantial number of customers.[41] Rosselli's manuscripts clearly demonstrate that this was not from a lack of curiosity, but from a clear sense of commercial imperative.

As importantly, while more work remains to be done, the Giglio's trajectory suggests considerable continuity across a sharp political divide. Far from being a dramatic break between one form of marketing within a communal republican environment, to another more élite form of court supply, the mechanisms were very similar. Indeed, from what the records suggest, the Medici were even reasonably efficient in paying their suppliers rather than using their power to create long-term credit arrangements.

Thus, while it is tempting to see the Medici as having introduced new networks of élite sociability, shops such as the Giglio acted as important intermediaries between the world of the court and its alchemical *fondaco* and the wider community. Rosselli's recipes – which were copied extensively by other contemporary apothecaries in Florence – indicate the strong links shared by the city's speziali and with their brethren in local monasteries and hospitals. The story of the Speziale al Giglio, therefore, is both a tale of a single shop, but at the same time it is a glimpse into a world of commerce, the Renaissance understanding of the body and of a social and political community that was flexible enough to withstand dramatic change.

Notes

1. P. Wallis, 'Apothecaries and the Consumption and Retailing of Medicines in Early Modern England', in L.H. Curth (ed.), *From Physick to Pharmacology: Five Hundred Years of British Drug Retailing* (Aldershot: Ashgate, 2006), 13–28; M. Fernandez-Carrion and J.L. Valverde, *Farmacia y sociedad en Sevilla en el siglo XVI* (Seville: Servicio de Publicaciones de Ayuntamiento de Sevilla, 1985).

2. J. Musacchio, 'The Medici Sale of 1495 and the Second-Hand Market for Domestic Goods in Late Fifteenth-Century Florence', in M. Fantoni, L.C. Matthew and S.F. Matthews-Grieco (eds), *The Art Market in Italy: 15th–17th Centuries. Il mercato dell'arte in Italia (secc. XV–XVII)* (Modena: Franco Cosimo Panini, 2003), 313–24.

3. G. Lazzi and M. Gabriele (eds), *Alambicchi di parole: il ricettario fiorentino e dintorni* (Florence: Polistampa, 1999).

4. R.B. Litchfield, *Florence Ducal Capital, 1530–1630* (New York: ACLS Humanities E-Book, 2008), para. 74–81.

5. J.E. Staley, *The Guilds of Florence*, (London: Methuen, 1906), 257.

6. ASF, MdP 1171, fo. 54, 2 June 1544, Agnolo Dovizi da Bibbiena to Pier Francesco Riccio: 'Me ne son venuto a stare qui in casa di ser Thomaso Bernj sin ch'io guarisca [...] È impossibile che io possa farmi le spese da me senza fare più debito, oltre a quello che io ho fatto per pagare il medico della malattia passata, et oltre a quello che mi converrà fare per pagare il medivo di nuovo, et le medicine che di due purgationi io devo a Viviano speciale.'

7. ASF, MdP 1170a, fo. 187, 28 October 1545, Lorenzo di Andrea Pagni to Pier Francesco Riccio: 'Io invio alla S. V. un pignattino di terra quale mi ha consegnato la Duchessa mia S.ra [Eleonora di Toledo] et secondo mi ha detto vi sono dentro certe lattuche [lattughe] in composta che hanno a serivre per la S.ra Donna Ysabella Figueroa. Et perchè lei, oltre alle lattuche ricercava ancora della zucca in composta dice S. Ex.a che la S. V. se ne facci dare da non so che monasterio, et gliela dia insieme con questo pignattino di lattuche. Inoltre dice S. Ex.a che la S. V. facci dare dalla p.ta s.ra Donna Ysabella tutto quello che ha bisogno dallo spetiale per questa sua malatia, a conto di S. E.x et che non se li manchi in cosa alcuna di quello che haverà di bisogno.'

8. A. Perifano, *L'alchimie à la cour de Come Ier de Medicis: savoirs, culture et politique* (Paris: Honore Champion, 1997), 75, 'Ma per camminare alla conclusione, voglio pur dire una cosa rara di questo príncipe, che di tutto

s'intende e ne fa professione, e ciascheduna cosa pare che sia sua propia. E specialmente delle erbe e dei semplici n'ha egli una grandissima cognitione, e n'ha i giardini ripieni, e ne fa tenere una particolare cura, con gradissima sua dilettatione in farli piantare, governare e sperimentare... e di continuo sopra questi fa lavorare d'acque e d'olii lambicati per esperimentarli in diverses infermita e ferite, ed ha ritrovato rimedii alla punta del fianco, alle strette di urina, et alle ferite della testa, che in Toscana per la sottilita dell'aria erano tutte mortali, ed ora sono fatte sanabili. Fa fare con diligenza il sopravvivo ed il mitridate, e con tanta perfezione, che se ne vede evidencte prova e salutífera alle acutezze dei veleni... e dove si fanno tante mirabili cose e un luogo grande, che si chiama la Fonderia del duca di Firenze, nella quale si lavora di continuo con infinite varieta di fuochi, di fucine, di fornelli e lambicchi, e il duca vi va spesso, e vi sta, e vi lavora di sua mano con grandissima sua dilettatione....'

9. A.M. Giusti, 'The Grand Ducal Workshops at the time of Ferdinando I and Cosimo II', in C. Acidini Luchinat (ed.), *Treasures of Florence: The Medici Collection 1400–1700* (Munich: Prestel, 1997), 115–41.

10. ASF, MdP 5119, fo. 79, 19 June 1570.

11. Litchfield, *op. cit.* (note 4). The profession represented just 2% of urban occupations in comparison with, for example, wool-workers (7%), shoemakers (8%) or goldsmiths (3%) but was on a par with barbers and stationers.

12. J. DeLancey, 'Dragonsblood and Ultramarine: The Apothecary and Artists' Pigments in Renaissance Florence', in Fantoni, Matthew and Matthews-Grieco (eds), *op. cit.* (note 2), 150, n.28.

13. Litchfield, *op. cit.* (note 4), para. 236–43.

14. Estranei 586, 'Questo libro sie di Lapino d'Agnolo d'Antonio Lapini proprio et chiamasi Debitori e creditori e ricordanze segnato A incominciato oggi questo dì di dicembre 1479 in nome di Dio e di buona ventura, tenuto per me Lapino sopraddetto.'

15. Estranei 904–6 covers the period supplying the Medici court from 1537–45.

16. Estranei 592–4, Libro Verde.

17. ASF, MdP 1175, Maestro Andrea Pasquale to Pier Francesco Ricci, 18 December 1549: 'Mia S.ra vuol' che Vostra Signoria le mandj oncie 4 . 5 di quella manna vecchia qual tiene Ang.lo Lapinj per darla al Cap.no Muchio de' Med' [Bartolomeo de' Medici] qual si amalò a Livorno a quelli freddi mortali. [...] E così manderete certa pasta di pillole vi darà Ang.lo Lapinj. Mandatele per persona fidata e ben sigillata.'

18. Perifano, *op. cit.* (note 8), 71; A. Corradi, *Le prime farmacopee italiane ed in particolare dei ricettari fiorentini* (Milan: Rechiedei, 1887).

19. Estranei, Processo 20, fo. 61v, 'A di ix di Giugno 1568: Questo è l'Inventario delle robbe della bottega detta Spetieria di detto Lorenzo Spetiale'. Our

thanks to Julia DeLancey who made her transcription of the inventory available to us.

20. Estranei, Processo 20, fo. 56v, lists 'dua putti di terra, un davitte, un' san girolamo di terra, un testa di x'po, un' crocifisso, una gocciola suvi un' san fran.o et un'altro santo di terra, una n'ra donna con fornimento dorato, un quadruccio d'una testa di x'po piccolo.'

21. Estranei, Processo 20, fo. 58v, 'tre pezzi di libri da leggere'.

22. Estranei, Processo 20, fo. 71r, 2 oz of 'p[illole] di M[aestr]o Franco Ruggieri'.

23. Estranei, Processo 20, fo. 75r, 100 lbs of 'Arsenico'.

24. T. Huguet Termes, 'New World Materia Medica in Spanish Renaissance Medicine: From Scholarly Reception to Practical Impact', *Medical History*, 45 (2001), 359–76; J. Henderson, 'Fracastoro, mal francese e la cura con il legno santo', in A. Pastore and E. Peruzzi (eds), *Girolamo Fracastoro: Fra medicina, filosofia e scienze della natura* (Florence: L.S. Olschki, 2006), 73–89.

25. D. Gentilcore, 'Charlatans, the Regulated Marketplace and the Treatment of Venereal Disease in Italy', in K. Siena (ed.), *Sins of the Flesh: Responding to Sexual Disease in Early Modern Europe* (Toronto: Centre for Reformation and Renaissance Studies, 2005), 57–80: 57. J. Flood and D. Shaw, 'The Price of the Pox in 1527: Johannes Sinapius and the Guaiac Cure', *Bibliothèque d'Humanisme et Renaissance*, LIV, 3 (1992), 691–707; R.S. Munger, 'Guaiacum, the Holy Wood from the New World', *Journal of the History of Medicine and Allied Sciences*, 4, 2 (1949), 196–229.

26. G. Fracastoro, *Il contagio, le malattie contagiose e la loro cura*, V. Busacchi (ed.), (Florence: L.S. Olschki, 1950).

27. ASF, MdP 7, fo. 128, 27 May 1546, Cosimo I to Pietro Camaiani: 'Habbiamo ricevuto il libretto che ci havete mandato del medico [Girolamo] Fracastoro, il quale vedremo et leggeremo volentieri sapendo che [cancelled: le] non posson essere l'opere sua se non buone, per la fama che tiene d'essere nella professione sua singulare. Ringratiatelo della parte che cen'ha fatto, co'l farli quelle offerte per nostra parte che convengono alla amorevolezza che ci ha [cancelled: demostro] ^usata^ et alle buone qualità et virtù sua....'

28. ASF MdP582, 20 December 1572, fo. 97, Antonio Serguidi to Francesco de' Medici: 'Doppo la partita di Vostra Altezza [Francesco de' Medici], il Granduca [Cosimo I de' Medici] è andato continuando nel miglioramento di maniera che agita molto meglio le mani et le braccia, et questa mattina ha cominciato a pigliare il legno et di già ha in corpo duoi sciloppi et ci si è accomodato assai bene [...] Dissi al Signor di Piombino [Iacopo VI Appiani d'Aragona] che tirasse avanti la pratica di quel pane incorruttibile che la vedde qua, et mi dice che non occorre farci altro havendomi dato la ricetta stessa [...]'

29. Gentilcore, *op. cit.* (note 25); D. Zanrè, 'French Diseases and Italian Responses: Representations of the *mal francese* in the Literature of Cinquecento Tuscany', in Siena (ed.), *op. cit.* (note 25), 187–208.

30. Estranei, Processo 20, fo. 93v, 'ordinati per la teriaca'.

31. E. Welch, 'Space and Spectacle in the Renaissance Pharmacy', *Medicina e Storia*, 15 (2008), 127–58.

32. Estranei, Processo 20, fo. 93v, 2 lbs 6 oz of 'Trocischi di vipera'.

33. Estranei, Processo 20, fo. 58v, 'camera d'agnolo' lists 'dua vasi da triaca'.

34. ASF, MdP 241, fo. 84, 7 January 1573, Cosimo to Francesco de' Medici: Maestro Baccio Baldini, 'sendo proposto del Collegio e veditore del'Arte delli Spetiali, dette licentia allo speciale del Moro che in certa triaca mettessi il balsamo del'Indie nuovamente ritrovato in cambio del'opobalsamo. Però sarei di parere, quando così anco paia a voi, che la querela stata posta al detto speciale non si termini insino a tanto che il detto maestro Baccio Baldini non venga in Fiorenza et vene ragguagli. Et in tanto sia loro renduto la triaca. Et sarei anco di parere che si determinassi che per l'advenire chi fa la triaca col'initridato o altro lattovaro dove vadia l'opobalsamo, si possa in tutti mettere il balsamo del'Indie, perchè pare che da questi medici sia approvato.'

35. G. Olmi, 'Farmacopea antica e medicina moderna: La disputa sulla teriaca nel cinquecento bolognese', *Physis. Rivista internazionale di storia della scienza*, 19 (1977), 197–246, 218: 'La magior parte de speciali che dovria haver cognitione in questa materia nondimeno si ritrovano tutti ignoranti che apena sanno legere e il più. Delle volte pongono un simplice per un altro di opposite e venenose qualità come mi potrei dir di molti; si trovano molto più essercitati li speciali in Fiandra, Bohemia e Germania che non son in Italia, intendendo almeno la lingua latina e facendo profession di cognoscer li semplici non vendendo cose vive cioè cere, olii, saponi e mille altre cose impertinenti come fanno li nostri, ma seperatamente facendo il medicinale distinto da l'altre droghe.' For a more extended discussion, see Welch, *op. cit.* (note 31).

36. J.S. Amelang, *The Flight of Icarus: Artisan Autobiography in Early Modern Europe* (Stanford: Stanford University Press, 1998), 68.

37. The only extensive investigation into Stefano Rosselli has been undertaken by S.B. Butters, *The Triumph of Vulcan: Sculptors' Tools, Porphyry, and the Prince in Ducal Florence*, 2 vols (Florence: L.S. Olschki, 1996), Vol. I, 219–23 and Vol. II, 454–5. She draws on A. Gotti, *Ricordanze della nobile famiglia Rosselli del Turco, tratte dai suoi archivi* (Florence: Tip. Calasanziana, 1890).

38. S. Rosselli, *Mes secrets: A Florence au temps des Medicis, 1593: patisserie,. parfumerie, medecine*, Rodrigo de Zayas (ed.), (Paris: J.-M. Place, 1996), 'libro pagonazo ferrato, insul quale scriverrà su diversi secreti non medicinali, come confetture azurrii, lache, cose di profumeria, lisci et simili et sul

pagonazo tucte cose medicinal et quello che sarà scripto sarà tucto provato
piú volte.'

39. *Ibid.*
40. Butters, *op. cit.* (note 37).
41. Welch, *op. cit.* (note 31).

Bibliography

Primary Sources

The Canons and Decrees of the Sacred and Oecumenical Council of Trent (London: Dolman, 1848), Hanover Historical Texts Project, 1995: http://history.hanover.edu/early/trent.htm

Liber Pandectarum (Vicenza, 1480).

Ricettario fiorentino (Florence: Compagnia del Drago, 1499).

Ricettario fiorentino (Florence, 1567).

G. Aiazzi (ed.), *Ricordi storici di Filippo di Cino Rinuccini dal 1282 al 1460 colla continuazione di Alamanno e Neri suoi figli fino al 1506 seguiti da altri documenti inediti di storia patria* (Florence: Stamperia Piatti, 1840).

S. Antoniano, *Educatione Christiana dei figliuoli* [1583], Biblioteca Italiana, Università degli Studi di Roma 'La Sapienza', 2005: http://www.bibliotecaitaliana.it/xtf/view?docId=bibit001008/bibit001008.xml

Antonius Guarnerinus de Padua, *Herbe pincte*, G. Silini (ed.), (Gorle: Iniziative Culturali, 2000).

P. Aretino, *Ragionamenti: Sei giornate* [1534], R. Marrone (ed.), (Rome: Newton Compton editori, 1993).

Q. Augusti, *Lumen apothecariorum* (Venice, 1498).

———, *Lumen apothecariorum cum certis expositionibus* (Venice, 1495).

D. Balestracci, *The Renaissance in the Fields: Family Memoirs of a Fifteenth-century Tuscan Peasant*, P. Squatriti and B. Merideth (trans.), (Pennsylvania: Pennsylvania State University Press, 1999).

F. Castellani, *Quaternuccio e giornale B (1459–1485)* (Florence: L.S. Olschki, 1995), Biblioteca Italiana, Università degli Studi di Roma 'La Sapienza', 2005: http://www.bibliotecaitaliana.it/xtf/view?docId=bibit000575/bibit000575.xml

313

G. Chellini, *Le ricordanze di Giovanni Chellini da San Miniato, medico, mercante e umanista (1425–1457)*, M.T. Sillano (ed.), (Milan: F. Angeli, 1984).

E. Conti (ed.), *Matteo Palmieri: Ricordi fiscali, 1427–1474* (Rome: Istituto storico italiano per il medio evo, 1983).

G. da Orta, 'Colloquies on the Simples and Drugs of India: Cinnamon, Cloves, Mace and Nutmeg, Pepper', in M.N. Pearson (ed.), *Spices in the Indian Ocean World* (Aldershot: Variorum, 1996).

L. Dolce, *Dialogo della istitutione delle donne* [1545], Biblioteca Italiana, Università degli Studi di Roma 'La Sapienza', 2006: http://www.bibliotecaitaliana.it/xtf/view?docId=bibit000361/bibit000361.xml

D. Erasmus, *Praise of Folly*, B. Radice (trans.), (Harmondsworth: Penguin, 1971).

E. Faccioli (ed.), *L'arte della cucina in Italia* (Turin: Einaudi, 1992).

M. Ficino, *Three Books on Life*, C.V. Kaske and J.R. Clark (trans.), (Binghampton: Medieval & Renaissance Texts & Studies, 1989).

L. Fioravanti, *Del compendio dei secreti rationali* (Venice: Vincenzo Valgrisi, 1564).

A. Firenzuola, *Ragionamenti* (Rome: Salerno editrice, 1971), Biblioteca Italiana, Università degli Studi di Roma 'La Sapienza', 2003: http://www.bibliotecaitaliana.it/xtf/view?docId=bibit000183/bibit000183.xml

G. Fracastoro, *Il contagio, le malattie contagiose e la loro cura*, V. Busacchi (ed.) (Florence: L.S. Olschki, 1950).

L. Frescobaldi, *Viaggio in Terrasanta* (Florence: Ponte alle Grazie, 1990), Biblioteca Italiana, Università degli Studi di Roma 'La Sapienza', 2004: http://www.bibliotecaitaliana.it/xtf/view?docId=bibit000795/bibit000795.xml

S. Gaddoni and B. Bughetti, *Giornale di una spezieria in Imola nel sec. XIV* (Imola: University Press Bologna, 1995).

T. Garzoni, *La piazza universale di tutte le professioni del Mondo*, P. Cherchi and B. Collina (eds), 2 vols (Turin: Einaudi, 1996).

A. Gotti, *Ricordanze della nobile famiglia Rosselli del Turco, tratte dai suoi archivi* (Florence: Tip. Calasanziana, 1890).

F. Guicciardini, 'Ricordanze', in C. Grayson (ed.), *Selected Writings* (New York: Harper & Row, 1965), 125–70.

T. Hobbes, *Leviathan* [1651] (London: J.M. Dent & Sons, 1914).

Bibliography

L. Landucci, *Diario fiorentino* (Florence: Sansoni, 1985), Biblioteca Italiana,
Università degli Studi di Roma 'La Sapienza', 2004:
http://www.bibliotecaitaliana.it/xtf/view?docId=bibit000998/bibit000998.xml

———, *A Florentine Diary from 1450 to 1516*, A. De Rosen Jervis (trans.),
(London: J.M. Dent & Sons, 1927).

B. Machiavelli, *Libro di ricordi* (Florence: Le Monnier, 1954), Biblioteca Italiana,
Università degli Studi di Roma 'La Sapienza', 2004:
http://www.bibliotecaitaliana.it/xtf/view?docId=bibit000830/bibit000830.xml

J. Mandeville, *The Foreign Travels of Sir John Mandeville* (London: Macmillan,
1900), Project Gutenberg, 1997: http://www.gutenberg.org/ebooks/782

P.A. Mattioli, *I discorsi di M. Pietro Andrea Matthioli Medico Sanese, ne i sei libri
della materia medicinale di Pedacio Dioscoride Anazarbeo* (Venice, 1557).

———, *I discorsi di M. Pietro Andrea Matthioli Sanese, Medico Cesareo, nei sei libri
di Pedacio Dioscoride Anazarbeo della materia medicinale* (Venice, 1585).

L. de' Medici, 'A Memoir and a Letter', in R.N. Watkins (ed.), *Humanism and
Liberty: Writings on Freedom from Fifteenth-Century Florence* (Columbia:
University of South Carolina Press, 1978).

C. Messisbugo, *Libro Nouo nel quale s'insegna a'far d'ogni sorte di viuanda secondo la
diuersità de i tempi, cosi di carne come di pesce* (Venice, 1564).

J. Mesue, *Opera* (Venice, 1497).

Molière, *The Imaginary Invalid* [1673], Project Gutenberg, 2005.
http://www.gutenberg.org/dirs/etext05/8mald10.txt

G. Morelli, *Ricordi* (Florence: Le Monnier, 1986), Biblioteca Italiana, Università
degli Studi di Roma 'La Sapienza', 2004: http://www.bibliotecaitaliana.it/
xtf/view?docId=bibit000286/bibit000286.xml

F.B. Pegolotti, *La pratica della mercatura*, A. Evans (ed.), (Cambridge: The
Medieval Academy of America, 1936).

G.G. Pontano, *Meteororum Liber* (Vienna, 1517), Bayerische Staatsbibliothek:
http://mdz10.bib-bvb.de/~db/bsb00005239/images/

S. Rosselli, *Mes secrets: A Florence au temps des Medicis, 1593: patisserie, parfumerie,
medecine*, Rodrigo de Zayas (ed.), (Paris: J.-M. Place, 1996).

G. Rucellai, *Giovanni Rucellai ed il suo zibaldone*, A. Perosa (ed.), (London:
Warburg Institute, 1960).

Bibliography

B. Sacchi, *Platina, On Right Pleasure and Good Health: A Critical Edition and Translation of De honesta voluptate et valetudine*, M.E. Milham (ed.), (Tempe: Medieval & Renaissance Texts & Studies, 1998).

G. Savonarola, 'The Ascension of Christ', in G. Kleiser (ed.), *The World's Great Sermons*, Project Gutenberg, 2004. http://www.gutenberg.org/etext/11981

M. Savonarola, *Libreto de tute le cosse che se manzano: un libro di dietetica di Michele Savonarola, medico padovano del secolo XV edizione critica basata sul Codice Casanatense 406*, J. Nystedt (ed.), (Stockholm: Almqvist & Wiksell International, 1988).

———, *Libreto de tutte le cosse che se magnano* (Stockholm: Almqvist & Wiksell international, 1988), Biblioteca Italiana, Università degli Studi di Roma 'La Sapienza', 2004: http://www.bibliotecaitaliana.it/xtf/ view?docId=bibit000989/bibit000989.xml

P. Suardo, *Thesaurus aromatariorum* [1536] (Milan, 1496).

G.B. Zapata, *Li maravigliosi secreti di medicina e chirurgia: nuovamente ritrovati, per guarire ogni sorte d'infirmita* [1577] (Turin, 1580).

Secondary Sources

Itinerario farmaceutico di Firenze (Milan: I.E.I., 1969).

Speziali aromatari e farmacisti in Sicilia: Convegno e mostra sulla storia della farmacia e del farmacista in Sicilia dal secolo XIII al secolo XIX, (Palermo: Associazione Culturale Apotheke, 1990).

D. Abulafia (ed.), *The French Descent into Renaissance Italy, 1494–5: Antecedents and Effects* (Aldershot: Variorum, 1995).

M.W. Adamson, *Medieval Dietetics: Food and Drink in 'Regimen Sanitatis' Literature from 800 to 1400* (Frankfurt-am-Main: P. Lang, 1995).

J. Agrimi and C. Crisciani, *Malato, medico e medicina nel medioevo* (Turin: Loescher, 1980).

I. Ait, *Tra scienza e mercato: gli speziali a Roma nel tardo medioevo* (Rome: Istituto Nazionale di Studi Romani, 1996).

K. Albala, *Eating Right in the Renaissance* (Berkeley: University of California Press, 2002).

Bibliography

G. Aleati and V. Bianchi, 'Farmacie pavesi nella prima metà del Quattrocento', in A.E. Vitolo (ed.), *Raccolta di scritti in onore di Giulio Conci* (Pisa: Arti Grafiche Pacini Mariotti, 1953), 7–50.

J.S. Amelang, *The Flight of Icarus: Artisan Autobiography in Early Modern Europe* (Stanford: Stanford University Press, 1998).

F. Ambrosini, 'Ceremonie, feste, lusso', in A. Tenenti and U. Tucci (eds), *Storia di Venezia, Vol. V, Il rinascimento. Società ed economia* (Rome: Istituto della Enciclopedia Italiana, 1996).

J. Arrizabalaga, 'Facing the Black Death: Perceptions and Reactions of University Medical Practitioners', in L. Garcìa Ballester (ed.), *Practical Medicine from Salerno to the Black Death* (Cambridge: Cambridge University Press, 1994).

J. Arrizabalaga, J. Henderson, and R.K. French, *The Great Pox: The French Disease in Renaissance Europe* (New Haven & London: Yale University Press, 1997).

L. Artusi and S. Gabbrielli, *Le feste di Firenze* (Rome: Newton Compton editori, 1991).

E. Ashtor, 'Spice Prices in the Near East in the 15th Century', in M.N. Pearson (ed.), *Spices in the Indian Ocean World* (Aldershot: Variorum, 1996).

———, 'The Volume of Mediaeval Spice Trade', *Journal of European Economic History*, 9, 3 (1980), 753–63.

A. Astorri, 'Appunti sull'esercizio dello speziale a Firenze nel quattrocento', *Archivio storico italiano*, 147 (1989), 31–62.

———, 'Il "Libro delle Senserie" di Girolamo di Agostino Maringhi (1483–1485)', *Archivio storico italiano*, 146, 3 (1988), 389–408.

M. Balard, 'Épices et condiments dans quelques livres de cuisine allemands (XIVe–XVIe siècles)', in C. Lambert (ed.), *Du manuscrit à la table: essais sur la cuisine au Moyen Age et repertoire des manuscrits medievaux contenant des recettes culinaires* (Montreal & Paris: Les presses de l'Université de Montreal, 1992).

J. Barbaud, 'Les formulaires médicaux du Moyen-âge: médicines savants et médicines populaires', *Revue d'histoire de la pharmacie*, 35, 277 (1988), 138–53.

L. Barton, 'The drugs didn't work' *The Guardian*, 24 September 2003. http://www.guardian.co.uk/news/2003/sep/24/food.foodanddrink

P. Battara, 'Botteghe e pigioni nella Firenze del '500: Un censimento industriale e commerciale all'epoca del granducato mediceo', *Archivio storico italiano*, 95, 2 (1937), 3–28.

Bibliography

R.M. Bell, *How to Do It: Guides to Good Living for Renaissance Italians* (Chicago: University of Chicago Press, 1999).

A. Benedicenti, *Malati, medici e farmacisti: Storia dei rimedi traverso i secoli e delle teorie che ne spiegano l'azione sull'organismo*, 2nd edn (Milan: Hoepli, 1947) [Milan, Hoepli, 1924–5].

J.-P. Bénézet, *Pharmacie et médicament en Méditerranée occidentale: (XIIIe–XVIe siècles)* (Paris: H. Champion, 1999).

C. Benporat, *Cucina italiano del quattrocento* (Florence: L.S. Olschki, 1996).

M. Beretta, *Il tesoro della salute: Dall'onnipotenza dei semplici all'atomizzazione del farmaco* (Florence: Giunti, 1997).

———, *The Treasure of Health: From the Omnipotence of Medicinal Herbs to the Atomization of Drugs*, A. Brierley (trans.), (Florence: Giunti, 1997).

G.C. Bergaglio, 'Gli speziali di due antichi ospedali di Genova', *Atti e memorie della accademia italiana di storia della farmacia*, 12, 3 (1995).

———, 'Inventario di una spezieria di Genova nel 1312', *Atti e memorie della accademia italiana di storia della farmacia*, 13, 3 (1996), 227–8.

———, 'A proposito di tre inventari di spezierie in Genova nel medio evo', *Atti e memorie della accademia italiana di storia della farmacia*, 15, 3 (1998), 220–2.

G. Bertoli, 'Librai, cartolai e ambulanti immatricolati nell'arte dei medici e speziali di Firenze dal 1490–1600. Parte 1', *Bibliofilia*, 94, 2 (1992), 125–64.

———, 'Librai, cartolai e ambulanti immatricolati nell'arte dei medici e speziali di Firenze dal 1490–1600. Parte 2', *Bibliofilia*, 94, 3 (1992), 227–62.

M.L. Bianchi and M.L. Grossi, 'Botteghe, economia e spazio urbano', in F. Franceschi and G. Fossi (eds), *La grande storia dell'artigianato* (Florence: Giunti, 1999), 27–64.

F. Binetti and C. Masino, 'La farmacia in Parma nei secoli XV–XVIII', *Atti e memorie della Accademia italiana di storia della farmacia*, 3, 1 (1986), 25–37.

A.R. Blumenthal, *et al.*, *Cosimo Rosselli Painter of the Sistine Chapel* (Winter Park, Florida: Cornell Fine Arts Museum, 2001).

G. Borghini, *et al.*, *Una farmacia preindustriale in Valdelsa : la spezieria e lo spedale di Santa Fina nella città di San Gimignano secc. XIV–XVIII* (San Gimignano: Città di San Gimignano, 1981).

E. Borsook, 'Cult and Imagery at Sant'Ambrogio in Florence', *Mitteilungen des Kunsthistorischen Institutes in Florenz*, 25 (1981), 147–202.

Bibliography

J. Bossy, *Christianity in the West, 1400–1700* (Oxford: Oxford University Press, 1985).

M. Brogi Ciofi, 'Malattie, mortalità dei fanciulli nei primi anni di vita nella Firence del '400: cause principali dei decessi. La medicina infantile', *Rivista di storia della medicina*, 2, 1 (1992), 3–15.

S. Broomhall, *Women's Medical Work in Early Modern France* (Manchester: Manchester University Press, 2004).

A. Brown, *Bartolomeo Scala, 1430–1497, Chancellor of Florence: The Humanist as Bureaucrat* (Princeton: Princeton University Press, 1979).

———, 'Bartolomeo Scala's Dealings with Booksellers, Scribes and Illuminators, 1459–63', *Journal of the Warburg and Courtauld Institutes*, 39 (1976), 237–9.

———, 'Florence, Renaissance and Early Modern State: Reappraisals', in *The Medici in Florence: The Exercise and Language of Power* (Florence: L.S. Olschki, 1992), 307–26.

———, 'Lorenzo de' Medici's New Men and their Mores: The Changing Lifestyle of Quattrocento Florence', *Renaissance Studies*, 16, 2 (2002), 113–42.

J.C. Brown, 'Prosperity or Hard Times in Renaissance Italy?' *Renaissance Quarterly*, 42 (1989), 761–80.

G.A. Brucker, 'Florentine Voices from the Catasto, 1427–1480', *I Tatti Studies*, 5 (1993), 11–32.

———, *The Society of Renaissance Florence: A Documentary Study*, Reprint edn (New York: Harper & Row, 1998) [1971].

A. Burmester, V. Haller and C. Krekel, 'Pigmenta et Colores: The Artist's Palette in Pharmacy Price Lists from Liegnitz (Silesia)', in J. Kirby, S. Nash and J. Cannon, *Trade in Artisis' Materials: Markets and Commerce in Europe in 1700* (London: Archetype, 2010).

S.B. Butters, *The Triumph of Vulcan: Sculptors' Tools, Porphyry, and the Prince in Ducal Florence*, 2 vols (Florence: L.S. Olschki, 1996).

D. Caffaratto Bordiglia, 'Un inventario del Cinquecento della spezieria dell'Ospedale Maggiore di S. Giovanni Battista e della città di Torino', *Atti e memorie della accademia italiana di storia della farmacia*, 6, 1 (1989), 55–74.

T.M. Caffaratto, 'Alcuni antichi documenti della spezieria dell'Ospedale Maggiore di San Giovanni Battista e della Città di Torino', *Atti e memorie della accademia italiana di storia della farmacia*, 3, 1 (1986).

S. Calonacci, 'Luca Landucci', in *Dizionario biografico degli italiani* (Rome: Istituto della Enciclopedia Italiana, 2004), 543–6.

E. Cameron, *The European Reformation* (Oxford: Clarendon, 1991).

P. Camporesi, *Bread of Dreams: Food and Fantasy in Early Modern Europe* (Cambridge: Polity, 1989).

G. Carbonelli, 'I conti di Giacomo Carlo speziale in Biella (1494–1523)', *Bollettino Storico Subalpino*, 14 (1909).

A.G. Carmichael, 'The Health Status of Florentines in the Fifteenth Century', in M. Tetel, R.G. Witt and R. Goffen (eds), *Life and Death in Fifteenth-Century Florence* (Durham: Duke University Press, 1989), 28–45.

————, *Plague and the Poor in Early Renaissance Florence* (Cambridge & New York: Cambridge University Press, 1986).

A.M. Carmona-Cornet, A. Corvi, and T. Huguet Termes, 'La farmacologia pratica nell'opera di Saladino d'Ascoli e la sua ripercussione nella farmacopea europea', *Atti e memorie della accademia italiana di storia della farmacia*, 12, 2 (1995), 132–6.

A.M. Carmona-Cornet and T. Huguet Termes, 'Traditional Herbal Medicine through the First Edition of the Florentine Receptair, 1498', in A. Guerci (ed.), *La cura delle malattie: itinerari storici: 3. Colloquio europeo di etnofarmacologia, 1. Conferenza internazionale di antropologia e storia della salute e delle malattie* (Genoa: Erga, 1998).

G. Carra, 'Speziali e spezierie nella Mantova dei Gonzaga', *Civiltà mantovana*, 12 (1978), 245–75.

B. Cassidy, 'The Financing of the Tabernacle of Orsanmichele', *Source: Notes in the History of Art* 8 (1988), 1–6.

J. Castle, 'Treatments & Medicines between 1400 & 1600', Doctoral Thesis, Diploma in the History of Medicine of the Society of Apothecaries (1999).

S. Cavallo, *Artisans of the Body in Early Modern Italy. Identities, Families, Masculinities* (Manchester: Manchester University Press, 2007).

S. Cavallo and D. Biow, *The Culture of Cleanliness in Renaissance Italy* (Ithaca: Cornell University Press, 2006).

D. Chambers and B. Pullan, *Venice: A Documentary History, 1450–1630* (Oxford: Blackwell, 1992).

J. Cherry, 'Healing through Faith: The Continuation of Medieval Attitudes to Jewellery into the Renaissance', *Renaissance Studies*, 15, 2 (2001), 154–71.

L. Chiappelli and A. Corsini, 'Un antico inventario dello Spedale di S. Maria Nuova in Firenze (a. 1376)', *Rivista delle biblioteche e degli archivi*, 32 (1921).

E. Chiaramonte and S. Tozzi, 'Un medico umanista fra dottrina e pratica', in S. Ferri (ed.), *Pietro Andrea Mattioli: Siena, 1501–Trento, 1578: la vita, le opere: con l'identificazione delle piante* (Ponte San Giovanni, Perugia: Quattroemme, 1997).

R. Ciabani, *Le famiglie di Firenze*, 4 vols (Florence: Bonechi, 1992).

G. Ciappelli, *Carnevale e quaresima: Comportamenti sociali e cultura a Firenze nel rinascimento* (Rome: Edizioni di storia e letteratura, 1997).

M.A. Ciasca, *Speziali e farmacopee nell'Italia del secolo XV* (Amatrice, Rieti: Tip. Orfanotrofio Maschile, 1951).

R. Ciasca, 'La cultura di un farmacista del '400', in A.E. Vitolo (ed.), *Raccolta di scritti in onore di Giulio Conci* (Pisa: Arti Grafiche Pacini Mariotti, 1953).

———, *L'arte dei medici e speziali nella storia e nel commercio fiorentino dal secolo XII al XV* (Florence: L.S. Olschki, 1927).

——— (ed.), *Statuti dell'arte dei medici e speziali* (Florence: L.S. Olschki, 1922).

E. Cingolani, 'Il Ricettario fiorentino e le disposizioni relative alla professione farmaceutica', *Atti e memorie della accademia italiana di storia della farmacia*, 16, 3 (1999), 122–32.

E. Cingolani and L. Colapinto, *Dagli antidotari alle moderne farmacopee* (Rome: Di Renzo, 2000).

C.M. Cipolla, *Cristofano and the Plague: A Study in the History of Public Health in the Age of Galileo* (London: Collins, 1973).

———, *Miasmi ed umori: ecologia e condizioni sanitarie in Toscana nel seicento* (Bologna: Il Mulino, 1989).

D. Clark, 'The Shop Within? An Analysis of the Architectural Evidence for Medieval Shops', *Architectural History*, 43 (2000), 58–87.

P.C. Clarke, *The Soderini and the Medici: Power and Patronage in Fifteenth-Century Florence* (Oxford: Clarendon, 1991).

E.S. Cohen, 'Miscarriages of Apothecary Justice: Un-separate Spaces of Work and Family in Early Modern Rome', *Renaissance Studies*, 21, 4 (2007), 480–504.

S.K.J. Cohn, *The Laboring Classes in Renaissance Florence* (New York: Academic Press, 1980).

L. Colapinto, 'La spezieria dell'Ospedale di S. Spirito in Saxia a Roma', *Atti e memorie della accademia italiana di storia della farmacia*, 12, 3 (1995).

————, 'The "Nuovo Receptario" of Florence', *Medicina nei secoli*, n.s. 5 (1993), 39–50.

L. Colapinto and G. Leopardi, *L'arte degli speziali italiani* (Milan: L'Ariete Edizioni, 1991).

H.J. Cook, *Matters of Exchange: Commerce, Medicine, and Science in the Dutch Golden Age* (New Haven: Yale University Press, 2007).

B.P. Copenhaver, 'Scholastic Philosophy and Renaissance Magic in the De vita of Marsilio Ficino', *Renaissance Quarterly*, 37 (1984), 523–54.

A. Corradi, *Le prime farmacopee italiane ed in particolare dei ricettari fiorentini* (Milan: Rechiedei, 1887).

————, *Le prime farmacopee italiane ed in particolare dei ricettari fiorentini. Memoria* (1966) [Milan, Ferro Edizioni, 1887].

L. Cortese and D. Cortese, 'Alle origini della farmacopea popolare', *Atti e memorie della accademia italiana di storia della farmacia*, Anno 3, 3 (1986), 173–96.

A. Corvi, 'La farmacia della Ca' Granda di Milano, fondata nel 1470', *Atti e memorie della accademia italiana di storia della farmacia*, 12, 3 (1995).

————, 'Le pillole nel XVI secolo: la riforma proposta dal pilluarium di Pantaleone da Confienza', *Atti e memorie della accademia italiana di storia della farmacia*, 18, 1 (2001), 11–16.

E. Coturri, 'Spunti di medicina e di farmacia nelle novelle di uno speziale toscano del trecento, Giovanni Sercambi (1348–1424)', in *Atti del IV convegno di studi AISF, Varese, 3–4 Ottobre 1959* (Pisa: Arti grafiche Pacini Mariotti, 1959).

D. Covi, 'A Documented Altarpiece by Cosimo Rosselli', *Art Bulletin*, 53, 2 (1971), 236–8.

D.L. Cowen and W.H. Helfand, *Pharmacy: An Illustrated History* (New York: Harry N. Abrams, 1988).

A.W. Crosby, *Ecological Imperialism: The Biological Expansion of Europe, 900–1900* (Cambridge: Cambridge University Press, 1986).

R.J. Crum and J.T. Paoletti (eds), *Renaissance Florence: A Social History* (Cambridge: Cambridge University Press, 2006).

E. Curi, 'Terapie e medicamenti del rinascimento', *Atti e memorie della accademia italiana di storia della farmacia*, 14, 1 (1997), 48–52.

Bibliography

F. De Vivo, *Information and Communication in Venice: Rethinking Early Modern Politics* (Oxford: Oxford University Press, 2007).

——, 'Pharmacies as Centres of Communication in Early Modern Venice', *Renaissance Studies*, 21, 4 (2007), 505–21.

T. Dean (ed.), *The Towns of Italy in the Later Middle Ages* (Manchester: Manchester University Press, 2000).

A. Debru, 'The Gardener and the Lady: Therapeutics and Society in the Age of Galen', in R. Pötzsch (ed.), *The Pharmacy: Windows on History* (Basel: Editiones Roche, 1996).

J. DeLancey, 'Dragonsblood and Ultramarine: The Apothecary and Artists' Pigments in Renaissance Florence', in M. Fantoni, L.C. Matthew, and S.F. Matthews-Grieco (eds), *The Art Market in Italy: 15th–17th Centuries. Il mercato dell'arte in Italia (secc. XV–XVII)* (Modena: Franco Cosimo Panini, 2003), 141–50.

E. Diana, 'Medici, speziali e barbieri nella Firenze della prima metà del '500', *Rivista di storia della medicina*, 4, 2 (1994), 13–27.

——, *San Matteo e San Giovanni di Dio: due ospedali nella storia fiorentina: struttura nosocomiale, patrimonio fondiario e assistenza nell Firenze dei secoli 15–18* (Florence: Le Lettere, 1999).

P. Dorveaux, *Inventaire de la pharmacie de l'Hôpital Saint-Nicholas de Metz (27 juin 1509)* (Paris: Wetter, 1894).

E. Duffy, *The Stripping of the Altars: Traditional Religion in England, c.1400–c.1580* (New Haven & London: Yale University Press, 1992).

W. Eamon, 'Books of Secrets in Medieval and Early Modern Science', *Sudhoffs Archiv fur geschichte der Medizin und der Naturwissenschaften*, 69, 1 (1985).

——, 'Medical Self-Fashioning, or How to Get Rich and Famous in the Renaissance Medical Marketplace', *Pharmacy in History*, 45 (2003), 123–9.

——, 'Plagues, Healers, and Patients in Early Modern Europe', *Renaissance Quarterly*, 52, 2 (1999), 474–86.

——, '"With the Rules of Life and an Enema": Leonardo Fioravanti's Medical Primitivism', in J.V. Field and F.A.J.L. James (eds), *Renaissance and Revolution: Humanists, Scholars, Craftsmen and Natural Philosophers in Early Modern Europe* (Cambridge: Cambridge University Press, 1993).

S.R. Ell, 'Governmental Regulation of Medicine in Late Medieval Venice', *Fifteenth-Century Studies*, 2 (1979).

Bibliography

M.S. Elsheikh and E. Coturri, 'Medici e medicina a Firenze fino alla metà del secolo XIX', in M.S. Elsheikh (ed.), *Medicina e farmacologia nei manoscritti della Biblioteca Riccardiana di Firenze* (Manziana, Rome: Vecchiarelli, 1990).

J.W. Estes, 'The European Reception of the First Drugs from the New World', *Pharmacy in History*, 37, 1 (1995), 3–23.

M. Fernandez-Carrion and J.L. Valverde, *Farmacia y sociedad en Sevilla en el siglo XVI* (Seville: Servicio de Publicaciones de Ayuntamiento de Sevilla, 1985).

S. Ferri, 'Il "Dioscoride", i "Discorsi", i "Commentarii": Gli amici e i nemici', in S. Ferri (ed.), *Pietro Andrea Mattioli: Siena, 1501–Trento, 1578: la vita, le opere: con l'identificazione delle piante* (Ponte San Giovanni, Perugia: Quattroemme, 1997).

P. Findlen, 'Inventing Nature: Commerce, Art and Science in the Early Modern Cabinet of Curiosities', in P.H. Smith and P. Findlen (eds), *Merchants & Marvels: Commerce, Science, and Art in Early Modern Europe* (New York: Routledge, 2002), 297–323.

J.-L. Flandrin, 'Le goût et la nécessité: sur l'usage des graisses dans les cuisines d'Europe occidentale (XIVe–XVIIIe siècle)', *Annales: E.S.C.*, 38, 2 (1983), 369–401.

———, 'Médecine et habitudes alimentaires anciennes', in J.-C. Margolin and R. Sauzet (eds), *Pratiques et discours alimentaires à la Renaissance. Actes du Colloque de Tours de mars 1979* (Paris: G.-P. Maisonneuve & Larose, 1982), 85–96.

———, 'Prix et statut gastronomique des viandes: réflexions sur quelques exemples des XVIe, XVIIe et XVIIIe siècles', in S. Cavaciocchi (ed.), *Alimentazione e nutrizione secc. XIII–XVIII: atti della ventottesima settimana di studi, 22–27 aprile 1996* (Florence: Le Monnier, 1997).

——— and M. Hyman, with P. Hyman, *Le Cuisinier François*, D. Roche (ed.), (Paris: Montalba, 1982).

——— and O. Redon, 'Les livres de cuisine italiens des XIVe et XVe siècles', *Archeologia medievale*, 8 (1981), 393–408.

J. Flood and D. Shaw, 'The Price of the Pox in 1527: Johannes Sinapius and the Guaiac Cure', *Bibliothèque d'Humanisme et Renaissance*, LIV, 3 (1992), 691–707.

C.M. Foust, 'Mysteries of Rhubarb: Chinese Medicinal Rhubarb through the Ages', *Pharmacy in History*, 36, 4 (1994), 155–9.

———, *Rhubarb: The Wondrous Drug* (Princeton, New Jersey: Princeton University Press, 1992).

F. Franceschi, 'La bottega come spazio di sociabilità', in F. Franceschi and G. Fossi (eds), *La grande storia dell'artigianato* (Florence: Giunti, 1999), 65–84.

D. Franklin, 'Rosso Fiorentino's Betrothal of the Virgin: Patronage and Interpretation', *Journal of the Warburg and Courtauld Institutes*, 55 (1992), 180–99.

J. Frith, 'Sweetness and Light: Evidence of Beeswax and Tallow Candles at Fountains Abbey, North Yorkshire', *Medieval Archaeology*, 48 (2004), 220–7.

G. Frosini (ed.), *Il cibo e i signori: La mensa dei priori di Firenze nel quinto decennio del secolo XIV* (Florence: Accademia della Crusca, 1993).

A.W. Frothingham, 'Apothecaries' Shops in Spain', *Notes Hispanic* (1941), 101–24.

P. Fumerton, 'Consuming the Void: Jacobean Banquets and Masques', in *Cultural Aesthetics: Renaissance Literature and the Practice of Social Ornament* (Chicago & London: University of Chicago Press, 1991).

R. Gascon, 'Un siècle du commerce des épices à Lyon: fin XVe–fin XVIe siècles', *Annales: E.S.C.*, 15 (1960), 647–8.

P. Gavitt, *Charity and Children in Renaissance Florence: The Ospedale degli Innocenti, 1410–1536* (Ann Arbor: University of Michigan Press, 1990).

D. Gentilcore, 'Apothecaries, "Charlatans", and the Medical Marketplace in Italy, 1400–1750 – Introduction', *Pharmacy in History* 45 (2003), 91–4.

———, '"For the Protection of Those who have both Shop and Home in this City": Relations between Italian Charlatans and Apothecaries', *Pharmacy in History* 45 (2003), 108–21.

———, *Healers and Healing in Early Modern Italy* (Manchester: Manchester University Press, 1998).

———, 'Charlatans, the Regulated Marketplace and the Treatment of Venereal Disease in Italy', in K. Siena (ed.), *Sins of the Flesh: Responding to Sexual Disease in Early Modern Europe* (Toronto: Centre for Reformation and Renaissance Studies, 2005), 57–80.

———, *Medical Charlatanism in Early Modern Italy* (Oxford: Oxford University Press, 2006).

M. Giagnacovo, 'Due "alimentazioni" del basso medioevo: la tavola dei mercanti e la tavola dei ceti subalterni', in S. Cavaciocchi (ed.), *Alimentazione e nutrizione secc. XIII–XVIII: atti della ventottesima settimana di studi, 22–27 aprile 1996* (Florence: Le Monnier, 1997).

S. Giovannini, 'La farmacia di Santa Maria Novella dalle origini al XVII secolo', in G. Mancini (ed.), *La farmacia de Santa Maria Novella* (Florence: Becocci Editore, 1987).

A. Giuffrida, 'La bottega dello speziale nelle città siciliane del '400', in *Atti del colloquio internazionale di archeologia medievale, Palermo-Erice, 20–22 settembre 1974* (Palermo: Istituto di storia medievale, Università di Palermo, 1976).

———, 'La bottega dello speziale nelle città siciliane del '400', in *Speziali aromatari e farmacisti in Sicilia. Convegno e mostra sulla storia della farmacia e del farmacista in Sicilia dal secolo XIII al secolo XIX* [1976] (Palermo: Associazione Culturale Apotheke, 1990).

A.M. Giusti, 'The Grand Ducal Workshops at the time of Ferdinando I and Cosimo II', in C. Acidini Luchinat (ed.), *Treasures of Florence: The Medici Collection 1400–1700* (Munich: Prestel, 1997), 115–41.

A. Goldgar, *Tulipmania: Money, Honor and Knowledge in the Dutch Golden Age* (Chicago: University of Chicago Press, 2007).

R. Goldthwaite and G. Mandich, *Studi sulla moneta fiorentina (secoli xiii–xvi)* (Florence: L.S. Olschki, 1994).

R.A. Goldthwaite, *The Building of Renaissance Florence: An Economic and Social History* (Baltimore: Johns Hopkins University Press, 1980).

———, 'The Economic and Social World of Italian Renaissance Majolica', *Renaissance Quarterly*, 42, 1 (1989), 1–32.

———, 'Local Banking in Renaissance Florence', *Journal of European Economic History*, 14, 1 (1985), 5–55.

———, *Wealth and the Demand for Art in Italy: 1300–1600* (Baltimore: Johns Hopkins University Press, 1993).

P.F. Grendler, *Schooling in Renaissance Italy: Literacy and Learning, 1300–1600* (Baltimore: Johns Hopkins University Press, 1989).

A.J. Grieco, 'From the Cookbook to the Table: A Florentine Table and Italian Recipes of the Fourteenth and Fifteenth Centuries', in C. Lambert (ed.), *Du manuscrit à la table: essais sur la cuisine au Moyen Age et repertoire des manuscrits medievaux contenant des recettes culinaires* (Montreal: Les presses de l'Université de Montreal, 1992).

S. Guaraldi, *et al.*, 'Su un trattato inedito di terapia medica del XV secolo: il codice Palatino 1045 (969-21,3) della Biblioteca Nazionale Centrale di Firenze', *Rivista di storia della medicina*, 5, 1 (1995), 39–63.

Bibliography

L. Haas, *The Renaissance Man and His Children: Childbirth and Early Childhood in Florence, 1300–1600* (New York: St Martin's Press, 1998).

M.B. Hall, 'Savonarola's Preaching and the Patronage of Art', in T. Verdon and J. Henderson (eds), *Christianity and the Renaissance: Image and Religious Imagination in the Quattrocento* (Syracuse: Syracuse University Press, 1990), 493–522.

S.K. Hamarneh, *Origins of Pharmacy and Therapy in the Near East* (Tokyo: Naito Foundation, 1973).

J. Henderson, 'Charity and Welfare in Early Modern Tuscany', in O.P. Grell, A. Cunningham and J. Arrizabalaga (eds), *Health Care and Poor Relief in Counter-Reformation Europe* (London: Routledge, 1999).

———, 'Healing the Body and Saving the Soul: Hospitals in Renaissance Florence', *Renaissance Studies*, 15, 2 (2001), 188–216.

———, 'The Hospitals of Late-Medieval and Renaissance Florence: A Preliminary Survey', in L. Granshaw and R. Porter (eds), *The Hospital in History* (London: Routledge, 1989).

———, *Piety and Charity in Late Medieval Florence* (Oxford & New York: Clarendon, 1994).

———, 'Women, Children and Poverty in Florence at the Time of the Black Death', in J. Henderson and R. Wall (eds), *Poor Women and Children in the European Past* (London: Routledge, 1994).

———, *The Renaissance Hospital: Healing the Body and Healing the Soul* (New Haven: Yale University Press, 2006).

———, 'Fracastoro, mal francese e la cura con il legno santo', in A. Pastore and E. Peruzzi (eds), *Girolamo Fracastoro: Fra medicina, filosofia e scienze della natura* (Florence: L.S. Olschki, 2006), 73–89.

D. Herlihy and C. Klapisch-Zuber, *I toscani e le loro famiglie: uno studio sul catasto fiorentino del 1427*, M. Bensi (trans.), (Bologna: Il Mulino, 1988).

———, *Tuscans and their Families: A Study of the Florentine Catasto of 1427* (New Haven: Yale University Press, 1985).

J.-C. Hocquet, 'Commercio e navigazione in Adriatico: Porto di Ancona, sale di Pago e marina di Ragusa (xiv–xvii secolo)', *Atti e memorie della deputazione di storia patria per le Marche*, 83 (1977), 221–54.

H.P. Horne, 'A Newly-Discovered Altarpiece by Alesso Baldovinetti', *Burlington Magazine* 8, 31 (1905), 51–53, 55–57, 59.

T. Huguet Termes, 'New World Materia Medica in Spanish Renaissance Medicine: From Scholarly Reception to Practical Impact', *Medical History*, 45 (2001), 359–76.

S.C. Humphreys, 'History, Economics and Anthropology: The Work of Karl Polanyi', *History and Theory*, 8 (1969), 165–212.

M. Hyman, 'Les "menues choses qui ne sont de neccessité": les confitures et la table', in C. Lambert (ed.), *Du manuscrit à la table: essais sur la cuisine au Moyen Age et repertoire des manuscrits medievaux contenant des recettes culinaires* (Montreal & Paris: Les presses de l'Université de Montreal, 1992).

P. Hyman and M. Hyman, 'Les livres de cuisine et le commerce des recettes en France aux XVe et XVIe siècles', in C. Lambert (ed.), *Du manuscrit à la table: essais sur la cuisine au Moyen Age et repertoire des manuscrits medievaux contenant des recettes culinaires* (Montreal & Paris: Les presses de l'Université de Montreal, 1992).

———, 'Table et sociabilité au XVIe siècle: l'example du sire de gouberville', *Revue d'Histoire Moderne et Contemporaine*, 31 (1984), 465–71.

V. Ignacii, 'Relazione commerciale tra Ragusa (Dubrovnik) e le Marche nel trecento e nel quattrocento', *Atti e memorie della deputazione di storia patria per le Marche*, 82 (1977), 197–219.

P. Jackson, 'Pomp or piety? The funeral of Pandolfo Petrucci', *Renaissance Studies*, 20, 2 (2006), 240–52.

D. Jacquart, 'Medical Practice in Paris in the First Half of the Fourteenth Century', in L. Garcìa Ballester (ed.), *Practical Medicine from Salerno to the Black Death* (Cambridge: Cambridge University Press, 1994).

———, 'Theory, Everyday Practice, and Three Fifteenth-Century Physicians', *Osiris: A Research Journal Devoted to the History of Science and Its Cultural Influence*, 2nd series, 6 (1990), 141–60.

J.D. Jensted, '"The City Cannot Hold You": Social Conversation in the Goldsmith's Shop', *Early Modern Literary Studies*, 8 (2002), 1–26.

C. Jones, 'The Great Chain of Buying: Medical Advertisement, the Bourgeois Public Sphere and the Origins of the French Revolution', *American Historical Review* 101, 1 (1996), 13–40.

M.A. Katritzky, *Women, Medicine and Theatre, 1500–1750: Literary Mountebanks and Performing Quacks* (Aldershot: Ashgate, 2007).

F.W. Kent, *Household and Lineage in Renaissance Florence: The Family Life of the Capponi, Ginori, and Rucellai* (Princeton: Princeton University Press, 1977).

J. Kirshner and A. Molho, 'The Dowry Fund and the Marriage Market in Early Quattrocento Florence', *Journal of Modern History*, 50 (1978), 403–38.

C. Klapisch-Zuber, 'Women Servants in Florence during the Fourteenth and Fifteenth Centuries', in B. Hanawalt (ed.), *Women and Work in Preindustrial Europe* (Bloomington: Indiana University Press, 1986).

——, *Women, Family, and Ritual in Renaissance Italy* (Chicago: University of Chicago Press, 1985).

A. Kolega, 'Speziali, spagirici, droghieri e ciarlatani: l'offerta terapeutica a Roma tra seicento e settecento', *Roma moderna e contemporanea*, 6, 3 (1998), 311–47.

E. Kremers, G. Sonnedecker, and G. Urdang, *Kremers and Urdang's History of Pharmacy*, 4th edn (Madison: American Institute of the History of Pharmacy, 1986).

T. Kuehn, *Law, Family and Women. Toward a Legal Anthropology of Renaissance Italy* (Chicago: Chicago University Press, 1993).

O. Lafont, 'Comptes d'apothicaires normands', *Revue d'histoire de la pharmacie*, 35 (1988), 135–37.

F.C. Lane, 'The Mediterranean Spice Trade" Further Evidence of its Revival in the Sixteenth Century', in B. Pullan (ed.), *Crisis and Change in the Venetian Economy in the Sixteenth and Seventeenth Centuries* (London: Methuen, 1968), 47–58.

——, 'Pepper Prices before da Gama', in M.N. Pearson (ed.), *Spices in the Indian Ocean World* (Aldershot: Variorum, 1996).

M. Laughran, 'Medicating without "Scruples": The "Professionalization" of the Apothecary in Sixteenth-century Venice', *Pharmacy in History*, 45 (2003), 95–107.

B. Laurioux, *Manger au moyen âge: pratiques et discours alimentaires en Europe aux XIVe et XVe siècles* (Paris: Hachette, 2002).

G. Lazzi and M. Gabriele (eds), *Alambicchi di parole: il ricettario fiorentino e dintorni: Firenze, Biblioteca Riccardiana, 18 ottobre 1999–15 gennaio 2000* (Florence: Polistampa, 1999).

M.L. Lenzi, 'Rabarbaro, manna e senna: la dolce medicina di Pietro Andrea Mattioli per il principe Ferdinando d'Asburgo, colpito da una crisi di melanconia', in S. Ferri (ed.), *Pietro Andrea Mattioli: Siena, 1501–Trento, 1578: la vita, le opere: con l'identificazione delle piante* (Ponte San Giovanni, Perugia: Quattroemme, 1997).

M. Lindemann, *Medicine and Society in Early Modern Europe* (Cambridge: Cambridge University Press, 1999).

R.B. Litchfield, *Florence Ducal Capital, 1530–1630* (New York: ACLS Humanities EBook, 2008).

C. Lury, 'Contemplating a Self-Portrait as a Pharmacist', *Theory, Culture and Society*, 22 (2005), 93–110.

E. Marchetti, 'Il Convento di San Marco a Firenze e la sua antica farmacia', *Notiziario farmaceutico*, 13, 3 (1951), 11–14.

M. Marighelli, 'L'arredo di una spezieria Ferrarese del trecento', *Atti e memorie della accademia italiana di storia della farmacia*, 14, 1 (1997), 25–8.

———, 'Un contratto inedito del XV secolo per la fornitura di generi di "speciaria" alla corte estense', *Atti e memorie della accademia italiana di storia della farmacia*, 9, 2 (1992), 109–19.

R.K. Marshall, *The Local Merchants of Prato: Small Entrepreneurs in the Late Medieval Economy* (Baltimore & London: Johns Hopkins University Press, 1999).

L. Martines, *Scourge and Fire: Savonarola and Renaissance Italy* (London: Jonathan Cape, 2006).

A. Martini, *Manuale di metrologia ossia misure, pesi e monete in uso attulamente ed anticamente presso tutti i popoli* (Turin: Loescher, 1883).

G. Martini, 'La spezieria dell'Ospedale Grande di Milano', *Notiziario Sandoz*, 1 (1958), 6–7.

E. Martinori, *La Moneta. Vocabolario generale* (Rome: Multigrafica editrice, 1977).

C. Masino, 'Interrogativi su Manlio di Bosco e Paolo Suardo speziali', *Atti e memorie della accademia italiana di storia della farmacia*, 5 (1988), 7–10.

L.C. Matthew, '"Vendecolori a Venezia": The Reconstruction of a Profession', *Burlington Magazine*, 144 (2002).

M.S. Mazzi, *Salute e societa nel medioevo* (Florence: La Nuova Italia, 1978).

M.S. Mazzi and S. Raveggi, *Gli uomini e le cose nelle campagne fiorentine del quattrocento* (Florence: L.S. Olschki, 1983).

R. Mazzucco, 'La data del primo Ricettario fiorentino', in *Actes du VIIIe Congrès international d'histoire des sciences, Florence/Milan 3–9 September 1956, Vol. 2* (Florence: G. Bruschi, 1958).

Bibliography

M.R. McVaugh, 'Medicine in the Latin Middle Ages', in I. Loudon (ed.), *Western Medicine: An Illustrated History* (Oxford: Oxford University Press, 1997).

F. Melis, *L'economia fiorentina del rinascimento*, B. Dini (ed.), (Florence: Le Monnier, 1984).

L. Meneghini, 'Breve analisi di alcune fra le piu significative raffigurazione dello speziale nella letteratura italiana', *Atti e memorie della accademia italiana di storia della farmacia*, 19, 3 (2001).

G. Metelli, 'L'alimentazione del ceto nobile e delle classi meno abbienti a Foligno tra cinque e seicento', in S. Cavaciocchi (ed.), *Alimentazione e nutrizione secc. XIII–XVIII: atti della ventottesima settimana di studi, 22–27 aprile 1996* (Florence: Le Monnier, 1997).

S.W. Mintz, *Sweetness and Power. The Place of Sugar in Modern History* (New York; & London: Sifton, 1985).

A. Molho, *Marriage Alliance in Late Medieval Florence* (Cambridge: Harvard University Press, 1994).

——, 'Names, Memory, Public Identity, in Late Medieval Florence', in G. Ciappelli and P.L. Rubin (eds), *Art, Memory, and Family in Renaissance Florence* (Cambridge: Cambridge University Press, 2000).

E. Muir, '"In Some Neighbours We Trust". The Exclusion of Women from the Public in Renaissance Italy', in D.E. Bornstein and D. Peterson (eds), *Florence and Beyond: Culture, Society and Politics in Renaissance Italy: Essays in Honour of John M. Najemy* (Toronto: Centre for Reformation and Renaissance Studies, 2008), 271–90.

C. Muldrew, *The Economy of Obligation: The Culture of Credit and Social Relations in Early Modern England* (London: Macmillan, 1998).

——, '"Hard Food for Midas": Cash and its Social Value in Early Modern England', *Past & Present*, 170, 1 (2001), 78–120.

R.S. Munger, 'Guaiacum, the Holy Wood from the New World', *Journal of the History of Medicine and Allied Sciences*, 4, 2 (1949), 196–229.

J. Musacchio, 'Conception and Birth', in M. Ajmar-Wollheim and F. Dennis (eds), *At Home in Renaissance Italy* (London: V&A Publications, 2006).

——, 'The Medici Sale of 1495 and the Second-Hand Market for Domestic Goods in Late Fifteenth-Century Florence', in M. Fantoni, L.C. Matthew and S.F. Matthews-Grieco (eds), *The Art Market in Italy: 15th–17th Centuries. Il mercato dell'arte in Italia (secc. XV–XVII)* (Modena: Franco Cosimo Panini, 2003), 313–24.

J. Musacchio (*cont...*), 'Weasels and Pregnancy in Renaissance Italy', *Renaissance Studies*, 15, 2 (2001), 172–87.

P. Musgrave, 'The Economics of Uncertainty: The Structural Revolution in the Spice Trade, 1480–1640', in M.N. Pearson (ed.), *Spices in the Indian Ocean World* (Aldershot: Variorum, 1996).

A.M. Nada Padrone, 'Trattati medici, diete e regimi alimentari in ambito piedemontano alla fine del medio evo', *Archeologia medievale*, 8 (1981).

J.M. Najemy, 'Guild Republicanism in Trecento Florence: The Successes and Ultimate Failure of Corporate Politics', *American Historical Review*, 84, 1 (1979), 53–71.

A. Nannizzi, 'L'arte degli speziali in Siena', *Bollettino senese di storia patria*, n.s. 10 (1939), 93–131.

G. Nardelli, *Farmacie e farmacisti in Umbria: dagli statuti degli speziali all'ordine* (Perugia: Umbrafarm, 1998).

G.M. Nardi, 'La medicina popolare in Toscana', *Lares*, 6, 4 (1935), 272–82.

I. Naso, *La cultura del cibo : alimentazione, dietetica, cucina nel basso Medioevo* (Turin: Paravia Scriptorium, 1999).

———, 'Sapori d'oriente alla corte sabauda: Le spezie in cucina al tempo di Amedeo VIII', in R. Comba, A.M. Nada Padrone, and I. Naso (eds), *La mensa del principe: cucina e regimi alimentari nelle corti sabaude (XIII–XV secolo)* (Cuneo: Società studi storici di Cuneo, 1997).

———, *Una bottega di panni alla fine del trecento: Giovanni Canale di Pinerolo e il suo libro di conti* (Genoa: Università di Genova, 1985).

M.E. Nicaise, *La pharmacie et la matière médicale au XIVe siècle* (Paris: Administ. des Deux Revues, 1892).

V. Nutton, 'Greek Science in the Sixteenth-Century Renaissance', in J.V. Field and F.A.J.L. James (eds), *Renaissance and Revolution: Humanists, Scholars, Craftsmen and Natural Philosophers in Early Modern Europe* (Cambridge: Cambridge University Press, 1993).

G. Olmi, 'Farmacopea antica e medicina moderna: La disputa sulla teriaca nel cinquecento bolognese', *Physis. Rivista internazionale di storia della scienza*, 19 (1977), 197–246.

M. O'Malley, *The Business of Art: Contracts and the Commissioning Process in Renaissance Italy* (New Haven: Yale University Press, 2005).

M. O'Malley and E. Welch (eds), *The Material Renaissance* (Manchester: Manchester University Press, 2007).

G. Ortalli, 'Cibi e cultura nel medioevo europeo', in A. Pertusi (ed.), *Civiltà della tavola dal medioevo al rinascimento* (Venice: Neri Pozza, 1983), 15–35.

I. Paccagnella, 'Cucina e ideologia alimentare nella Venezia del rinascimento', in A. Pertusi (ed.), *Civiltà della tavola dal medioevo al rinascimento* (Vicenza: Neri Pozza, 1983).

R. Palmer, 'Pharmacy in the Republic of Venice in the Sixteenth Century', in A. Wear, R.K. French, and I.M. Lonie (eds), *The Medical Renaissance of the Sixteenth Century* (Cambridge: Cambridge University Press, 1985).

————, 'Physicians and the State in Post-Medieval Italy', in *The Town and State Physician in Europe from the Middle Ages to the Enlightenment* (Wolfenbuttel: Herzog August Bibliothek, 1981).

K. Park, 'Country Medicine in the City Marketplace: Snakehandlers as Itinerant Healers', *Renaissance Studies*, 15, 2 (2001), 104–20.

————, *Doctors and Medicine in Early Renaissance Florence* (Princeton: Princeton University Press, 1985).

————, 'Healing the Poor: Hospitals and Medical Assistance in Renaissance Florence', in J. Barry and C. Jones (eds), *Medicine and Charity before the Welfare State* (London: Routledge, 1991).

————, 'Medicine and the Renaissance', in I. Loudon (ed.), *Western Medicine: An Illustrated History* (Oxford: Oxford University Press, 1997).

K. Park and J. Henderson, '"The First Hospital among Christians": The Ospedale di Santa Maria Nuova in Early Sixteenth-Century Florence', *Medical History*, 35 (1991).

M.N. Pearson, 'Introduction', in M.N. Pearson (ed.), *Spices in the Indian Ocean World* (Aldershot: Variorum, 1996).

M. Pelling, 'Occupational Diversity: Barbersurgeons and the Trades of Norwich, 1550–1640', *Bulletin of the History of Medicine*, 56, 4 (1982), 484–511.

M. Pelling and C. Webster, 'Medical Practitioners', in C. Webster (ed.), *Health, Medicine and Mortality in the Sixteenth Century* (Cambridge: Cambridge University Press, 1979).

S. Pennell, 'Perfecting Practice? Women, Manuscript Recipes and Knowledge in Early Modern England', in V.E. Burke and J. Gibson (eds), *Early Modern Women's Manuscript Writing* (Aldershot: Ashgate, 2004), 237–58.

333

Bibliography

A. Perifano, *L'alchimie à la cour de Come Ier de Medicis: savoirs, culture et politique* (Paris: Honore Champion, 1997).

S. Pezzella, *Gli erbari: I primi libri di medicina (Le virtù curative delle piante)* (Perugia: Grifo, 1993).

G. Phillips, *Seven Centuries of Light: The Tallow Chandlers Company* (London: Book Production Company, 1999).

L. Polizzotto, *'The Elect Nation': The Savonarolan Movement in Florence, 1494–1545* (Oxford: Clarendon, 1994).

G. Pomata, *Contracting a Cure: Patients, Healers, and the Law in Early Modern Bologna*, G. Pomata, R. Foy, and A. Taraboletti-Segre (trans.), (Baltimore: Johns Hopkins University Press, 1998).

R.A. Pratt, 'Giovanni Sercambi, Speziale', *Italica*, 25, 1 (1948), 12–14.

F. Raspadori (ed.), *I maestri di medicina ed arti dell'Università di Ferrara, 1391–1950* (Florence: L.S. Olschki, 1991).

O. Redon, 'La réglementation des banquets par les lois somptuaries dans les villes d'Italie (XIIIe–Xve siècles)', in C. Lambert (ed.), *Du manuscrit à la table: essais sur la cuisine au Moyen Age et repertoire des manuscrits medievaux contenant des recettes culinaires* (Montreal & Paris: Les presses de l'Université de Montreal, 1992).

N. Reynolds, 'Pickled Sheep off the menu as Hirst opens' *The Daily Telegraph*, 15 January 1998. http://www.telegraph.co.uk/ htmlContent.jhtml?html=/archive/1998/01/15/nbaa15.html

J.M. Riddle, *Dioscorides on Pharmacy and Medicine*, 1st edn (Austin: University of Texas Press, 1985).

———, *Quid Pro Quo: Studies in the History of Drugs* (Aldershot: Variorum, 1992).

———, 'Theory and Practice in Medieval Medicine', *Viator*, 5 (1974).

R. Romanelli, 'La spezieria dell'ospedale di S. Giovanni di Dio di Firenze', *Notiziario Sandoz*, 3 (1959), 6–7.

D. Romano, 'Aspects of Patronage in Fifteenth- and Sixteenth-Century Venice', *Renaissance Quarterly*, 46 (1993), 712–33.

———, *Housecraft and Statecraft: Domestic Service in Renaissance Venice, 1400–1600* (Baltimore & London: Johns Hopkins University Press, 1996).

R. Romano, 'Farmacie e farmacisti a Venezia', in R. Romano and A. Schwarz (eds), *Per una storia della farmacia e del farmacista in Italia. Vol 2. Venezia e Veneto* (Bologna: Edizioni Skema, 1981).

S. Rosati, 'Benedetto di Tacco da Prato speziale, 1345–1392: Vita, attività, ambiente sociale ed economico' (unpublished graduate thesis: Università di Firenze, 1971).

D. Rosenthal, 'The Spaces of Plebeian Ritual and the Boundaries of Transgression', in R.J. Crum and J.T. Paoletti (eds), *Renaissance Florence: A Social History* (Cambridge: Cambridge University Press, 2006).

B. Rossignol, *Médecine et médicaments au XVIe siècle à Lyon* (Lyon: Presses universitaires de Lyon, 1990).

V. Rotolo, 'La storia medica dello zucchero', *Rivista di storia della medicina*, 8, 1 (1998), 15–25.

P.L. Rubin, *Images and Identity in Fifteenth-Century Florence* (New Haven: Yale University Press, 2007).

N. Rubinstein, *The Government of Florence under the Medici (1434 to 1494)* [1966], 2nd edn (Oxford: Clarendon, 1997).

———, 'Oligarchy and Democracy in Fifteenth-Century Florence', in S. Bertelli and N. Rubinstein (eds), *Florence and Venice: Comparisons and Relations. Volume 1: Quattrocento* (Florence: La Nuova Italia, 1980), 99–112.

L. Sandri, *L'archivio dell'Ospedale San Giovanni di Dio di Firenze (1604–1890). Inventario* (Cernusco, Milano: Fatebenefratelli, 1991).

L. Sandri and A.J. Grieco, 'Appunti per una storia dell'aquavite in Italia: da Taddeo Alderotti alla Fonderia Medicea di Palazzo Pitti (1280–1591)', in *Grappa e alchimia: Un percorso nella millenaria storia della distillazione* (Rome: Agra Editrice, 1999), 33–48.

B. Santich, 'The Evolution of Culinary Techniques in the Medieval Era', in M.W. Adamson (ed.), *Food in the Middle Ages: A Book of Essays* (New York: Garland Pub., 1995).

G. Savonarola, 'On the Renovation of the Church', in J.C. Olin (ed.), *The Catholic Reformation: Savonarola to Ignatius Loyola* (New York: Fordham University Press, 1992).

J. Scarborough, 'The Opium Poppy in Hellenistic and Roman Medicine', in R. Porter and M. Teich (eds), *Drugs and Narcotics in History* (Cambridge: Cambridge University Press, 1995), 4–23.

J. Schönfeld, 'Pharmacy in the Medieval Arab World', in R. Pötzsch (ed.), *The Pharmacy: Windows on History* (Basel: Editiones Roche, 1996).

A. Schwarz, 'Intorno all'origine a allo sviluppo dell'arte farmaceutica a Venezia e nel Veneto', in R. Romano and A. Schwarz (eds), *Per una storia della farmacia e del farmacista in Italia. Vol 2. Venezia e Veneto* (Bologna: Edizioni Skema, 1981).

T. Scully, 'The Sickdish in Early French Recipe Collections', in S.D. Campbell, B.S. Hall, and D. Klausner (eds), *Health, Disease and Healing in Medieval Culture* (Basingstoke: Macmillan, 1992), 132–40.

———, 'Tempering Medieval Food', in M.W. Adamson (ed.), *Food in the Middle Ages: A Book of Essays* (New York: Garland Pub., 1995).

M.M. Serena, *Prostitute e lenoni nella Firenze del quattrocento* (Milan: Il Saggiatore, 1991).

L. Sguanci. 'Dante, l'arte dei medici e speziali e le spezierie della Firenze medioevale', *Relazione presentata al 5. Congresso della Società italiana di farmacia ospitaliera, tenuto a Firenze nel 1960* (Florence: 1960).

J.E. Shaw, *The Justice of Venice: Authorities and Liberties in the Urban Economy, 1550–1700* (Oxford: Oxford University Press, 2006).

H.C. Silberman, 'Les formulaires des pharmaciens Manlius di Bosco Quiricus de Augustis et Paulus Suardus et la place importante qu'y prennent les sucreries', *Atti e memorie della accademia italiana di storia della farmacia,* 18, 1 (2001), 17–22.

———, 'Sugar in the Middle Ages', *Pharmaceutical Historian*, 28, 4 (1998), 59–65.

———, 'Superstition and Medical Knowledge in an Italian Herbal', *Pharmacy in History*, 38, 2 (1996), 87–94.

G. Silini, 'La cultura medica e farmaceutica', in G. Silini (ed.), *Herbe pincte* (Gorle: Iniziative Culturali, 2000).

———, *Umori e farmaci: terapia medica tardo-medievale* (Gandino: Servitium, 2001).

N.G. Siraisi, *Medieval & Early Renaissance Medicine: An Introduction to Knowledge and Practice* (Chicago: University of Chicago Press, 1990).

———, *Taddeo Alderotti and His Pupils. Two Generations of Italian Medical Learning* (Princeton: Princeton University Press, 1981).

Bibliography

V.A. Sironi, 'La farmacologia a Milano dagli erbari alle biotecnologie', in F. Berti (ed.), *Uomini e farmaci: la farmacologia a Milano tra storia e memoria* (Rome: Laterza, 2002).

P. Skinner, *Health and Medicine in Early Medieval Southern Italy* (Leiden: Brill, 1997).

P. Slack, 'Mirrors of Health and Treasures of Poor Men: The Uses of the Vernacular Medical Literature of Tudor England', in C. Webster (ed.), *Health, Medicine and Mortality in the Sixteenth Century* (Cambridge: Cambridge University Press, 1979).

A. Spicciani, 'Aspetti finanziari dell'assistenza e struttura cetuale dei poveri vergognosi fiorentini al tempo del Savonarola (1487–1498)', in *Studi di storia economica toscana nel medioevo e nel rinascimento: In memoria di Federigo Melis* (Pisa: Pacini, 1987).

P. Spufford, *Handbook of Medieval Exchange* (London: Royal Historical Society, 1986).

R. Staccini, 'L'inventario di una spezieria del quattrocento', *Studi medievali*, 22, 1 (1981), 377–420.

J.E. Staley, *The Guilds of Florence* (London: Methuen, 1906).

J. Stannard, 'Dioscorides and Renaissance Materia Medica', in M. Florkin (ed.), *Materia Medica in the XVIth Century: Proceedings of a Symposium of the International Academy of the History of Medicine, held at the University of Basel, 7th September 1964* (Oxford ; New York: Pergamon Press, 1966).

———, 'The Herbal as a Medical Document', *Bulletin of the History of Medicine*, 43 (1969), 212–20.

———, *Herbs and Herbalism in the Middle Ages and Renaissance* (Aldershot: Ashgate, 1999).

———, 'Hippocratic Pharmacology', *Bulletin of the History of Medicine*, 35 (1961).

S.T. Strocchia, *Death and Ritual in Renaissance Florence* (Baltimore & London: Johns Hopkins University Press, 1992).

———, 'Death Rites and the Ritual Family in Renaissance Florence', in M. Tetel, R.G. Witt and R. Goffen (eds), *Life and Death in Fifteenth-Century Florence* (Durham: Duke University Press, 1989), 120–45.

———, 'Funerals and the Politics of Gender in Early Renaissance Florence', in M. Migiel and J. Schiesari (eds), *Refiguring Women: Perspectives on Gender and the Italian Renaissance* (Ithaca: Cornell University Press, 1991), 155–68.

S.T. Strocchia (*cont...*), 'Sisters in Spirit: The Nuns of S. Ambrogio and their Consorority in Early Sixteenth-Century Florence', *Sixteenth Century Journal*, 33, 3 (2002), 735–67.

J. Styles, 'Product Innovation in Early Modern London', *Past & Present*, 148 (2000), 124–69.

I. Szmigin, 'The Aestheticization of Consumption: An Exploration of "brand.new" and "Shopping"', *Marketing Theory*, 6 (2006), 107–18.

P.M. Teigen, 'Taste and Quality in 15th- and 16th-Century Galenic Pharmacology', *Pharmacy in History*, 29, 2 (1987), 60–8.

O. Temkin, *Galenism: Rise and Fall of a Medical Philosophy* (Ithaca: Cornell University Press, 1973).

A. Thomas, *The Painter's Practice in Renaissance Tuscany* (Cambridge: Cambridge University Press, 1995).

———, 'The Workshop as the Space of Collaborative Artistic Production', in R.J. Crum and J.T. Paoletti (eds), *Renaissance Florence: A Social History* (Cambridge: Cambridge University Press, 2006).

P. Thornton, *The Italian Renaissance Interior, 1400–1600* (London: Weidenfeld & Nicolson, 1991).

S. Tognetti, 'Prezzi e salari nella Firenze tardomedievale: un profilo', *Archivio storico italiano*, 153, 2 (1995), 263–333.

A.P. Torresi, *Il ricettario Bardi: cosmesi e tecnica artistica nella Firenze medicea* (Ferrara: Liberty house, 1994).

B.J. Trexler, 'Hospital Patients in Florence: San Paolo, 1567–8', *Bulletin of the History of Medicine*, 48 (1974), 41–59.

R.C. Trexler, *Public Life in Renaissance Florence* (New York: Academic Press, 1980).

L. Valls and L. Dulieu, 'A propos d'un compte d'apothicaire montpelliérain', *Bulletin de liaison de l'Association des amis du Musée de la pharmacie*, 9 (1984).

N.-E. Vanzan Marchini, *Le leggi di sanità della repubblica di Venezia* (Vicenza: Neri Pozza, 1995).

T. Vecchi, 'Piante medicinali nel trattato salernitano "Curae Magistri Ferrarii"', *Atti e memorie della accademia italiana di storia della farmacia*, 15, 3 (1998), 223–7.

C. Vincent, *Fiat Lux: Lumière et luminaires dans la vie religieuse du XIIIe au XVIe siècle* (Paris: Editions du Cerf, 2004).

Bibliography

A.E. Vitolo, 'Evoluzione della figura dello speziale', *Notiziario Sandoz*, 6 (1960), 2–4.

C.H.H. Wake, 'The Changing Patterns of Europe's Pepper and Spice Imports, ca. 1400–1700', in M.N. Pearson (ed.), *Spices in the Indian Ocean World* (Aldershot: Variorum, 1996) [1979].

——, 'The Volume of European Spice Imports at the Beginning and End of the Fifteenth Century', *Journal of European Economic History*, 15, 3 (1986), 621–35.

P. Wallis, 'Apothecaries and the Consumption and Retailing of Medicines in Early Modern England', in L.H. Curth (ed.), *From Physick to Pharmacology: Five Hundred Years of British Drug Retailing* (Aldershot: Ashgate, 2006), 13–28.

——, 'Consumption, Retailing and Medicine in Early Modern London', *Economic History Review*, 61 (2008), 26–53.

G. Watson, *Theriac and Mithridatium: A Study in Therapeutics* (London: Wellcome Historical Medical Library, 1966).

R.F.E. Weissman, *Ritual Brotherhood in Renaissance Florence* (New York: Academic Press, 1982).

——, 'Taking Patronage Seriously: Mediterranean Values and Renaissance Society', in F.W. Kent and P. Simons (eds), *Patronage, Art and Society in Renaissance Italy* (Oxford: Clarendon, 1987).

E. Welch, *Shopping in the Renaissance: Consumer Cultures in Italy 1400–1600* (New Haven: Yale University Press, 2005).

E. Welch, 'Space and Spectacle in the Renaissance Pharmacy', *Medicina & Storia*, 15 (2008), 127–58.

A. West Vivarelli, 'Giovanni Sercambi's Novelle and the Legacy of Boccaccio', *MLN: Modern Language Notes*, 90, 1 (1975), 109–27.

T.D. Whittet, 'Pepperers, Spicers and Grocers: Forerunners of the Apothecaries', *Proceedings of the Royal Society of Medicine*, 61 (1968), 801–6.

F.A. Yates, *Giordano Bruno and the Hermetic Tradition* [1964] (London: Routledge, 2002).

D. Zanetti, 'Farmacie e farmacisti di Lombardia', in C.M. Cipolla, A. Russo, and D. Zanetti (eds), *Per una storia della farmacia e del farmacista in Italia. Vol. 6. Milano e Lombardia* (Bologna: Edizioni Skema, 1992).

D. Zanrè, 'French Diseases and Italian Responses: Representations of the *mal francese* in the Literature of Cinquecento Tuscany', in K. Siena (ed.), *Sins of the*

Flesh: Responding to Sexual Disease in Early Modern Europe (Toronto: Centre for Reformation and Renaissance Studies, 2005), 187–208.

Index